HOME
CARE
OF THE
ELDERLY

HOME CARE

OF THE

ELDERLY

♦

♦

♦

Sheryl Mara Zang, RN, MS, FNP

Assistant Professor
College of Nursing
SUNY Health Science Center at Brooklyn
State University of New York
Brooklyn, New York

♦　♦　♦

Judith A. Allender, RN C, MSN, EdD

Professor
Department of Nursing
School of Health and Human Services
California State University
Fresno, California

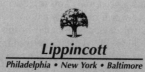

Lippincott

Philadelphia • New York • Baltimore

Acquisitions Editor: Susan M. Glover, RN, MSN
Coordinating Editorial Assistant: Bridget Blatteau
Production Editor: Virginia Barishek
Production Manager: Helen Ewan
Production Service: Berliner, Inc.
Printer/Binder: R. R. Donnelley & Sons Company/Crawfordsville
Cover Designer: Melissa Walter
Cover Printer: Lehigh Press

9 8 7 6 5 4 3 2 1

Library of Congress Cataloging-in-Publication Data

Home care of the elderly / [edited by] Sheryl Mara Zang, Judith A. Allender.

p.   cm.

Includes bibliographical references and index.

ISBN 0-7817-1542-3

1. Geriatric nursing. 2.Home nursing. 3. Aged—Home care. I. Zang, Sheryl Mara. II. Allender, Judith Ann.

[DNLM: 1. Home Care Services nurses' instruction.   WY 115 H7642 1999]
RC954.H575 1999
610.73'65—dc21
DNLM/DLC
for Library of Congress   98-22344
                                                                        CIP

Care has been taken to confirm the accuracy of the information presented and to describe generally accepted practices. However, the authors, editors, and publisher are not responsible for errors or omissions or for any consequences from application of the information in the book and make no warranty, express or implied, with respect to the contents of the publication.

The authors, editors, and publisher have exerted every effort to ensure that drug selection and dosage set forth in this text are in accordance with current recommendations and practice at the time of publication. However, in view of ongoing research, changes in government regulations, and the constant flow of information relating to drug therapy and drug reactions, the reader is urged to check the package insert for each drug for any change in indications and dosage and for added warnings and precautions. This is particularly important when the recommended agent is a new or infrequently employed drug.

Some drugs and medical devices presented in this publication have U.S. Food and Drug Administration (FDA) clearance for limited use in restricted research settings. It is the responsibility of the health care provider to ascertain the FDA status of each drug or device planned for use in clinical practice.

This book is dedicated to my mother,
Mrs. Renee Cohen,
who is always there for me.

Sheryl Mara Zang

♦   ♦   ♦

This book is dedicated in memory of my mother,
Elizabeth A. Schuepp,
who lived by the saying: "Count that day lost whose low descending
sun views from thy hand no worthy action done."

November 12, 1915–August 19, 1997

Judith A. Allender

CONTRIBUTORS

Judith A. Allender, RN C, MSN, EdD
Professor
Department of Nursing, School of Health and Human Services,
California State University, Fresno, California

Vilma Baltazar, RN, MSN
Director of Resident Care Services
Hebrew Home for the Aged at Riverdale, Riverdale, New York

Flora R. Bienstock, MSSW, CSW, ACSW
Clinical Director
New Horizon Counseling Center, Far Rockaway, New York

Mark D. Bienstock, MPA
Executive Director
Bronx Children's Psychiatric Center, Bronx, New York

Henry Cohen, BS, MS, PharmD
Associate Professor of Pharmacy Practice
Arnold & Marie Schwartz College of Pharmacy and Health Sciences,
Long Island University
Coordinator of Clinical Pharmacy Services
Departments of Pharmacy and Medicine, Kingsbrook Jewish
Medical Center
Associate Professor of Pharmacology and Medicine
College of Nursing, SUNY Health Science Center at Brooklyn,
Brooklyn, New York

Rae Lord Crowe, RN, PhD, CS, GNP
Associate Professor
College of Nursing, SUNY Health Science Center at Brooklyn,
Brooklyn, New York

Dianna D'Amico-Panomeritakis, RN C, MA, CRRN
Home Care Rehabilitation Supervisor
New York Methodist Hospital, Brooklyn, New York

Ann Marie D'Angelo, RN, C, MSN
Nurse Psychotherapist
Nurse Geriatric Care Manager/Consultant, Garden City, New York

Frank G. D'Angelo, Esq.
Attorney
Law Offices of D'Angelo and Begley, LLP, Garden City, New York

Maureen Dailey, RN, MSN, CETN
Director of the Centers for Excellence and Disease Management
Visiting Nurse Service of New York,
New York, New York

Instructor
Molloy College, Continuing Education in Transitions to Home Care,
Community Health Nurse Training Program,
Rockville Centre, New York

Andrew J. Devlin, RRT
Respiratory Care Program
New York University (Bellevue), Administrator of Clinical Services,
Metropolitan HomeCare, Bronx, New York

Donna Diamantopulos, RN, MS, FNP
Clinical Nurse Specialist
Comprehensive Stroke Center, Beth Israel Medical Center,
New York, New York

Elaine Edelstein, RN, MS, CDE
Diabetes Clinical Nurse Specialist
Visiting Nurse Service of New York,
New York, New York

Herminia B. Nueva Espana, RN, MED, MA
Nurse Practitioner in Gerontology
Section of Geriatrics, St. Agnes Hospital, Our Lady of Mercy
Healthcare System, White Plains, New York

Mary Farren, RN, MSN
SPHN, Grant Program Manager
Metropolitan Jewish Health System, Brooklyn, New York

Eileen Garry, RN, BSN, CNOR
Nurse Educator
Hospital for Special Surgery, New York, New York

Janice H. Hentgen, RN, MS, MA
Rehabilitation Clinical Nurse Specialist
Hebrew Home for the Aged at Riverdale, Riverdale, New York

Olivia Babol Ibe, RN C, MSN
Dementia Special Care Coordinator; Nursing Care Coordinator
Hebrew Home for the Aged at Riverdale, Riverdale, New York

Mary Ellen McCann, RN, MA
Cardiopulmonary Clinical Nurse Specialist
Visiting Nurse Service of New York,
New York, New York

Patrice Kenneally Nicholas, RN, DNSc, CS
Associate Professor
MGH Institute of Health Professions, Graduate Program in Nursing,
Boston, Massachusetts

Marilyn Oppong-Addae, RN, BSN
Rehabilitation Nurse
Hebrew Home for the Aged at Riverdale, Riverdale, New York

Alexandra Paul-Simon, RN, PhD
Assistant Professor; Associate Director, Generalist Level
Institute of Health Professions, MGH,
Boston, Massachusetts

Vivian Schulkin, RN, MS
Assistant Director of Patient Services
Family Care Certified Services, Brooklyn, New York

Joan Kurtz Sommer, RN, MA, CRRN
Nurse Specialist
Rehabilitation Educational Consultants, Rutherford, New Jersey

Victoria D. Tanico, RN, MSN
Rehabilitation Nurse Clinician
Hebrew Home for the Aged at Riverdale, Riverdale, New York

Anne Walsh, RN, MS
Continuous Quality Improvement Manager
Metropolitan Jewish Health Systems, Brooklyn, New York

Margaret Walsh, RN, MS, CS
Clinical Nurse Specialist/Consultant
Visiting Nurse Service of New York,
New York, New York

Bettina Bentley Willis, RN, MS, OCN
Associate Director of Nursing
SUNY Health Science Center at Brooklyn, Brooklyn, New York

Sheryl Mara Zang, RN, MS, FNP
Assistant Professor
College of Nursing, SUNY Health Science Center at Brooklyn,
Brooklyn, New York

REVIEWERS

Jo-Ann D. Barrett, RN, BSN, CDE
Consultant
Creative Health Care, Westwood, Maryland

Nora Bashian, RD, BS, CDE
Director of Nutrition
Central Valley Indian Health, Clovis, California

Jane G. Frankenfield, RN, BSN, CPHQ
Healthcare Consultant
Managed Care Strategies, Baltimore, Maryland

Linda J. Hewett, PsyD
Co-Director
Alzheimer's Disease Center,
University of California–San Francisco, Fresno, California
Assistant Clinical Professor
University of California–San Francisco, Fresno, California

Charlotte Ryan, RN, MSN, CS, OCN
Oncology Staff Nurse/Clinical Specialist
St. Agnes Medical Center, Fresno, California
Lecturer
Department of Nursing, California State University,
Fresno, California

Nina M. Smith, RN C, MEd
President
Integrated Behavioral Health Consultants, Fort Collins, Colorado

P R E F A C E

Most nurses have worked very effectively with elderly clients in the structured environment of the hospital or nursing home. In this environment, clients are seen as being quite ill. They are dependent on the staff and services of the facility to regain a state of wellness, which hopefully leads to a higher level of wellness, discharge to home, and independent functioning.

For most younger clients, this is the pattern for them. Once they are discharged from an inpatient setting they usually need no additional care or are able to provide their own care. Their illnesses are most often acute, and recovery is swift. For older adults, chronic illnesses, compounded with multiple effects of aging, cause these clients to need the expertise of an interdisciplinary team of caregivers to meet healthcare needs through the services of a home health agency. The home care nurse is the most involved professional team member and is the one professional who sees the client on a regular and continuous basis. It is the home care nurse, along with the physician, who develops the plan of care and directs services provided by home health aides. Other agency team members include physical, speech, and occupational therapists, social workers, and nutritionists. However, the most *important* team members are the clients and their primary caregivers.

Elderly clients make up about 85 percent of the home care population, so home care nurses need to be prepared to meet the demanding and special needs of these people. The goal of the plan of care is that clients regain or maintain a wellness state or are comforted while experiencing a peaceful death. Goals might include preventing skin breakdown, promoting continence or wound healing, and teaching family members and other health care personnel to effectively manage clients with limiting and potentially debilitating or terminal illnesses.

Some nurses may be new to home care nursing and have limited experience with elders at home. Depending upon the nurses' education and professional experiences, they may have never before worked so directly and intimately with clients and family members in an environment outside of the familiar inpatient setting.

Home Care of the Elderly will help the nurse new to home care, and the nurse not so new to home care, deal more effectively with the elderly client at home. It is designed to help nurses create strategies that provide a safe and wellness-focused environment that promotes healing and prevents or solves problems occurring among elders at home.

The book is divided into four units. In Unit I, three chapters focus on fundamental and foundational information useful to nurses who work with the homebound elder. The chapters focus on managing elders at home; financial, legal and ethical issues; and the unique characteristics of conducting a physical assessment on elders.

In Unit II, the four chapters discuss home safety, promotion of mobility and safe use of ambulatory aids, principles of nutritional adequacy and adaptations needed by some elders, and promotion of healthy sexual expressions among older adults. Points covered in this unit apply to all elders regardless of their medical or surgical conditions.

Unit III has five chapters filled with information that is applicable to most elders visited through home health agencies. Elders are frequently on several medications, and the safe administration, side effects, and potentially detrimental side effects need to be recognized and taught to clients and caregivers. In addition, many elders experience hearing and vision changes, and the home care nurse can offer effective ways to manage the frustrations caused by changes in these senses. Some elders or family members may be physically or verbally abusive, and the home care nurse needs to know how to recognize and constructively deal with such abuse. Frequently elders experience temporary or permanent bladder or bowel problems, including continence and constipation issues or even managing and coping with medically or surgically altered elimination patterns. Protecting skin from damage and promoting pressure ulcer healing is the focus of the last chapter in this unit.

Unit IV is lengthy, containing ten chapters. The intensity of these chapters reflects specific social, medical, and surgical conditions that are especially common to the elderly and helps guide the nurse in providing excellent care. The topics include postoperative considerations, rheumatic diseases, diabetes care, cardiac and respiratory conditions, neurological conditions, psychiatric disorders, cancer care, Alzheimer's disease and related dementias, and finally palliative caregiving.

By including all aspects of the possible range of conditions and issues the home care nurse may encounter with older homebound clients, *Home Care of the Elderly* becomes essential reading for the home care nurse and other health care professionals.

Sheryl Mara Zang, RN, MS, FNP
Judith A. Allender, RN C, MSN, EdD

ACKNOWLEDGMENTS

First, we want to thank all the contributors and reviewers for sharing their expertise, their dedication, and a part of their lives. We are all richer for their clinical expertise and excellent caregiving to our elderly population.

We want to thank our elderly home care clients for sharing their lives and homes with us. At each encounter we feel that we are experiencing a part of history. These clients' values, beliefs, and strengths have always guided us and taught us that the richness of life is measured by experiences and relationships with others.

A special thanks goes to the staff, clients, and residents of:

The Metropolitan Jewish Geriatric Center Home Health Care Systems and Visiting Nurse Service of New York

Menorah Nursing Home in Manhattan Beach, New York

The Gerontology Program and Geriatric Education Center at California State University, Fresno, California

Comfort Care Residential Care Facility, Fresno, California

Our thanks would not be complete without recognizing the special efforts of Susan M. Glover, senior editor, and Bridget Blatteau, editorial assistant, at Lippincott Williams & Wilkins. Their faith in this project and invaluable assistance are appreciated.

Finally, a special thanks to our wonderful husbands, Steven Zang and Gilbert Allender, for always being there for us during every facet of this book. And a very special thanks to the Zang children, Ivy and Andrew, for all their support.

C O N T E N T S

UNIT IV

Home Care Management of Elderly Clients With Specific Medical and Surgical Diagnoses

FOUNDATIONAL ISSUES IN HOME CARE FOR THE OLDER ADULT

n this first unit, the reader is presented with a set of three chapters that are foundational to practice in home healthcare, especially with the elderly. The nurse entering home health nursing will find that these chapters are designed to augment skills already developed for the acute care setting.

However, in home care, there are additional considerations the nurse must address. These include working in an environment familiar to the client but not necessarily to the nurse and dealing with family members, lay caregivers, and community resources. Working within a different financial structure and time frame will also be a new experience for the nurse. Home care nurses must modify traditional physical, mental, and emotional assessments to accommodate the nature of the home environment and age of the client.

These differences from the acute care setting are addressed in the context of working with older adults in their homes. We anticipate that the reader will be able to use these foundational chapters to "set the scene" for effective practice in home health.

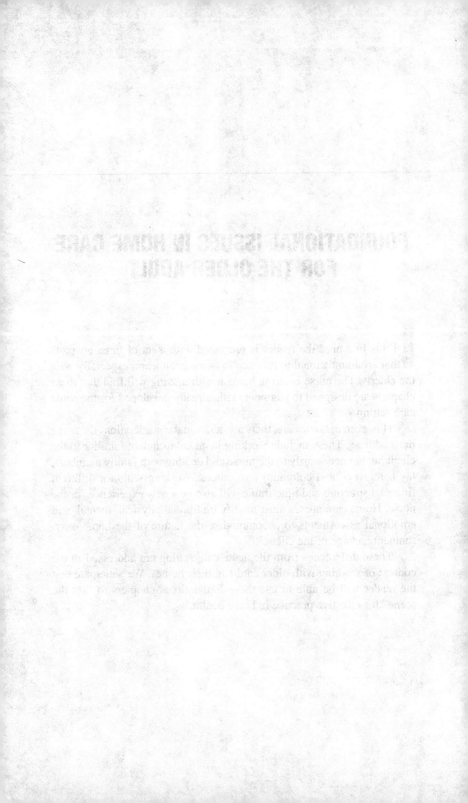

EFFECTIVELY MANAGING THE ELDERLY CLIENT IN THE COMMUNITY

Ann Marie D'Angelo

◆ ◆ ◆

The Discharge Plan
Issues Related to the Home Environment
Role of the Primary Informal Caregiver
Involving Other Informal Caregivers
Identifying Community Resources
Housing Options for Elders
The Long-Term Planning Process
Summary

The home care nurse plays a central role in identifying and managing the 24-hour care of the elderly client at home. The role entails understanding the multifaceted needs of diverse clients as they exist in the home and community setting. It is through a detailed assessment and evaluation of each client's physical, psychosocial, environmental, and financial needs that this can be accomplished. As the coordinator or care manager of the client, the home care nurse is responsible for developing a client and family centered plan of care, which includes a realistic discharge plan that is mutually developed with the client and significant family members and also includes follow-up care supported mainly by community resources.

THE DISCHARGE PLAN

The ideal discharge plan begins when the client enters the acute care setting with a plan for care to be continued through the acute care stay, discharge to another appropriate facility as necessary, or discharge to home with care provided by community support or from a home care agency. A realistic discharge plan should entail a long-term care plan that helps the client and family identify community resources that will help maintain the client at home as long as possible. In most inpatient facilities, a discharge planner (who is usually a registered nurse or social worker) identifies clients who may need home health services upon discharge and integrates home care in the discharge planning process. In some communities, home health agencies have agreements with acute care centers and have a staff member attending discharge planning meetings. In either case, providing such continuity from hospital stay through to appropriate discharge insures no interruption in services and makes the transition to home as safe and supportive as possible.

ISSUES RELATED TO THE HOME ENVIRONMENT

Home care staff members' visits will be limited by the extent of insurance coverage and the family's ability to pay for services. Therefore an important role of the home care nurse is to identify community services the family can tap into to meet caregiving needs when home care services are discontinued. This long-term care planning process should begin with identifying issues that confront the client at home. Particulars about financing home care are covered in Chapter 2.

Knowing the client's income sources, which may include Social Security, retirement benefits, savings, investments, or Supplemental Security Income (SSI), gives the nurse information necessary to determine eligibility for services that are based on the client's resources. The nurse also needs to know if the client has Medicare and Medicaid benefits— allowances within these two programs can determine what services and supplies will be paid for by insurance instead of by the client. A client's private funds become relevant and necessary issues to discuss in order to institute appropriate services. Nurses are not used to gathering this information from clients in the acute care setting, and it may be harder for the nurse to ask these questions than it is for the client to answer.

There are many issues the home care nurse deals with when providing care outside of a structured facility, and several are mentioned here but will be dealt with in depth in later chapters. For example, issues such as safety take on a greater meaning for the home care nurse, who must consider the safety of the neighborhood as well as the apartment or house where the client resides. Does the client live with relatives, friends, in a congregate living center, foster home, or residential care facility? How do safety factors differ in each situation?

Understanding the client's cultural and religious affiliations and how they might dictate healthcare regimens and dietary restrictions are important both to client teaching and compliance. Culture and religion have overwhelming influences on everyday practices, which are strongly health-related when the practices are assessed. For example, if a client believes in fate and that the control of her health is in the hands of the gods, noncompliance issues take on a different meaning than with a client who believes her health is in her hands but who does not have the knowledge base to help herself. In each case the nurse has an important, but different, role.

Assessing community resources that are available to assist the client and family in maintaining the client at home are essential to any long-term care plan. The home care nurse must be knowledgeable about community resources, how to access them, and how to explain their services to the client and family members. This is necessary to maintain the level of wellness when services are discontinued through the home care agency.

There are also times, despite thorough planning, that the client can no longer realistically remain at home safely. This is again a time when the home care nurse helps the client and family by knowing about the alternative housing and caregiving options available in the community and how they fit with the client's needs, desires, and financial resources.

ROLE OF THE PRIMARY INFORMAL CAREGIVER

It is important to understand the role of the informal caregiver. The primary caregiver and the client are the central players in maintaining the client at home. In many instances, without the assistance of the primary informal caregiver, the client would not be able to do well at home. This is a different concept for most nurses who are used to working only with professionals, paraprofessionals, and occasionally volunteers.

The primary caregiver is often an elderly spouse, an adult child, or a close relative of the client. These caregivers are physically and emotionally involved family members. They have attachments to the client that are overwhelmingly beneficial, but at times the attachments can cloud the caregiving needed by the client. There are occasions when the need for care services has more to do with competing demands on the caregiver's time than actual changes in the condition of the client. When the caregiver is feeling overburdened, it will directly effect the care of the client. It is, therefore, the responsibility of the home care nurse to identify other resources that may assist in the direct or indirect care of the client. This will permit the client to receive the care needed at home, as well as give the primary caregiver much needed relief.

INVOLVING OTHER INFORMAL CAREGIVERS

Involving others in the care of the client gives the primary caregiver time to renew energy and to lessen or eliminate the possibility of caregiver burnout. Very often the primary caregiver has difficulty in asking others to help with any tasks. However, the home care nurse can suggest and encourage the involvement of others. The home care nurse needs to help the client and primary caregiver to (1) identify other family members or friends that are willing to help, (2) identify tasks that they are willing to allow others to do, and (3) have a family meeting or telephone conference with the client, primary caregiver, family, and friends to request assistance.

The discussion about requesting help must remain goal-oriented. However, by nature of identifying certain people, the client and primary caregiver are indicating those people in their lives whom they feel comfortable reaching out to. This can be facilitated by directing the client and caregiver to (1) list which family and friends live close by, (2) who visits them, and (3) with what community agencies they are affiliated. If there are relatives the nurse is aware of that the client does not mention, such as a daughter or a grown grandson, it is appropriate for the home care nurse to explore why these people were not mentioned. Listening to their reasons is important, and the exercise would not be complete if the nurse did not take the discussion further and perhaps unravel miscommunication or unresolved family issues. It is important to remind the client and caregiver that they need help now and to ask for it if at all possible.

It is essential to help the client and caregiver to identify tasks that they are willing to allow others to do. This is an important issue because there may be traditional tasks that are part of their roles that they want to maintain. To facilitate the client and primary caregiver to make the decisions, ask them what tasks or activities are becoming more difficult due to either competing demands or a change in medical condition. Competing demands on the caregiver may range from having to do something outside the house and not feeling comfortable leaving the client alone to being unable to prepare a meal because the client needs frequent attention. A change in medical condition can increase the need for assistance with basic activities of daily living (ADL), such as eating, drinking, repositioning, getting out of bed, transferring, or toileting. This can be very frustrating to any independent individual and very frightening if it is not likely to improve. The home care nurse must determine with the client and caregiver if the informal support of family and friends will be enough help.

The nurse can suggest a family meeting or telephone conference with the client, caregiver, family, and friends. This can be more successful if the caregiver has a "to do" list of specific tasks or activities. The list should be developed prior to the family meeting and include both realistic and specific requests that are time limited. This could include asking for help two times a week from 3:00 to 5:00 p.m. so the caregiver can prepare dinner without interruption, or from 1:00 to 3:00 p.m. so the caregiver can go out shopping. This list can also include assistance with personal care, financial tasks, grocery shopping, dog walking, home maintenance tasks and repairs, yard work, and transportation, depending on the client's and caregiver's needs and the others' willingness to help.

This process will ensure the active participation of all involved. It also gives potential caregivers ideas for specific tasks they may be willing to do without feeling overburdened themselves. The out-of-town daughter may be willing to visit on Saturdays so the primary caregiver can go out shopping, the grown grandson may agree to mow the lawn once a week, and members from the family's church may agree to bring the family a hot meal on Tuesday evenings. This shares some of the burden of caregiving, and it gives the primary caregiver some relief and possibly less worry.

IDENTIFYING COMMUNITY RESOURCES

An important role of the home care nurse is to educate the client and caregivers about local community resources available to lessen the caregivers' burden and perhaps enrich the client's life. These resources include local programs and services offered to seniors and caregivers. There are outreach programs in many churches and synagogues that provide weekly visits and phone calls that will help keep the client connected to the community. Local pharmacies, food stores, and some supermarkets will deliver medicines and groceries free of charge or for a nominal fee. The yellow pages of the local phone book lists resources that offer services for the elderly and for caregivers.

As a beginning home care nurse, knowledge about the availability of services may be limited. As time in this type of nursing continues, the nurse learns from fellow staff members, supervisors, and personal experiences what is available in the region for present and potential clients. The expert home care nurse keeps a file (in an address book or a small notebook) with business cards, phone numbers, and information about agencies or people who can provide a bevy of needed services for elders. Several categories of agencies and services specific to elders are highlighted below. Most communities have these available to their members. The names of agencies may be different and the services may vary, but they are an essential place to begin when developing a community resource file.

Area Agency on Aging

This nonprofit agency can guide callers to a broad listing of services for elders, including legal (for abuse, neglect, exploitation issues), housing, and healthcare placement options. Information about individual concerns with elders can be gathered from agency staff.

National Organizations

There are several national organizations whose primary goals are to inform the lay and professional public on social, medical, and environmental issues and to promote the health and well-being of elders. Some resources in this category include the American Society on Aging (ASA), the American Association of Retired Persons (AARP), and the Gerontological Society of America (GSA). Each has publications, annual and regional informative or scientific meetings, and other benefits for members.

Disease-Specific Support Groups

There are support groups available for clients and caregivers that focus on many disease- or injury-related health problems. Local telephone books and newspapers may list dates and times of meetings. These groups can be educational in nature, providing health information specific to the clients' problems. They also provide emotional support, helping clients realize that they are not alone. Similar groups are available for caregivers to support them in this difficult role. These groups can help caregivers verbalize concerns, express feelings, meet others in the same position, and develop new friendships, as well as provide a means of becoming aware of other community services. Support groups are sponsored by adult daycare programs, libraries, churches, synagogues, and Alzheimer's or other illness-oriented organizations, such as the American Diabetic Association (ADA) or the American Heart Association (AHA), as well as by adult education programs and senior citizen centers.

Meal Delivery Programs

Meal delivery programs come with many names and offer different types of service, region to region. One name that may be familiar is Meals on Wheels. It is a service for the homebound client who lives alone, and it provides one to two meals a day depending on the region. Accessing these services occurs by calling local senior centers, Catholic charities, or the Jewish Association for Services for the Elderly.

Caregiving Supportive Programs

Adult daycare programs. These programs provide more services for the frail elderly client than local senior centers. There are two types of adult daycare: (1) the social or social club model and (2) the medical model. The social model provides socialization, recreation, transportation, and meals. There are adult daycare centers that design activities specifically for dementia or Alzheimer's clients. The medical model provides outpatient services in a community setting, including medical, nursing, rehabilitation, and social services. Some adult daycare programs may be covered by Medicaid or partially covered by Medicare Part B. The social models that have no medical component are not covered by

Medicare or Medicaid, but they often offer services at a nominal fee or request only a contribution.

Respite programs. These provide short-term and infrequent care. Their services can involve in-home supervision, adult daycare, or overnight stays at the client's home, at a residential care facility, or at a skilled nursing facility. The purpose of a respite program is to provide caregiver relief. Respite services are a very important method of temporary relief from the continuous burden of caregiving. It can provide time for caregivers to focus on their own needs. Respite services can be provided on a daytime, overnight, weekend, or one or more week basis (to allow the caregiver a vacation), depending on the needs of the caregiver. Respite care may be paid for by Medicare, Medicaid, or private pay. Medicare will provide up to 80 hours of respite care per year.

Hospice care programs. These provide comprehensive palliative medical care and supportive services for terminally ill clients and their families. These services can be provided at home, in a participating skilled nursing facility, or for a limited stay in an acute care facility. It is an important long-term care option for the terminally ill client and family (see Chapter 22).

Personal Emergency Response Systems

A personal emergency response system is an emergency communication system that provides a device with a call button. The device can be worn as a bracelet or necklace. When the call button is pressed, an electronic signal is sent and brings outside help. This can give the caregiver peace of mind when leaving the client alone to run an errand. It also gives the client who lives alone some reassurance because of the emergency contact. These systems have a cost involved that is not covered by insurance.

HOUSING OPTIONS FOR ELDERS

For a variety of reasons, elderly clients may not be able to remain in the home they once occupied. A large, multilevel house is too large and expensive to care for; a second-floor apartment is too difficult to reach by the stairs; assistance is needed with showering or to remember medications. Fortunately, housing options for elders are many, and more will become available as our aging population grows.

Older adults need safe housing options that offer the least restrictive and most independent living along with the potential for increased services as health needs change. For this reason, home care nurses need to know the community resources available to clients in all phases of the health continuum. Clients should be living in a setting that best meets their needs and that allows them to remain as independent as possible for as long as possible. The home care nurse may be instrumental in offering other alternatives if the client's present living situation becomes unsafe.

The times when the home care client can no longer remain at home can be as diverse as the client population that the home care nurse services. However, there are indicators that will identify some of these times. These indicators include but are not limited to: (1) the client lives alone and can no longer direct his own care; (2) the primary caregiver is no longer able, willing, or available to take responsibility for the client's care; (3) the client needs assistance with activities of daily living (ADL); (4) the place the client lives in is no longer available and no other suitable arrangements can be made; (5) the client prefers to live in a senior congregate living center, an adult home, or a residential care facility. These indicators will direct the home care nurse to discuss other options with the client and family. It is important for the home care nurse to assist in long-term planning with detailed knowledge of available services. In addition, it is important to understand and realize the complex and difficult decision this is for all involved.

Congregate Living Centers

The congregate living center option, which is becoming very popular among older adults, provides a supervised apartment setting with support services that enable elderly residents to continue to live in the community with as much independence as they can manage. The resident needs to be in stable health and not in need of continuous medical, nursing, or personal care services unless the congregate living center is licensed to provide an assisted living program. The centers provide assistance with housekeeping, laundry, group or aggregate dining, and some personal care services, as well as transportation for medical appointments and shopping. Residents can rent a studio or a one- or two-bedroom apartment. Some congregate living centers offer only long-term contracts with a significant buy-in cost; others rent on a month-to-month basis.

If such housing options offer *assisted living* and this is what the client needs or wants, clients may elect to share a two- or three-bedroom apartment. Assisted living offers a minimal level of care where medications are administered by the staff and assistance with personal care is available as needed. Staff in congregate living centers, even in the sections offering assisted living, are not required to be licensed, so if a resident needs definitive skilled care on a short-term basis, home care nursing service can be initiated. If the skilled needs are greater, alternative housing options may need to be considered.

Many congregate living centers are run by public and not-for-profit agencies. They are rich with aesthetic amenities and often have long waiting lists. Home care nurses can be proactive with clients and help them make long-term housing option plans by getting on waiting lists for preferred centers before the need arises, for indeed, some popular housing option choices may have a five- to ten-year waiting list.

Adult Foster Care

This is a program for the elderly administered by the Department of Social Services. The elderly client lives in a home with a nonrelated family that provides meals, supervision, laundry service, and limited personal care. They often have to share a room with another elderly client, and they cannot need skilled nursing care on an ongoing basis. The foster care home may accept SSI or private pay. This is usually a less-expensive option for elders. Home care nurses visit in these settings when needs for skilled care arise.

Residential Care Facilities (RCFs)

These long-term residential facilities provide room, board, housekeeping, supervision, and limited personal care services to five or more adults not related to the administrator. They are usually small and homey, with residents frequently sharing a bedroom and using the common rooms along with other residents. They can be proprietary (for profit), public, or voluntary (not-for-profit) facilities. There are a wide range of RCFs in the country. Their populations can be frail elderly, psychiatric, or mixed. Unless an adult home is affiliated with an assisted living program, their admission criteria includes (1) a medical evaluation, including TB skin test; (2) a psychiatric evaluation if the client has a psychiatric history; and (3) an admission interview. The home care nurse frequently visits clients in these facilities.

These facilities make very comfortable homes for frail, elderly clients who enjoy the smaller, home-like setting the RCF provides. Some of the large congregate living centers appeal to hardy, elderly clients who are physically active and for whom walking to a dining room hundreds of feet from their apartments is desirable and accomplishable.

The surge in building various types of senior housing is a sign of the times in the United States. Decades of a productive economy, years of women in the workplace, work settings offering retirement benefits, families being physically and emotionally separated, and people living longer have set the stage for such housing options. In addition, these varying options help maintain the older adult in the community longer at a substantially decreased cost compared to living in a skilled nursing facility (SNF). Since many of the newer, hotel-like facilities only accept private pay, the client and family must be prepared to investigate all of the housing options available in their price range.

THE LONG-TERM PLANNING PROCESS

Long-term care planning is a process that entails consideration of issues and options for elderly clients and their family members. The home care nurse is uniquely qualified to assist in this process because of specialized training in community health issues and long-term care needs of the elderly client. As the home care nurse discharges a client from agency services, part of that discharge process should be a comprehensive discharge plan that includes long-term arrangements indicating community resources for the client and primary caregiver. Most elderly clients discharged from home healthcare services continue to live in their present environment, hopefully at a higher level of wellness. For others, alternative options need to be discussed and choices be made.

At the point of discharge from home health services, the home health nurse terminates client caregiving. If the client is transferred to a skilled nursing facility (SNF), the professional staff in that facility will provide skilled services, as the home health nurse did when the client was at home.

Some of the issues that become important during a long-term care-planning process include: (1) the prognosis of the client's overall health status and the possibility of the client remaining in place with additional support, (2) the way the client and caregiver view home care in their current residence versus moving to a senior housing facility, (3) the nurse's ability to discuss the client's and caregiver's concerns and options openly, (4) facilitating realistic discussions regarding the client's health status and prognosis and the caregiver's ability as caregiving needs increase or change, (5) informing and educating the client and family about the services of SNFs and reinforcing that SNFs have many specialized services that can improve the quality of life for the elderly, including adult daycare programs and short-term rehabilitation. This can be especially important since there are many negative ideas and feelings that people have about SNFs.

Feelings of sadness, anger, guilt, inadequacy, and helplessness may all be expressed by the client and family during this process. In fact, their feelings may be similar to how the home care nurse feels about having to redirect the client and family toward these options. It is important for home care nurses to come to terms with their own feelings in order to support and direct the client and family to the next best possible step.

Based on family resources and client needs, a SNF placement may be the best option available. Families need to know that long-term SNF placement is not the worst placement option. Although it is the least independent of the options, it is the best in meeting the complex needs of the client. It can offer socialization to lonely isolated clients and give 24-hour care for clients who can no longer care for themselves.

Central to the planning process are payment considerations. Medicaid covers long-term care in assisted living programs and skilled nursing facilities, but only a minority of elders are eligible for Medicaid benefits. Even those elders with limited resources must first spend them before becoming eligible for Medicaid (see Chapter 2).

Other benefits, such as Medicare, pay for limited, short-term care for the homebound client. Long-term care insurance is a viable payment source depending on the amount of coverage. However, coverage varies considerably regarding home care and skilled nursing care, and very few elders have such policies, as they are expensive, especially if purchased later in life. Private pay is always the most flexible payment form because all healthcare services will accept private funds. However, most people's private funds are limited. Costs for SNFs vary by region and amenities, but it is not unusual for monthly fees to exceed $3,500.

Managed care affects the client's Medicare benefits, including home care and extended care services. This means the home care nurse will be coordinating care with a case manager, who is often a registered nurse, to obtain needed services. Managed care creates contracts with certain facilities for short-term rehabilitation to decrease costs and provide closer monitoring of their clients. This will influence placement decisions and severely limit the client's and family's choices of facilities.

The last and most important consideration for any senior housing option or skilled nursing facility placement is whether the facility is the right one for the client and family. All residential facilities have their own culture and personality, and therefore it is important for the family and client, if possible, to explore several facilities. It is important to remember that placements are not always available at the time of need, especially in skilled nursing facilities, so temporary alternative plans need to be made.

There are many considerations in choosing any housing option or skilled nursing facility, including: (1) proximity to family, (2) ability to address the client's special needs, (3) similar cultural and religious backgrounds among staff and residents, (4) having a solid reputation in the community, (5) maintaining all state and local licenses, certifications, and assessments, (6) being in a safe area with transportation and parking available. These are just a few of the important considerations for any senior living arrangement. Each family will need to personalize its own list of concerns with the assistance of the home care nurse.

SUMMARY

Home care clients need supportive caregivers in order to be effectively managed at home. When informal caregivers are nonexistent or limited, community resources need to be included in the caregiving plan. Even when available, the caregivers may need the services of different resources in the community in order to cope with the physically and emotionally demanding role of caregiver. Home care clients live in a variety of settings and home care nurses visit in all of them. If and when a client needs the services of a skilled nursing facility, the home care nurse does not provide care, the agency staff does. However, this does not eliminate the home health nurse's role as an educator and counselor while the client and family considers options they must make. Making a decision to move into a skilled nursing facility is not an easy one, but it can be made as pleasant as possible with the help of an expert home care nurse who listens to and processes the client's needs. The home care nurse is uniquely qualified to assist the client and family in the long-term planning process. This process should be part of any discharge plan from home health services to help clients and their families prepare for future needs.

2

FINANCIAL, LEGAL, AND ETHICAL ISSUES WHEN PROVIDING HEALTHCARE FOR ELDERLY CLIENTS AT HOME

Frank G. D'Angelo, Esq.
Ann Marie D'Angelo

◆　◆　◆

Home care in the United States is a diverse and growing service industry. Many nurses who thought their careers would always be in the acute care setting are now entering the home care field. Making this change is exciting and challenging. There are many unanswered questions that nurses have who are new to home care. Invariably, some of them will pertain to the financial structure of this specialty area of nursing, because in no other healthcare setting are nurses so involved with the paperwork related to reimbursement issues. Two of the systems most elders are a part of are Medicare and Medicaid. These two programs are the primary funding sources for older adults, and the ones with which the home care nurse will need to be the most familiar. There are other funding mechanisms that will also be mentioned in this chapter.

Other aspects of healthcare delivered in clients' homes that may be different from those in the acute care setting include legal and ethical issues. The most common concerns are presented here. It is the intention of this chapter to orient the new home care nurse to a variety of financial, legal, and ethical considerations. There are over 17,000 providers delivering home care to over 7 million individuals in the community, and billions of dollars are spent each year on the bevy of services provided (National Association for Home Care [NAHC], 1995). This is an area that employs nurses in increasing numbers. The more knowledgeable the new home care nurse is, the easier the transition will be.

FINANCING HOME CARE THROUGH ENTITLEMENT/BENEFIT PROGRAMS

Medicare Covered Home Healthcare

Medicare is a federally funded, federally administered health insurance program designed primarily to guarantee the provision of healthcare to the elderly and to some others who are permanently disabled, regardless of age. It is administered by the Health Care Financing Administration (HCFA) of the federal government. Participation in the Medicare program is completely voluntary and must be applied for prior to the 65th birthday. All persons over the age of 65 who have paid the allotted quarters of eligibility in Social Security taxes are entitled to participate in the Medicare program. Any person entitled to Medicare benefits is free to obtain necessary health services from any institution, agency, or person participating in the program.

Medicare consists of two separate programs. Part A covers hospital insurance benefits, which include home healthcare. Part B provides supplementary medical insurance for items and services that are either not fully covered or not covered at all by Part A hospital insurance. Part A hospital insurance is provided to eligible persons without charge. By contrast, there is a monthly premium ($43.80 in 1997) for Part B medical insurance coverage. For persons receiving Social Security benefits, the fee for Medicare Part B is deducted from their monthly check before they receive it.

Medicare Part A hospital insurance helps pay for four types of services:

- Inpatient hospital care for a limited number of days in any benefit period.
- Post-hospital extended care services for up to 100 days per benefit period.
- Home health services.
- Hospice care for limited periods in cases of terminal illness, by election of the beneficiary and in lieu of the standard Medicare benefits noted above.

The Medicare program considers citizenship or legal alien status, eligibility for Social Security benefits, and permanent disability status. To determine if a client is eligible for Medicare, the nurse can have the client or family contact the nearest Social Security Administration (SSA) office for information. It is important to note that at times the rules and requirements for Medicare enrollment change, and all clients and their families should know the nearest SSA office phone number. Once persons are receiving Medicare, they are eligible for all hospital and/or home care services covered by the program.

There are many services covered by Medicare Part A for an elderly client receiving care in acute care settings. Those services will not be covered in this chapter. This chapter focuses on benefits or entitlements to people receiving care outside of the acute care setting, namely those at home and needing home healthcare services. Home health eligibility rules under Medicare are set forth in detail in the *Medicare Health Insurance Manual* (HCFA pub. 11), known as the *HIM 11*. Once enrolled, to qualify for Medicare home health coverage, five conditions must be met:

1. *The client's primary care provider must have determined that medical care in the home is needed, and the primary care provider must prepare a plan of care.* This can happen in a variety of ways. Usually the need for home care is determined while the client is hospitalized, and plans are set in motion prior to discharge through the efforts of the healthcare provider and the discharge planner. Clients can also enter home care via a telephone call from the client or concerned family member or friend. The home care agency contacted will have a registered nurse make an assessment visit; the client's primary care provider will be contacted and a plan of care initiated. The primary care provider has to sign and agree to the plan of care developed by the nurse but usually does not design the plan.

2. *The client must remain under the care of a primary care provider.*

3. *Care needed must include intermittent (not full-time) skilled nursing care, physical therapy, or speech language pathology services (speech therapy).* The medical provider in collaboration with a registered nurse (either the discharge planner or a home care nurse) can determine if a specific client meets these criteria.

4. *The client must be homebound. Homebound status is considered when the client can leave the home only with considerable and taxing effort. Absences from home must be infrequent and of short duration, or to get medical care.* This is a difficult conditional requirement to explain to clients and at times to verify. The home care nurse uses well-developed skills of listening and assessing when determining this status.

5. *The home care agency must be approved by the Medicare program.* Even though there are over 17,000 home care agencies, only about half of them are Medicare-certified agencies. For a variety of reasons, the other agencies remain outside of the Medicare program. Usually it is because they are involved primarily in the provision of homemaker–home health aide services, in services to pediatric or other non-elderly populations, or in high-tech services.

Once eligibility for Medicare-approved home health services has been established, caregiving can begin. If the client meets all five of the conditions, Medicare will pay for:

- Skilled nursing care—on an intermittent or part-time basis
- Home health aide services—on an intermittent or part-time basis for personal assistance
- Physical therapy
- Speech language pathology (speech therapy)
- Occupational therapy
- Medical social services—to assess the social and emotional factors related to the client's illness, for counseling, and to search for available community resources
- Medical supplies—disposable products such as dressings and disposable pads
- Medical equipment—durable medical equipment (DME), such as a wheelchair, walker, or oxygen equipment

Nurses need to be aware that Medicare does NOT cover:

- 24-hour care at home (unless it is only necessary for one day)
- Prescription drugs (exceptions may apply to drugs administered by a pump)
- Blood transfusions
- Ambulance transportation
- Dental care, eyeglasses, and hearing aides
- Meals delivered to the home
- Homemaker services, such as shopping, cleaning, and laundry (except home health aides may do a small amount of these chores at the time they are providing covered services)
- Personal care provided by home health aides, such as bathing, toileting, and providing help in getting dressed—if this is the *only* care the client needs. This service alone is classified as "custodial" because it could be provided safely and reasonably by people without professional skills and training.

Unlike inpatient hospital and skilled nursing facility benefits, Medicare hospital insurance pays the entire cost of most covered home health services, without regard to the number of visits to the home as long as skilled services are needed. Although the regulations provide for visits in the home, the visits are limited. The weekly maximum of 28 hours for skilled nursing and home health aide care combined is the general limit of part-time or intermittent care. The services can be provided seven days a week as long as they are provided for less than eight hours per day.

The only exception to the rule in which Medicare pays the entire cost of home health services is for new durable medical equipment, for which there is a copayment of 20 percent of the reasonable cost of such equipment, as determined by Medicare. This would include walkers, wheelchairs, and oxygen equipment. The client is not responsible for any deductibles or copayments on any other covered items and services.

The Medicare program significantly helps elders receive needed care and services through home health agencies, but there are many services not covered and a good portion of the costs must be picked up by the client. The Medicare program can also be quite complex. Billing staff in home health agencies can be of great assistance to both new and experienced nurses who need current Medicare information or clarification on numbers of covered hours of services that particular clients can receive as the plan of care is being formulated. The nurse must take into account the client's condition; the client's potential for learning and assisting in self-care; what needs to be achieved; who is available, able, and willing to help, such as significant others, family, and friends; and accessibility of community resources. It is only then that an effective plan of care can be established within the structure of Medicare guidelines that meets client needs without costing the client unnecessary out-of-pocket expense.

Medicare Covered Hospice Care

Medicare Part A hospital insurance has been providing coverage for care received from a hospice since 1983. The hospice philosophy of terminal care requires that clients choose to forego active treatment and receive only palliative care. Hospices provide palliative medical care and supportive social, emotional, and spiritual services to the terminally ill and their families. There are about 1,800 Medicare-certified hospices in the United States (NAHC, 1995).

A client wishing to receive care from a hospice must obtain a doctor's certification that he or she is "terminally ill." For purposes of qualifying for hospice care benefits, a client is considered to be terminally ill if life expectancy is estimated by a primary care provider to be about six months. The client's attending primary care provider must also formulate a written plan for providing hospice care and periodically review that plan to ensure that hospice care is being provided in accordance with it.

If the client qualifies for hospice care and chooses it in lieu of all other Medicare hospital insurance benefits, the following items and services are included:

- Nursing care by or under the supervision of a registered nurse
- Primary care providers' services
- Physical or occupational therapy or speech pathology
- Medical social services under the direction of a primary care provider
- Drugs and biologicals, including outpatient drugs

- Home health aide and homemaker services
- Medical supplies, such as dressings and casts
- Use of medical equipment such as wheelchairs and crutches
- Counseling, including dietary counseling, with respect to terminal illness and adjustment to death
- Short-term inpatient care, including "respite care"— short-term inpatient stays to temporarily relieve a person who normally provides hospice care to the client. Note that respite care periods to be covered under Part A must not exceed five consecutive days at a time.

These services are available on a 24-hour, continuous basis during crises periods and as necessary to maintain terminally ill patients at home. About 90 percent of hospice clients have cancer, while the remaining clients have illnesses other than cancer, namely cardiac diagnoses and chronic lung disease (Rosenzweig, 1995).

Medicaid Covered Home Healthcare

Medicaid needs to be distinguished from Medicare, and often the two programs are confused when referring to them. While Medicare is a form of health insurance with eligibility not depending on the recipient's level of assets, Medicaid covers certain categories of individuals with very low income and resources. Medicaid is a joint federal and state program, funded half by the federal government and half by the state.

Federal legislation and regulations set forth the general requirements that states must follow, making coverage of some categories of individuals and some benefits mandatory and some optional. Since Medicaid is administered by individual states, this allows for flexibility in choosing which services to cover under each Medicaid program. Each state can use the money for its medically indigent residents as the state so desires. Because the needs of individual residents in each state may fluctuate and differ and agendas may vary with changing political leadership, the Medicaid program has more frequent changes than the Medicare program. Each state covers healthcare services for its residents in need with a varying focus, length of time, and amount. To discuss what is covered for whom and for how long in one state would be neglecting the differences in 49 others. Again, this is a time when the billing staff in the home health agency or personnel in the local office of the Department of Social Services can give the nurse the most current Medicaid coverage information for that state.

The Medicaid program covers the medically indigent of all ages, but for the purposes of this book only elders eligible for Medicaid are focused on. Older adults enrolled in Medicare may also be eligible for Medicaid benefits because they have become or are medically indigent. Each client's assets are assessed and if the "means testing" supports eligibility, then the Medicaid program supplements home healthcare services needed and not covered by Medicare. Certain assets are considered exempt and so do not have to be spent by the applicant in order to qualify for Medicaid. Nonexempt assets have to be spent to pay for care before the applicant can qualify. For example, there is a limit on the amount of cash in checking or savings accounts and a limit on the amount of life insurance a person can have. The value of a client's vehicle is also considered, and at times clients may need to sell an expensive car for a less expensive one. (See Box 2-1 for an eligibility example from one state.)

The in-home services that clients may qualify for under Medicaid may be more generous than what the Medicare program alone covers. Home care nurses should be aware that for all clients receiving home care from a certified home health agency (CHHA) a fiscal assessment is required. A fiscal assessment is applied to every case on a predetermined basis, regardless of the duration of care on an hourly or daily basis. In addition, recertification must also be done as determined by the state's Medicaid program on a regular basis, such as every six months, or in the case of a change in the client's medical condition or mental state.

Medicaid Covered Hospice Care

Hospice care is an optional Medicaid service that is currently offered by most of the states (36 in 1995). Since Medicare has been covering a major portion of the cost of hospice care for older adults, the bulk of Medicaid-paid hospice care recipients are younger than 65 years old. During the 15-plus years Medicare has been covering hospice care for older adults, their needs through a hospice philosophy have been met. The states have optional plan services through the Medicaid program. Essentially this allows states to determine what special groups they will cover through specific Medicaid options. Often the frail elderly, functionally disabled

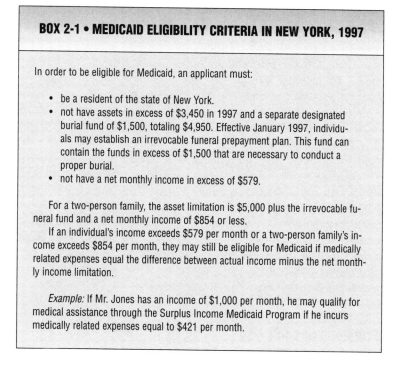

BOX 2-1 • MEDICAID ELIGIBILITY CRITERIA IN NEW YORK, 1997

In order to be eligible for Medicaid, an applicant must:

- be a resident of the state of New York.
- not have assets in excess of $3,450 in 1997 and a separate designated burial fund of $1,500, totaling $4,950. Effective January 1997, individuals may establish an irrevocable funeral prepayment plan. This fund can contain the funds in excess of $1,500 that are necessary to conduct a proper burial.
- not have a net monthly income in excess of $579.

For a two-person family, the asset limitation is $5,000 plus the irrevocable funeral fund and a net monthly income of $854 or less.

If an individual's income exceeds $579 per month or a two-person family's income exceeds $854 per month, they may still be eligible for Medicaid if medically related expenses equal the difference between actual income minus the net monthly income limitation.

Example: If Mr. Jones has an income of $1,000 per month, he may qualify for medical assistance through the Surplus Income Medicaid Program if he incurs medically related expenses equal to $421 per month.

persons, ventilator-dependent individuals who would otherwise require institutionalization, and clients requesting a hospice program are the main options states choose. Younger, terminally ill clients benefit most from the Medicaid covered hospice program. The largest group receiving care through the Medicaid hospice care program is AIDS clients. Unfortunately they are often younger than the Medicare eligible population, yet are a big part of the home health nurse's case load.

OTHER WAYS TO FINANCE HOME CARE

Veteran Benefits

Persons eligible for veteran medical benefits through the Veterans Administration Medical Center (VAMC) system also have access to VAMC's system of home care services. There is at least one VAMC in each state, and in most states there are several. In this system, clients receive comprehensive care through a bevy of outpatient clinics, acute care services, and in most facilities a well-developed home care and hospice program.

Those eligible for Veterans Administration healthcare services include all men and women who served in the armed services, were honorably discharged, and choose to enter this system of caregiving as their primary healthcare provider. In some situations, they may enter this system after using up benefits from other health insurance programs they have. Because of its comprehensive nature, clients may enter the system at a younger age and continue to receive care as they grow older.

This system of caregiving often manages clients who suffer from chronic conditions, such as respiratory, psychiatric, and cardiac conditions. Because clients with these conditions may be managed for years in other systems of caregiving and come to the Veterans Administration healthcare system later in the illness, it is not unusual for clients in the home care component of this system to be middle aged or older. Thus, information in this book is valuable to nurses both employed in this system and in other systems of healthcare delivery.

Private Insurance

There are many private insurance companies that cover home care services for their policy holders. For older adults, it is recommended that they buy supplemental insurance to use with Medicare. This will help eliminate large out-of-pocket expenses. These Medicare supplemental insurances are frequently advertised in the media, and often older adults ask the home care nurse about the benefits of different policies. The nurse will need to act as an advocate and help the client sort through the actual and touted benefits as compared to cost of each policy. Unfortunately, there are people offering supplemental insurance policies that are worthless. Checking with the Better Business Bureau or Area Agency on Aging on behalf of clients will give them some direction to help with appropriate decision making.

Out of Pocket

When all healthcare insurance resources have been applied to incurred home care costs, out-of-pocket resources must be used. This can be very disconcerting for older adults who live on fixed incomes and perhaps have not budgeted or cannot budget for additional healthcare costs.

Most elders will try to "stretch" their dollars by cutting back in other critical areas, such as food, heat, and routine medications. It is important for the home care nurse to assess the client's financial situation, make appropriate suggestions to apply for specific programs designed to give eligible clients relief from some expenses, and refer clients to the medical social worker on staff. Some programs available in most communities that elders may be eligible for include reduced gas and electric costs, free home energy saving changes, and reductions in basic telephone service costs. Taking advantage of these savings may make the difference in an elder taking a daily blood pressure medication or skipping it every other day to pay the telephone bill. Advocacy is interwoven throughout the care given by home care nurses.

ETHICAL AND LEGAL ISSUES

Facing Issues Proactively

Home care nurses are likely to encounter ethical and legal dilemmas in the course of their work. For example, a client's health changes and a primary care provider cannot be reached, a client falls in the presence of a home health aide, or a client has a do not resuscitate order (DNR) and arrests while the nurse is present. If these situations occur, the home care nurse needs a legal framework from which to work. All registered nurses should work within the scope of nursing practice in their state. The contractual relationship between the home care agency and the client spell out actions that will be taken in specific circumstances. In other cases, legal documents the client prepares through the help of a lawyer give direction when health conditions change.

Living wills and healthcare proxies are legal documents in which a client expresses his or her wishes regarding future medical and healthcare treatment and are primary examples of proactive healthcare planning. Home care agencies require older adults to have these documents prepared in advance or during the planning process when beginning care provided by the agency.

The living will pertains to end-of-life decision making, such as the withdrawal or discontinuance of treatment when the person is found to be terminally ill and death is near. The type of treatment that is desired or not desired can be specified. For example, individuals may express their feelings about the withdrawal or withholding of life-prolonging treatment, such as the use of respirators, dialysis, artificial nutrition, or hydration. The withholding of this type of treatment usually becomes particularly relevant when a patient is in a persistent vegetative (permanently unconscious) state. The courts in most states will use the living will as evidence to determine the intentions of the individual.

Generally, the living will must be signed by the client in the presence of two witnesses, just as a last will and testament is signed. In any event, the person's wishes must be established by "clear and convincing proof" of their intentions before they become incompetent. Their wishes must be clear and unequivocal. The witnesses will help establish the intentions of the individual at any hearings that may be necessary. If a hearing is required, the person's wishes may be established orally or in writing. However, a written expression is preferable because it is easier to determine a person's wishes and has greater validity. However, any expression by the afflicted individual will be used to establish his or her intentions regarding healthcare directives.

A living will can express general wishes or can be as specific as the client wants. If a client has specific desires or wishes, they should be written in the document, especially those wishes concerning (1) cardiac resuscitation (CPR), (2) artificial respiration, and (3) artificial nutrition and hydration.

Rather than a living will, some states recommend a document called a healthcare proxy. This is a written document that appoints a healthcare agent to make healthcare decisions in the event of the client's loss of decision-making capacity. It is a legal document recognized by hospitals, doctors, healthcare providers, and healthcare facilities. The healthcare proxy is an easy document to execute. The client simply appoints a primary and an alternate agent. The signing of the document is witnessed by two individuals other than those two appointed as representatives under the proxy. Once appointed, the healthcare proxy agent may make broad-range decisions about the client's course of treatment. The proxy agent's authority becomes effective only if the client is unable to make decisions. In addition to general care management, the proxy agent is also empowered to make decisions about the termination or withholding of life support consistent with the client's wishes if it is determined that the client is terminally ill and that death is imminent.

Clients should give careful thought to their wishes regarding the withholding of artificial nutrition and hydration. The Public Health Law requires that the agent "clearly and convincingly" know the client's wishes regarding the administration or withholding of artificial nutrition and hydration. It is advisable to state these particular wishes in the health proxy instrument.

Once the healthcare proxy has been executed, the original should be kept in a safe and retrievable place, such as a fireproof document box in the client's home. The healthcare proxy should not be kept in a bank safe deposit vault because it is difficult to retrieve in the event of an emergency. Additionally, in the event of hospitalization or involvement with a home care agency, the original should not be given to the agency; only copies should be given. In the case of a home care agency, one copy is given to the nurse to place in the client's chart in the agency and one made available in a folder where home care visits are documented in the home. This is helpful because frequently more than one nurse or home health aide visits the client. The original should, however, be available for comparison when needed. Any documents placed in the home care agency's client record become the property of the agency and it will be difficult for clients to obtain these documents from the agency upon discharge.

Home care nurses should be mindful of implementation concerns regarding the use of living wills, healthcare proxies, and other advance directives, such as a non–hospital do not resuscitate order (NHDNR) in the community setting. Home care nurses must make the client and family aware of the procedures and policies that are consistent with the Federal Patient Self-Determination Act of 1990 and any state regulations governing patient healthcare decision making.

All advance directive documents, such as a living will, healthcare proxy, or NHDNR, should be made part of the client's medical record. This information should be "flagged" so the home care nurse can respond appropriately in the event of an emergency.

Clients who have not implemented advance directives should be encouraged to do so and instructed as needed regarding the options as set forth above. It is necessary for the home care nurse to document that advance directive information was given to the client or family and an acknowledgment should be signed by the client or family. In addition, if the client has amended, modified, or revoked an advance directive, this change should be documented and the appropriate health providers and family members should be notified promptly.

Clients who were diagnosed as terminally ill and who are discharged to the community should give careful consideration to the implementation of a NHDNR order. This order should provide that if a client goes into cardiac or respiratory arrest, no cardiac or pulmonary resuscitation will be initiated. However, all other treatment from the home care nurse or the agency personnel must still be provided unless the client indicates an intent to refuse treatment. The NHDNR order may be executed while the client is in the hospital or in the community. Regardless, the document must deal specifically with the issue of non-intervention in the community.

Home care nurses should utilize the following procedures when a NHDNR order is being implemented:

1. Explain the policy clearly to the client.
2. Be sure the order is signed by the client or treating primary care provider and that it is incorporated in the home care record.
3. Any competent adult over 18 years of age may give approval for a NHDNR order by signing a consent before two witnesses over 18 years of age. These witnesses must also sign the order.
4. It is possible to consent orally if the client does so to an attending primary care provider in the presence of two witnesses over the age of 18. If the order is made orally in the hospital, one of the witnesses must be a primary care provider affiliated with the hospital.
5. Consent may also be gotten through the healthcare proxy agent to the attending primary care provider. This type of order must contain a medical determination that the client lacks decision-making capacity.
6. The general procedure for surrogate consents (i.e., someone other than the client acting as representative) is as follows: the client lacks capacity, the client is terminally ill or presently unconscious, resuscitation would be medically futile, and resuscitation would impose an extraordinary burden on the client. Such surrogate consents must be accompanied by two primary care providers determining that the client lacks the requisite capacity to consent personally.
7. Home care nurses should be mindful that an on-hand copy of the NHDNR is required. It should be in standard form and signed by the primary care provider.
8. Progress notes containing the date, time, and place of the decision, as well as identification of the individuals present, must also be collected. The notes should indicate the level of the client's understanding of these decisions.
9. The NHDNR order must be reviewed and renewed every 60 days by the attending primary care provider.
10. The order is not effective until the primary care provider signs it and it is received by the home care agency.

11. Clients may revoke their NHDNR at anytime, and notice must be given to the primary care provider, the home care agency, and the home care nurse.

Malpractice

Being sued for malpractice is a concern of all nurses in all settings in which they work, especially in the home care setting where nurses work more independently. It is required by some home care agencies and recommended by most that nurses have their own malpractice insurance in addition to any malpractice insurance the agency may have on the nurse. This insurance is readily available from several sources, including professional nursing organizations. Cost is reasonable (and tax deductible) considering the amount of coverage it provides. Most policies cost under a hundred dollars a year and cover the nurse for one million dollars per suit, up to three suits per policy year. This provides adequate insurance coverage. The vast majority of registered nurses, fortunately, never need to use the benefits of their policies. Nonetheless, being vulnerable to a malpractice suit is a reality of professional nursing.

Malpractice is defined by four distinct elements, all of which must be proven by the plaintiff. Elements of malpractice include the following:

1. Duty: established by a professional relationship
2. Breach of duty: an act or omission in violation of the standard of care
3. Injury to the client
4. Causation: nurse's breach of duty causes client's injury

First, duty must be established. Home care nurses are legally obligated to care for assigned clients while visiting them. If a home care nurse is "off duty" and comes upon a neighbor having a medical crisis, stopping to help may be the ethically proper thing to do but there is no legal requirement to assist.

Breach of duty requirements are established by agency policy and procedures that are based on a standard of care. A standard of care is determined by what is expected of the profession from another nurse who acts reasonably as compared to the policies and procedures of the agency. In home care, as with care given in hospitals, breach of duty can occur by commission as well as omission. The nurse may do (commission) something wrong or may omit (omission) doing something right. Either can result in injury and a malpractice suit.

The third requirement is that the client suffers harm or injury. Omitting one dose of digoxin 0.25 mg may not harm the client, but administering 25.0 mg can be a lethal dose of medication. Many nursing activities will not cause injury to a client despite being performed improperly or omitted entirely. For example, a nurse misreads an order for a client to bathe his feet for 20 minutes three times a day. The nurse instructs the client to soak his feet for 30 minutes twice a day. Despite this error, the client is not injured. When an error of this type is identified, the right time and duration are instituted, the primary care provider is notified, and an incident report is placed on file in the agency.

Finally, causation must be established. It must be proven that the nurse's breach of duty caused the client's injury. It might be difficult to prove that feet soaked two times a day for 30 minutes rather than three times a day for 20 minutes caused the client to lose his toe; it would not be difficult to determine that if a client was given 100 times the normal medication dose, the overdosage is the cause of the harm incurred.

Provision for a Safe Work Environment

There are several proactive safety measures the profession of nursing and agencies hiring nurses must take to reduce, if not eliminate, risks to clients and risks to the nurse's license. First, registered nurses must be licensed by the state they work in, after the satisfactory completion of a rigorous educational program that is followed by a comprehensive examination process. Second, all agencies—inpatient and home care—should offer a thorough orientation for new nurses.

In addition to a comprehensive review of how nursing is conducted in the particular agency, orientation should include a review of policies and procedures (which should also be reviewed each year by all nurses in the agency). Educational in-services should be offered whenever new products, treatments, or procedures are introduced in the agency. Also, nurses are mandated in most states to receive a certain number of continuing education units per licensing period in order to remain licensed. It is the responsibility of the nurse to be knowledgeable about all aspects of client care and to ask for assistance or training when approaching a new or unfamiliar situation.

Safety, as a primary prevention strategy, begins with the basics mentioned above, which should be expected components of all nurses' work regardless of location or agency. It continues into the home with nursing care using safety principles when dealing with people (personal safety, see Chapter 4), using universal precautions in any dealings with bodily fluids (personal and client safety), and in assessing for and teaching home safety to elderly clients (client safety, see Chapter 4).

SUMMARY

Financing healthcare in the home setting has similar rules and regulations to financing in the acute care setting. however in the home care setting the nurse becomes more intimately involved in the process. Knowledge of Medicare, Medicaid, veteran benefits, and private pay through insurance policies and self-pay best prepares the nurse to act as a client advocate. Legal and ethical issues in home care exist and cannot be ignored. Again, the home care nurse may become more intimately involved in these issues because of the nature of nursing in the home and the intimacy this role requires. The use of the living will, healthcare proxy, or other form of advance directive, such as the non–hospital do not resuscitate order, is a right and responsibility of elders when contracting for home healthcare. It is also an essential component to good care management and will certainly help to insure that clients are not treated unnecessarily and that they are treated in a humane manner, thus assuring quality of care. Malpractice concerns can be lessened or eliminated through a comprehensive orientation and training program for nurses and through nurses taking responsibility to keep knowledge of nursing and elder healthcare issues current.

REFERENCES

National Association for Home Care. (1995). *Basic statistics about home care, 1995*. Washington, DC: Author.

Rosenzweig, E. P. (1995). Trends in home care entitlements and benefits. *Journal of Gerontological Social Work, 24*(3/4), 9–29.

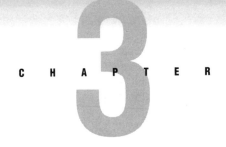

ASSESSMENT OF THE ELDERLY CLIENT IN THE HOME

Herminia B. Nueva Espana

◆ ◆ ◆

Geriatric Health Assessment
Geriatric Physical Assessment
Health Risk Appraisal: Recognizing Acute/Emergency Situations

The uniqueness of this chapter is that it focuses on an in-home assessment of elders receiving home care services. As a result, this chapter can be used to guide the home care nurse in assessing the general health of the homebound elderly client and in identifying potential as well as chronic health problems.

While more detailed assessments are covered in specific clinical chapters, this chapter assists the nurse in completing a comprehensive home, social, psychological, and physical assessment of the client. This comprehensive assessment aids the nurse in working with the older client, family, and caregiver to plan strategies that assist with maintaining optimal health within the limitations of chronic illness. This chapter also serves as a guide in recognizing emergency home situations that require immediate intervention.

The reader is most likely an experienced nurse, adept at physical and mental assessment, who is new to home care and working for the first time with a significant number of homebound older adults. Caregiving at home differs greatly from caregiving in the acute care setting.

Assessing the client's and caregiver's ability to provide care with safety in the home situation is an additional assessment skill the home care nurse must have.

GERIATRIC HEALTH ASSESSMENT

There are many facets to assessing elders at home as experienced home health nurses know. The home care nurse who visits a client for the first time may know that the client is female, 84 years old, lives alone, and has just been discharged from the hospital for an exacerbation of congestive heart failure. The primary care provider wants a home care nurse to visit and assess medication compliance and signs and symptoms of recurring heart failure. This might sound simple enough, but immediately questions should come to mind about the client's health history, functional ability, social support system, psychological status, financial resources, physical health (perceived and objective), medication regimen (including prescriptions, over the counter and home remedies, and folk medicine practices), nutritional status, and risks to her future health status. As a result, a complex web of assessment parameters unfold. Conducting a health history interview begins this data gathering process.

Health History Interview

The health history is the client's own account of his health. The components of the health history include a client's profile, religious affiliation and values, family history, past medical and surgical history, previous hospitalizations, medications, food and drug allergies, immunizations, and a review of past and current symptoms.

Eliciting information from the elderly client is an art in itself. It requires communication skills that project a genuine interest in and respect for the client. The initial encounter with the client has a powerful and lasting value. Aside from being the tool to gather data, the interview initiates the development of a client-nurse relationship that will impact on the attainment of desired goals.

Information gathered from the client must be accurate and reliable. It is important to ascertain the cognitive status of the client. A formal mental status test is not necessary at this time. Asking simple questions that will yield information regarding the client's orientation and memory will suffice. Even the mildly demented client may give a satisfactory history. Unless the client prefers another person to be present, it is best to conduct the interview with the client alone. Vital information may be withheld by the elderly person if a family member or a friend is present. With the client's permission, family members may be interviewed separately to get a better and more comprehensive perspective of existing client health problems and family support.

Special consideration should be given to the initial home visit. Simple courtesies such as promptness and proper decorum are expected; the nurse is now in the client's domain. You should introduce yourself using your full name, the agency which you represent, and the official reason for the visit. Ideally, the interview should take place in a well-lit and comfortable room in the home. If there are extraneous noises, such as from a radio or television, ask permission to lower the volume. You should sit at eye-level facing the light so the client can see your face clearly. If there is some hearing impairment, speak loudly but avoid shouting. An inexpensive voice amplifier sold at electronic stores can be useful. A stethoscope can also be used to amplify sound by placing the ear pieces on the client's ears and talking directly to the diaphragm. If the client has a hearing aid, check to see that it is being worn, is turned on, and the battery is good. Before starting the interview, determine whether the client is ready and has no pressing needs, such as to go to the bathroom or to turn off a stove.

The nurse initiates the interview by asking open-ended questions, ones that are not answerable by yes or no but require a narrative response. Allow the client to take time to answer a question, but gently focus attention back to the subject as necessary. Allowing a client to direct the interview can give the nurse a "window" to the innermost feelings of the client and to understanding the client better. Because elders have so much more "history" than younger clients, the interview may be lengthy. The nurse may need to filter out important information from a rich tapestry of reminiscence when open-ended questions are used. A client's values and beliefs—including perceptions of good and evil, moral and ethical beliefs, and a sense of self—can be incorporated in responses to open-ended questions. An individual's pattern of valuing and believing is shaped from childhood and continues to evolve throughout life. A discussion of values and beliefs should include perceptions of mortality, religious beliefs, and plans for the future, all of which may be included in the beginning of the geriatric assessment interview.

Close-ended questions are answered by yes or no and are useful in extracting specific answers. An important key to interviewing is the ability to phrase a question that yields the most information. Other verbal strategies such as reflection (repetition of the words used by the client), clarification, and summarization also enhance the interview. Nonverbal strategies that facilitate the process of interviewing include leaning toward the client, eye-to-eye contact, smiling, and nodding.

Special considerations to be mindful of when interviewing elders include:

- Language barriers: Some older adults may not speak the same language as the nurse, or they may have a speech impediment due to a cerebral vascular accident (CVA), a strong accent, or no dentures. With these clients, an interpreter may be essential or helpful. During the interview, the nurse should speak directly to the client (not the interpreter), using expressiveness and gestures to enhance establishing rapport.

- Memory impairments: Be selective about the kinds of information asked, arrange for a family member to fill in missing information, and consult other data sources for confirmation.

- Rambling speech: Some clients may be so lonely and ready to talk to someone that they seem pressured to talk on and on. Gently interrupt and redirect them back to the subject. Some reminiscence can be shared along the way to gain an understanding of the client's past and values. When allowed to be shared, it may increase rapport and enrich the client-nurse relationship.

- Under-reporting: Many older adults may not mention a symptom they are experiencing because they may feel it is a normal part of aging or because of embarrassment. Gently ask questions in ways that will make it comfortable to give a truthful response. For instance, if a question is phrased, "You don't have any urinary incontinence do you?" the answer will probably be no. However, if the question is phrased, "Do you ever have any urinary incontinence when you cough, laugh, or sneeze?" the client will be more likely to admit if the problem exists.

- Additional communication barriers: Using medical terminology may or may not be appropriate. It is useful to back

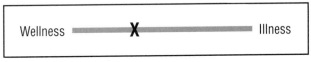

FIGURE 3-1 • The Wellness–Illness Continuum

up medical terms with lay terms to assist the client in understanding the questions asked. For instance, when the nurse asks about urinary incontinence, the same information can be gathered without offending the most sensitive or educated clients by asking about "loss of bladder control" or an "inability to hold water." Even a client who uses "street terms" such as pee or piss, which might be uncomfortable for the nurse to initially use, will understand more generally accepted lay terms.

During the interview, it is best to cover all necessary areas systematically and proceed with questions from the less-personal to the more-sensitive. Demographic data is a safe area with which to begin. The identifying data includes the client's name, date and place of birth, marital status, ethnic group, and previous occupation. Ethnicity is included in the identifying data to give the nurse a perspective on where the client's views originate. Health and care-seeking behavior is to a large extent determined by one's ethnicity.

Further along in the interview, it is important for the nurse to assess the client's health-illness perception. A good tool to use is the wellness and illness continuum. Ask clients to determine how healthy they believe they are on a scale of one to ten, with one being the most ill and ten being the most healthy. Likewise, the nurse can use a bar with wellness on one end and illness on the other and have clients place an X where they feel they fit best. To glean more information, have clients explain why they placed the X where they did (see Figure 3-1).

The elderly client's self-evaluation, in general, is influenced by the ability to do self-care. For example, a client who experiences debilitating arthritis may claim to be not healthy because of limitations and increasing dependence on others for help. An elder's perception of wellness or illness often mirrors an ability to perform tasks of daily living as compared to ability that existed in the past. As the parts of the geriatric health assessment unfold, recording the data needs to be done as efficiently as possible. The home care nurse's and the client's time is valuable, and the client may tire if there are long pauses between questions because the nurse is recording data. It is helpful if the home care agency uses a checklist-type form for geriatric assessment data. A useful classification system (adapted from Staab and Lyles, 1990) for recording data is as follows:

1 = No symptoms present when observed, absent, none, no problem
2 = Mild symptoms, no limitation or distress, or a history of inactive symptoms
3 = Symptoms present, distressing or limiting
4 = Severe, incapacitating symptoms
5 = Very severe or totally restricting symptoms
6 = Ambiguous, questionable
7 = Not asked, not required, not relevant

If number 7 is recorded, the reason should be noted in the "Narrative."

Functional Assessment and Mobility

Once the initial demographic information is collected, an assessment of perceived level of wellness established, and an efficient data gathering tool adopted, obtaining information about other aspects of the client's health follows. Multiple physiologic changes affect the older client's level of activity. For many clients, compounding chronic diseases involving various systems markedly reduce their ability to be as active as they once were or as they would like to be. Ask about the client's ability to do activities of daily living (ADL) and instrumental activities of daily living (IADL). Follow a pattern of progressively more active or more limiting questions to determine the extent of endurance and independence. An in-depth clinical focus on mobility and tools to assess mobility appears in Chapter 5.

Home Safety Assessment

Ideal geriatric assessments of elderly clients take place in the clients' living environments. Nothing else demonstrates quite so clearly the ability to maintain independent living. This is an advantage the home care nurse has over the nurse in the acute care setting. As part of the initial home visit, most home health agencies require the nurse to conduct a home safety assessment. If an agency does not require this, it should be suggested for inclusion in the admission packet by a nurse who is thinking of the client's holistic health and well-being. Home assessments can provide valuable perspectives on clients, their life-styles, values, and relationships, as well as health and safety risk appraisals.

The nurse needs to ask permission to tour any client's home, but most elderly clients will be willing to show the nurse around. Experienced home health nurses have found that homes come in varying degrees of tidiness and cleanliness. Housekeeping standards are personal and may be vastly different from the nurse's own. Cluttered, dusty, or disorganized households are not automatically a health hazard, and the nurse must be careful not to impose personal standards on the client's ability to manage in the environment. What is important about the condition of the home is if it signals a recent decline or is an early sign of a change in health status.

If safety is an issue, the nurse can incorporate ways to create a safer environment without altering a client's "casual" lifestyle. Target areas in the home, where safety is especially important, include the kitchen, bathroom, stairways, halls, all pathways throughout the home, and the garage. Primary prevention of accidents should be uppermost in the nurse's mind as efforts to make improvements in home safety are worked on with clients. It is a sad scenario when an older adult follows medical regimens, eats properly, gets enough rest and exercise, and then falls over a telephone cord and fractures a hip. The home safety assessment should also include an assessment of the availability of emergency phone numbers, working smoke and carbon monoxide detectors, a fire extinguisher in the kitchen, and an emergency home evacuation plan in case of fire or other regional disaster situation, such as a tornado or flood.

Social Support Assessment

It is important to determine strengths and weaknesses in the social support systems of elderly clients. As people become frail and more dependent on others for assistance, a strong support system can mean the difference between remaining at home or needing a more protective environment. Social isolation is also a risk to the well-being of many elderly clients. A useful tool for the home care nurse to use is the Sociogram (see Figure 3-2). With this device, the nurse is able to depict the richness and voids in a client's social support system, the quality of the support, and if there is conflict in relationships. Once a client's

Place a circle in the middle of a piece of paper, depicting the client. Place other smaller circles around the client's circle at varying distances to depict persons in the client's support system. The further away the support person's circle, the more distanced the emotional tie is to the client (e.g., a daughter's circle may be closer than a grandchild's). Connect the circles using the following legend:

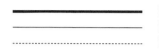

indicates a strong connection
indicates a weak connection
indicates a troubled connection

Double the lines if the connection is mutual. Place an arrow in the direction of the support.

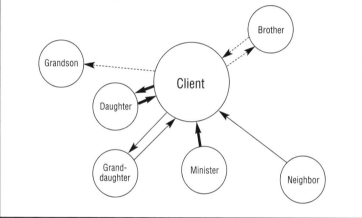

FIGURE 3-2 • Sociogram

Sociogram is developed with the client, both the nurse and client can see the strengths and weakness in the system and it can be used as a catalyst for discussion that guides the nurse and client to appropriate changes as needed.

Many factors may severely affect the normal expression of a client's sexuality. Throughout life, the capacity and need for sexual enjoyment in both male and female clients remains. Chronic debilitating illness, medications, depression, and social isolation may adversely affect the capacity to engage in sexual activities. Open discussion of clients' perceptions of their own sexuality should be encouraged (see Chapter 7).

Psychological Assessment

During a comprehensive assessment, the home health nurse gains many clues to cognitive and behavioral functioning. Clues such as dress, hygiene, affect, speech, attention span, appropriateness of answers, ability to place events in time, general functioning, judgment, and life satisfaction are observed and assessed. Unless there is an obvious abnormality, a psychological assessment through the use of a mental status examination (MSE) usually is performed in the middle of the interview, after the client is more comfortable with the interview process. There are several versions of MSEs designed to screen for depression, phobias, paranoia, compulsiveness, and dementia. Ten items are commonly used as an easy measure of orientation for future comparison, quantifying the mental status quotient (MSQ):

1. Current day of month?
2. Current month?
3. Current year?
4. Immediate past president of the United States?
5. Name of this place?
6. Where is it located?
7. How old are you?
8. Month of birth?
9. Year of birth?
10. Current president of the United States?

This tool should be used for periodic reassessment, because an older person's mental status can alter rapidly with the general state of health. A decrease in the MSQ may be the first sign of an onslaught of problems in an older person living alone. Early recognition and intervention can be critical (Staab and Lyles, 1990).

Financial Assessment

This information can be gathered earlier in the interview if it is agency policy to have it included with demographic data. Financial assessment information includes the amount and sources of income, the client's perception of adequacy of income, and assets such as savings, homes, and vehicles owned. Also pertinent are any forms of public assistance the client is receiving or is eligible to receive, including Supplemental

Security Income (SSI), Medicaid, food stamps, rent credit, and fuel or telephone assistance. Responses to financial questions give clues to clients' attitudes regarding assistance programs or perceived comfort or ability to manage with their present income. Many elders have lived through the depression of the 1930s and "belt-tightening" during World War II and may come from a work ethic background where you "don't take handouts" and "you work for what you have." When elders are truly in need of resources to meet even basic necessities, these attitudes are difficult to overcome. It is the skillful home care nurse who can explain to clients that they have already paid for many of these benefits or services through years of paying taxes and that the programs were originally designed to meet the future needs of those taxpayers.

Medication Assessment

Polypharmacy is common with the elderly. The nurse needs to be aware of all the current prescribed medications, over-the-counter medications, home remedies, and use of folk medicine practices. A listing of medications and practices alone is not enough. The home care nurse must discuss medications one at a time after looking at all medicines taken. A client may often see more than one primary care provider and go to more than one pharmacy. Hence, the client may be taking a generic-named drug and a trade-named drug not knowing they are the same. A comprehensive overview of managing medications with an elderly population follows in Chapter 8.

Nutrition Assessment

Nutrition in the elderly is affected by various factors, such as the presence of chronic diseases, reduction in the level of exercise and activity, medications that affect the gastrointestinal system, social isolation, depression, inability to prepare food, and unavailability of food due to poverty or occasionally due to elder abuse/neglect. It is important to ask the client about usual diet and food preferences. It is also important to find out who shops for food and prepares meals for the client, what the client's and caregiver's understanding of a healthy diet for older adults is, and if there are any dietary restrictions. See Chapter 6 for a detailed review of maintaining optimum nutrition in the homebound elderly.

GERIATRIC PHYSICAL ASSESSMENT

Review of Systems

During the review of systems, the home care nurse may uncover symptoms or complaints that otherwise would remain unreported if not specifically elicited. Addressing these symptoms/syndromes in a timely manner may prevent morbidity and mortality in an elderly client. In this age group, disease conditions may present atypically and, therefore, nonspecific symptoms may not be perceived as a problem. Vague abdominal pain, for example, may be considered an annoying sensation rather than a symptom of an impending cardiac event, and this can lead to a catastrophic situation.

Review of systems in the elderly does not differ from that of younger adults. However, it may be time consuming due to slowness of the client's responses, but meticulous attention to details will be beneficial in the long run. Emphasis will be given to specific organ systems that manifest more symptoms commonly occurring in the elderly population. By this time in the geriatric assessment process, the client may be fatigued. Reassure the client that the physical examination can be completed on a second home visit if necessary. Since the home care nurse often visits over a period of weeks, this is not an unusual occurrence. Also, the nurse may need to include client teaching in this visit, and having an alert client for the teaching is more important. This is an example of how the home care nurse has to prioritize activities.

The Physical Examination

The home care nurse uses the basic techniques of physical examination when conducting an examination on a client in the home. However, the examination may not be comprehensive, including all systems, unless the client's condition so requires. Usually the physical examination focuses on systems that the client has specific complaints about (discerned from information shared during the interview) and on systems related to the purpose of the referral. With congestive heart failure, the lungs, heart, extremities, and mobility are fully assessed. On all home visits, the nurse assesses temperature, blood pressure, and apical and radial pulse. The client may be used to the assessment of these parameters. They can be done quickly and reveal important information.

In some elderly clients, especially frail, bed- or chair-bound, and demented clients, following a head-to-toe and total assessment in sequence may not be feasible. In this case, the nurse may need to modify the process to accommodate the client's ability to cooperate and execute required motions. Occasionally, it may require two or more visits to complete a comprehensive physical examination. It is worth investing the time and effort in gathering objective data through physical examination as it provides the nurse a baseline with which to compare future physical findings on subsequent visits.

Basic equipment needed for conducting a physical examination in a client's home remains unchanged from what is used in other settings. The physical examination should be carried out in a comfortable, well-lit room, such as a bedroom or livingroom (with a couch). Always provide privacy and comfort. Loose clothing is preferable, and use of a bathrobe or sweatsuit is best. They preserve modesty, warmth, and accessibility to body parts that need to be examined.

The home care nurse needs to explain to the client the purpose of the physical assessment. This alleviates anxiety that the client may be experiencing. Help the client relax by explaining the procedure and then allowing the client to ask questions. A calm, unhurried, and friendly manner conveys professionalism and provides reassurance.

Vital Signs

Vital signs should be taken on each home visit. If a home health aide is visiting on a regular basis between home care nurse visits, a record of vital sign changes for past days and weeks is available to the home care nurse. Variances in vital signs that are normal for elders include:

Body temperature. It is not unusual for an elderly client to register 35°C because of slow metabolism and decreased activity. Changes in temperature may be due to infectious states, central nervous disease, or injury. Infection may manifest as hyperthermia, while severe sepsis may manifest as hypothermia.

Pulse. The normal pulse of adults and elders is 60 to 100 beats per minute. The most common pulse taken is the radial pulse. When this is not accessible, the nurse may use other peripheral sites, such as the brachial and carotid. When using the carotid pulse, take it on one side. If taken on both sides simultaneously, it can cause bradycardia in the client.

Respiratory rate. Observe the rate, pattern, and depth of respiration. Note the ease of respiration or the use of an accessory muscle for breathing, such as the sternocleidomastoid, scalene, or trapezius muscle. Flaring of the ala nasi must also be noted if present. A respiratory rate of 12 to 20 breaths per minute is considered normal. Aside from counting the respiratory rate, observe the depth of respiration and chest expansion. Note for adequacy and symmetry. Respiratory patterns can be altered by the presence of infection or neurologic conditions. Metabolic derangement also affects respiratory pattern.

Blood pressure. In the elderly, blood pressure must be taken while the client is lying down and again while standing or sitting to determine orthostatic hypotension, which can cause unsteadiness upon arising and lead to a fall.

System Variances

Variances in the physical examination of an elder's systems include:

Skin. An elder's skin is thinner and more translucent. Inspect for lesions, moles, ulcers, and pressure sores. Note location and color of bruises and abrasions. Look for signs of dehydration such as skin moisture and turgor.

Nails. Fingernails and toenails must be inspected and palpated. Special attention should be given to the feet and toenails of diabetic clients. Inspect for fungal infection. With immobile clients, the circulation may be impaired and the client may develop stasis dermatitis and stasis ulcers.

Eyes. Inspect the eyes and note for physiologic changes with aging. The eyes may be seated deeply because of loss of fatty tissues. Upper eyelids may look droopy because of loss of tissue elasticity (blepharochalasis). Symmetrical blepharochalasis is normal in the elderly. However, if a unilateral droopy lid is observed, it may indicate a problem. The eye may look dry due to decrease in tear production. The lacrimal apparatus and its ducts may become plugged causing watery eyes. The conjunctiva thins, becomes pale, and appears slightly yellowed. The pupils may appear irregularly shaped after cataract removal. Examine for pterygium, a fleshy fold of conjunctiva onto the cornea. Pterygium is slow growing and may not present any problems until it covers a large portion of the cornea and pupil.

A slowing of the response to light (pupillary reflex) and accommodation occurs in the elderly. This is what causes a slower and less-effective dark adaptation. The lens increases in size and thickens. This causes a decrease in glare tolerance and lessened visual acuity. Test vision by asking the client to read from a newspaper (first assess if the client is literate). If unable to see and read from regular print, ask the client to read from a large-print book or magazine. The client should be tested wearing eyeglasses if regularly worn. Any problems noted with vision should be referred to an ophthalmologist. By age eighty, average visual acuity is 20/30 to 20/40 due to the loss of accommodative power, called "farsightedness" or presbyopia.

Ears and hearing. The quality of life of elderly clients is diminished by the loss of the sense of hearing. The ability of the client to communicate is to a large extent affected by the ability to hear. Hearing loss in the elderly can further aggravate their sense of isolation. Use an otoscopic exam to detect problems associated with the tympanic membrane and middle and outer ear. Use the tuning fork examination to differentiate between conductive and sensorineural hearing losses (Rinne's or Weber's tests).

It is not uncommon for the elderly client to complain of difficulty hearing. This condition is most often caused by presbycusis, a slowly progressive degenerative condition of the whole auditory system that accompanies aging. Transient conductive hearing loss may be due to middle ear infections, impacted ear wax, or a blocked eustachian tube.

Dizziness and vertigo have a multifactorial etiology, which includes pathology of the inner ear. It is important to ask the client when the vertigo/dizziness starts, how long it lasts, and if it causes nausea or vomiting.

Tinnitus is a sensation of ringing in the ear, which can be annoying or distressing. It is associated with fluid in the middle ear accompanying an upper respiratory infection or nasal allergies, perforation of the eardrum, or wax build-up. Some medications are known to cause damage to the 8th cranial nerve, which may lead to tinnitus and deafness. As a result, an assessment of the side effects and compounded effect of several medications is warranted.

Pain in the ear can be due to middle ear pathology or from other structures, such as the mouth, teeth, nose, or paranasal sinuses. Ask if the client has mouth sores, tooth cavities, upper respiratory infection, or nasal discharge.

Frequently the symptoms of hearing loss, vertigo, dizziness, tinnitus, or ear pain are caused by an outer, middle, or inner ear obstruction, which can be treated in the primary care provider's office. This information may be welcomed by the client and assessment of hearing changes should be part of an initial physical assessment and included whenever the client has complaints.

At the time of the initial geriatric interview the home care nurse has already started assessing the client's hearing. The client may not volunteer being hard of hearing. Notice if the client focuses on the nurse's mouth while talking or if the client cups a hand over the better ear.

Two simple tests can be done to check the gross hearing of the client: the watch-tick and whispered speech tests. For the watch-tick test, instruct the client to say "yes" when ticking is heard and to say "no" as soon as the sound is no longer heard. The nurse might need to repeat this test several times on each ear if the client tends to forget the instructions. Be careful not to blow air on the client's ears and not to touch the client's hair as the client may respond to the sense of touch.

If hearing loss is suspected, discuss with the client and primary care provider the need for further consultation and examination. Audiometry is used to classify and quantify hearing loss. These tests tend to be confusing to elderly clients, and results may be unreliable in demented clients.

Respiratory system. The aging individual experiences declines in lung function, efficiency and effectiveness of gas exchange, and vital capacity. The rib cage becomes more stiff and rigid with an increased anterior/posterior diameter.

To conduct a respiratory assessment, the ideal position for examining the thorax is to have the client sit on the edge of a bed, chair, or couch and lean forward. If this position is not tolerated, place the client in a semi-Fowler's position by using several pillows and exposing the anterior thorax. To examine the posterior chest, have the client lean forward. For a debilitated client who cannot assume either maneuver, position the client laterally, perform the examination on the upper side first, then roll the client on the opposite side and continue the examination.

Observe for cyanosis of lips, nail beds, and buccal mucosa. Feel the skin for dryness or diaphoresis. Inspect the nose for swelling, bleeding, and congestion. Listen for audible wheezing or gurgly sounds of accumulated mucus or sputum. Ideally, if the client has dentures, they should be removed before the inspection. Examine the oropharynx for lesions, inflammation, white patches, bleeding, and exudates. Check for a gag reflex by touching both sides of the posterior pharynx with an applicator. Offer a small amount of water and ask the client to drink it, then observe for coughing. If the client coughs repeatedly, it may indicate difficulty in swallowing solid and liquid food and saliva (see Chapter 6).

Inspect the posterior and anterior chest for scars, wounds, lesions, and masses. Observe retraction of intercostal spaces during inspiration and expiration. Inspect for spinal deformities such as scoliosis, lordosis, and kyphosis.

If a client is too frail or debilitated to sit or stand, position the client on the lateral decubitus side. Percuss one side, roll the client to the other side, and repeat the procedure.

When auscultating, observe carefully how the client tolerates the procedure. Some clients tire easily with deep breathing and may also experience lightheadedness. When it is suspected that the client has crackles at the bases, reverse the sequence of auscultation by starting at the bases and ending at the upper thorax before the client tires. If the client is tired midway through the auscultation, allow the client to rest.

Dyspnea is not a normal symptom of the aging respiratory system. It exists as a symptom of an underlying health problem, such as congestive heart failure (CHF), chronic obstructive pulmonary disease (COPD), or coronary heart disease. Types of dyspnea observed are exertional, at-rest, and orthopnea. If the client complains of exertional dyspnea, inquire how much activity triggers a shortness of breath. Dyspnea at rest does not require activity for it to be manifested. Orthopnea requires an elevation of the head and thorax to a vertical (sitting or standing) position for relief. Severity of orthopnea is gauged by how many pillows the client uses when reclining, thus the term two-pillow and three-pillow orthopnea. Clients may not volunteer this information. It should be asked specifically. Use these parameters to assess good or bad management of chronic health conditions. Dyspnea may not be eliminated, but it can be significantly reduced if an effective medication regimen is followed.

Cardiovascular system. The most common cause of rehospitalization and death among the elderly is cardiovascular disease. It is essential that the home care nurse have mastery of cardiac assessment and an extensive understanding of the cardiovascular system. Normal age-associated alterations in the heart and vascular system are manifested by a progressive functional decline, particularly in the ability to adapt and appropriately deal with stress or increased physical demands. The heart works harder but is less efficient and cardiac valves become thicker and less elastic, causing increased resistance to diastolic filling. these changes cause a slower circulation with a slower transport of nutrients and oxygen, and slower elimination of wastes. Examine the client for peripheral edema. The home care nurse should measure any edema in inches and document exactly where the edema is measured and any changes in existing edema.

Chest pain. Ask the client to describe the pain (squeezing, burning, pressure) and point to the area. Ask if the pain is stationary or if it moves or radiates to any other body parts. It is important to ask how long the client has been having this pain, how long the pain lasts, and what the client has done or taken to relieve the pain.

Palpitation. This is a sensation of being aware of one's heartbeat. Palpitations are described as bounding, pounding, fluttering, jumping, or "skipping a beat." This may seem a trivial symptom, but it needs to be reported to the primary care provider. Inquire about the actions of medications, as some drugs can cause palpitations.

Cardiac assessment. Assess for cyanosis in the lips and nail beds. Take the radial pulse and compare it with the apical pulse to check for pulse deficit. Observe respirations as described in the previous section. Take the blood pressure in both arms, sitting and standing. Inspect for jugular vein distention. Ask the client to lie down in a semi-Fowler's position of 45-degree elevation with head turned slightly away from you. If the right heart function is normal, the jugular veins will not be prominent. Jugular veins are prominent in congestive heart failure.

To inspect the precordium, sit or stand at the client's right side. The precordium is the area of the anterior chest, close to the heart, bounded by the 2nd to the 5th intercostal space and the right border of the sternum to the left midclavicular line. Observe the apical impulse, usually located at the 5th intercostal space, midclavicular line. Note for visible right ventricular impulse, usually located at the 3rd to the 5th intercostal space medial to the apex. This may indicate pathology as the right ventricular muscle is not strong enough to generate a visible impulse on the precordium. Feel for thrills over the precordium and note the location.

Note gross distortion of the thorax, such as funnel, pigeon, or barrel chest. The funnel chest is a depression of the lower sternum, which may not be related to cardiac pathology. The pigeon chest is a protrusion of the sternum and is associated with cardiovascular and respiratory disorders. The barrel chest is an enlargement of the anteroposterior and transverse chest dimension and is associated with chronic respiratory disorder.

Palpate the peripheral pulses for rate, rhythm, amplitude, and symmetry. Feel for the brachial, ulnar, and radial pulses on the arms. Feel for the femoral, popliteal, posterior tibial, and dorsalis pedis pulses on the legs. Except for the carotid pulse, palpate peripheral pulses simultaneously. Indicate the pulse volume by using a 0 to 3 scale, where 0 is absent, 1 is weak or thready, 2 is normal, and 3 is bounding or increased.

The home care nurse checks for capillary refill by pressing a finger on the client's fingernail or toenail. As pressure is released, observe the blanching. Normal capillary refill is seen as an immediate return in the color of the nails and is an indication of good arterial supply.

Auscultation. S_1 and S_2 are normal heart sounds. S_1 is the lub. S_2 is the dub. The diaphragm of the stethoscope is used to listen to these sounds. Use the bell side of the stethoscope to listen to abnormal heart sounds S_3 and S_4. Appearance of S_3 is an important sound that may indicate a cardiac problem such as congestive heart failure. S_4 is heard preceding S_1 and is also a sign of a cardiac problem. With the bell of the stethoscope, listen for heart murmurs. Murmurs are sounds produced by the flow of blood through a stenotic valve. These abnormal heart sounds are difficult to identify. It is a skill that is developed by listening to numerous normal and abnormal heart sounds. Listen also to the mid-epigastric area for bruits, which may indicate aortic pathology.

Breast examination. Inspect the client's breasts for shape, scars, and nipple symmetry and color. Note for orange-rind skin present when there is edema. Palpate the breast with the client in a supine position. Use the pads of the index and middle fingers to palpate the entire breast area in a circular motion. Palpate the axillary region. If there are suspicious areas, mark the area with a pen and ask client to sit with her arms over her head and palms pressed together. (In elderly clients, the breasts have lost fat and supporting tissues, making the breasts pendulous.) Repeat palpation and note findings. If any suspicious area is noted, follow up with the primary care provider. In addition to conducting a thorough breast examination, the home care nurse should instruct the client in doing monthly self–breast exams.

Breast cancer is the second most common malignancy in the United States and accounts for a fourth of all cancers in women. Monthly self–breast examinations and yearly mammography for women over 50 are recommended. Early detection is a woman's best chance to become a cancer survivor.

Gastrointestinal system. Some signs and symptoms of pathology seem to originate from the gastrointestinal system but actually originate from other systems, such as the genitourinary or cardiovascular system. A thorough abdominal examination is useful in differentiating the source of the problem. Because of skeletal changes and thoracic rigidity, abdominal organs may shift and clients may complain of pain in a different location than expected. Signs and symptoms such as pain, nausea and vomiting, dysphagia, diarrhea, and constipation are the most common gastrointestinal complaints. In elders, each complaint needs to be assessed thoroughly by asking a variety of pertinent questions and using the steps of abdominal assessment as needed (i.e., inspection, palpation, percussion, and auscultation).

Musculoskeletal system. Most of the disabling conditions in the elderly can be attributed to the musculoskeletal system. Ability to walk and perform activities of daily living are limited by muscle and joint problems. Falls that occur with elderly clients are also often due to musculoskeletal problems.

Pain is the most common complaint related to pathology of joints, as in osteoarthritis, gout, and degenerative disease of the spine. Ask the client about the location and characteristic of the pain, what exacerbates it, and what treatments or medications relieve it.

Inspection and palpation are the major physical examination techniques used for the musculoskeletal system. With the client in a sitting position, inspect and palpate all joints for swelling, redness, and tenderness. Inspect spine for deformities. If possible, do range of motion on all major joints. The elderly client may be unable to do all range of motion of the joints, so focus on joints that are affected. The range of motion of the cervical spine must be checked. Some elderly clients have kyphosis so severely that the chin almost touches the chest. In this case, check ability to swallow, breathe, and ambulate, as such anatomical deformities may impede many normal functions.

The shoulders should be inspected for swelling and redness. Range of motion and muscle strength should be assessed. Pathology in the shoulder limits activities such as grooming and bathing. Fingers and wrists should be inspected for deformities and swelling. Gait is observed for balance, posture, rhythm, and length of stride. A waddling gait may indicate congenital abnormality, hip dislocation, or fracture.

Ask the client to assume a supine position to assess the hips and knees. Align the legs together and note whether the legs are equal in length. Check for hip deformity or pelvic fracture by bending one knee toward the chest. Flexion on the other hip may indicate hip deformity, while pain may indicate fracture. The knees should be observed for redness or swelling. Palpate around the knee joint and note tenderness and presence of fluid. Check range of motion and test for muscle strength.

Poor circulation to the extremities may cause discomfort in the arms and legs. Ask if the client feels pain or cramping while walking, if the client needs to rest after walking several blocks, or if pain is increased with prolonged standing or sitting.

Nervous system. Pathology of the nervous system accounts for the etiology of a number of functional limitations in the elderly. The effects of a cerebrovascular accident (CVA) that occurred years earlier may continue to negatively and progressively impact on the client's quality of life. Some neurologic disorders tend to primarily affect the elderly, such as Parkinson's and Alzheimer's diseases. It is no surprise that many elderly clients have a combination effect from previous and current neurologic disorders.

The most common neurologic syndromes include motor disturbances (weakness, paresis, paralysis, tremors), seizures, and dementia. Inquire about the progression of motor disturbances and how it has affected the client's lifestyle.

If dementia is present, ask a family member, friend, or caregiver (someone who knows the client intimately) what the client's baseline cognitive function was.

Neurologic examination. A complete neurologic examination includes tests for cerebral, cranial, motor, and sensory functions and reflexes. It may not be feasible or necessary to do a complete neurologic examination on one visit. Cerebral function includes general appearance, behavior, level of consciousness, orientation, general knowledge, abstraction, and judgment. Several mental function tests are available to assess most of these functions. Detailed discussion can be found in Chapter 21.

The technique of examining the twelve cranial nerves can be found in Chapter 18. Physiologic changes related to aging that affect the cranial nerves include loss of function of the olfactory, optic, facial, auditory, glossopharyngeal, and hypoglossal nerves. It is not unusual for elderly clients to show loss of smell discrimination, presbyopia, decreased taste sensation, presbycusis, poor or absent gag reflex, and some tongue sluggishness.

Motor system. Note body position. Hemiplegic clients assume a characteristic posture. Observe for abnormal movements such as tremors, fasciculations, and tics. Inspect for muscle bulk and tone. Examine for muscle strength. Check for coordination and examine for gait. Ask the client to walk away, turn, and return. Check if the client can do "heel and toe." Other techniques include walking on toes, hopping in place with one foot, and knee bends. The nurse should use discretion with these techniques depending on the goals of the examination and the client's ability to perform the tests. These tests can provoke undue anxiety and may put a client whom the nurse does not know well at risk.

The Romberg test is an important test for position sense. Ask the client to stand with feet together and eyes open, then to stand with eyes closed for 20 seconds. A positive Romberg sign (loss of balance when eyes are closed) suggests poor position sense. Also test the client for pronator drift. Ask the client to hold arms straight out with eyes closed for 20 seconds. In hemiplegia, flexion and pronation are present at the elbow and the arm drifts down.

Sensory system. Assess for sensation of touch, pain, and temperature of the arms and legs. A decrease in sensation may indicate peripheral neuropathy. It is important to test these sensations as a decrease or loss puts clients at risk for burning, scalding, and wounding themselves.

There are other tests for fine and discriminative sensation. They will not be discussed in this chapter, but the reader is encouraged to refer to an extensive physical examination textbook.

Genitourinary system. Problems related to the genitourinary system can cause not only discomfort but also embarrassment to the client. Both male and female clients react to urinary incontinence with emotional distress. A verbal assessment of urinary and bowel patterns can gather the most useful information. Questions about urinary and bowel habits are quite personal. However, the elderly can be very distressed by their problems and so appreciate the nurse's interest in their dilemma. Urinary and bowel concerns and assessments are discussed in detail in Chapter 11.

Examination of the genitalia completes the physical assessment. As stated earlier, not all aspects of a physical assessment need to be conducted by the home care nurse. Primarily the client's complaints and the focus of the referral will guide the nurse to conduct the appropriate parts of a physical examination. The client may complain of a new problem during a home visit, and so the physical assessment may become more comprehensive. If examining the genitalia of an elderly client is required, steps to the assessment remain the same as those for any adult. However, elders may be more embarrassed and reticent to participate in an examination. Elderly female clients may never have had a vaginal examination, and exposing themselves to anyone may be a foreign experience. The same may be true for elderly male clients.

It is best to first conduct a verbal assessment by having clients explain and describe their concerns. In most cases, an in-depth verbal assessment will provide enough information to guide the nurse to the appropriate actions. If the nurse believes a physical assessment is necessary, the nurse should provide privacy and inspect only the part of the perineal area or genitalia the client has concerns about. For example, if you suspect the client is describing hemorrhoids, have the client lay done on his or her side, facing away from you; the client should be covered with a blanket or towel, with only the lower buttocks exposed. If a client describes a rash on the mons pubis, the rest of the client's body should remain covered. The client should be in a comfortable position and one that allows the nurse to clearly see the affected area.

HEALTH RISK APPRAISAL: RECOGNIZING ACUTE/EMERGENCY SITUATIONS

Quick reaction of the nurse to emergency situations is the key to preventing unnecessary morbidity and mortality. Skills in observation sharpen the nurse's awareness to potentially debilitating or fatal situations. This acute sensitivity is demonstrated by the home care nurse responding to clues that "something is wrong" or to "a gut feeling" and is frequently called the "clinical eye."

Preventing crisis situations is an ongoing role of the home care nurse. Finding subtle changes in vital signs, recognizing the need for making necessary adjustments in medication dosages, and being vigilant to take every opportunity to teach safety in the home prevents many potential crisis situations.

At times, a client's health status may unpredictably change for the worse. Acute respiratory distress, severe chest pain, or gastrointestinal bleeding occurring at home necessitates an emergency telephone call. The home care nurse should teach the client, family, and caregivers which signs and symptoms may signal an impending health change and precipitate a dangerous situation. This training also includes who they should call and what they should do in an emergency.

Because people experience stress during an emergency, they may have trouble locating misplaced telephone numbers or even dialing the telephone. On an initial visit, the nurse can prepare a list of important numbers and attach them to the telephone. Some home health agencies provide a sticker for the telephone with the agency's telephone number and places to add several emergency numbers.

Infrequently the nurse will make a home visit to a client who lives alone and find the client in a crisis. Once the nurse determines that the client needs definitive medical care, a call to 911 should be placed. While waiting for the ambulance, the nurse should make the client comfortable and take vital signs. If there are other people in the house, the nurse can get more facts about the current situation. The nurse reassures the client and any others present by being calm and by explaining that help is on the way.

Most illnesses in the elderly present in an atypical way. It is easy to take action when clients experience "classic" signs and symptoms of illness. Taking appropriate action may be more difficult when it is reported that the client is not acting normally, is refusing to eat, is sleeping most of the time, is agitated and confused, or was "found on the floor." The nurse's assessment data and the family's recollection of the crisis event are shared with the paramedics when they arrive.

In the elderly, many diseases or conditions such as congestive heart failure, pulmonary edema, stroke, infection, and metabolic derangement (e.g., hypo- and hyperglycemia) present as delirium. Failure to recognize delirium may lead to death. Delirium should therefore be treated just like "classic" signs and symptoms.

REFERENCE

Staab, A., & Lyles, M. (1990). *Manual of Geriatric Nursing*. Glenview, IL: Scott, Foresman.

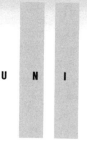

PROMOTING WELLNESS AMONG ELDERLY HOME CARE CLIENTS

Unit II continues the look at elderly home care clients' needs. There are topics that are common among all elders, regardless of specific healthcare issues, such as safety, mobility, nutrition, and sexuality.

Chapters 4 and 5 are companion chapters. Chapter 4 introduces the reader to causes, effects, and prevention of falls and other risk factors common to elders in the home. Appropriate nursing interventions in primary and secondary prevention are shared. In Chapter 5, modifications in mobility due to chronic or debilitating illnesses is discussed. With an underlying message of safety and promotion of an elder's independence at home, this chapter reflects on ways for the home care nurse to assist clients with progressive and safe mobility.

At all ages, what is consumed and how much is consumed influences wellness. In old age, good nutrition becomes critical to the quality of life and to life itself. In Chapter 6, an elder's nutritional well-being is explored. Basic nutrition, dietary modifications, and ways to help the homebound elder enhance eating patterns are shared.

The last chapter in this unit, Chapter 7, focuses on the topic of sexuality in old age. This is an often-neglected topic of discussion with clients by all healthcare workers, due mostly to unfamiliarity or embarrassment. It is, however, a very vital part of people's lives, including elders. This chapter helps the nurse discuss sexuality issues with the homebound elder.

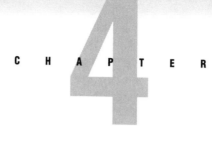

ENSURING SAFETY FOR THE ELDERLY CLIENT AT HOME

Mary Farren

◆   ◆   ◆

Assessing a Client's Health and Functional Ability
Environmental Assessment
Primary Prevention
Secondary Prevention
Use of Restraints in Home Care
Summary

One of the most important assessments the home health nurse is called upon to perform in community-based nursing is the assessment of client safety in the home environment. The issue of safety is broad and encompasses many factors and situations.

This chapter assists the nurse by providing information and insight into how to conduct a safety assessment. The safety assessment entails assessing the client, the caregivers, and the identification of factors in the environment that put the client at risk for falls, injury, or harm. The environment includes both the home and surrounding community. Every home care client, regardless of age, should be assessed for risks to safety and potential for falls. The very fact that a client has had a health problem and requires home care services places the client in a category and situation that increase potential risk factors.

Identifying risk factors and hazards is a fundamental and essential step in the prevention of falls and injuries. "Prevention" is a healthy, cost-effective nursing intervention that is the best way of promoting and ensuring safety.

Falls present a serious threat to the health of the elderly and unfortunately are a common occurrence. Falls and resulting injuries are a major cause of hospitalization, institutionalization, and mortality among the elderly. The fear of falling itself can significantly affect the ability of the client to function independently in the community setting and the client's quality of life. In this chapter, a "Home Safety Checklist" tool is presented; it guides the nurse in the assessment and is useful as a teaching tool when working with clients and their caregivers.

ASSESSING A CLIENT'S HEALTH AND FUNCTIONAL ABILITY

The reality is anyone can fall, but research has shown that there are factors that place some people at greater risk for falling. Elders are among this group. The nurse must make a careful clinical evaluation of the client to assess the risk for falling and formulate a care plan with client-specific interventions.

Common factors indicative of a high safety risk include being over 65 years old, female, and having a health history of a condition that affects coordination and balance. Conditions such as osteoporosis, arthritis, degenerative joint disease, prior stroke, vertigo, Parkinson's disease, seizure disorders, a history of falls, pathological fractures, foot disorders, and peripheral neuropathies increase safety risks. Included also is any malady that has left the client with residual functional limitations, such as an unsteady gait, paralysis, or weakness of the upper or lower extremities.

Information about the client's functional status and living arrangements are provided on the primary care provider's order form when the referral for home care services is generated. The description of the client's health status and functional ability on the referral can sometimes be quite different than what the nurse actually encounters on the initial visit. Every home care nurse has probably had this experience and should be prepared to "expect the unexpected" and make decisions based on sound judgment, nursing knowledge, and agency policy (see Box 4-1).

BOX 4-1 • CASE STUDY

The home care nurse is to make an initial visit to Mr. Fields, who lives alone and has been discharged from the hospital after an exacerbation of congestive heart failure. The MD order form states he is independent in ambulation but will require short-term assistance from a home health aide for assistance with personal care and some IADL. When the nurse rings the doorbell, Mr. Fields calls, "Come in. The door is open." The nurse finds an elderly, frail looking man seated on a chair. He tells the nurse he cannot get up from the chair. The ambulette driver had helped him into the house, but he has not been able to get up since then as he has no strength to push up from the chair. The nurse is able to help him stand up but discovers he is unable to ambulate without total assistance. The nurse at this point must decide if he is an appropriate candidate for home care services, as he is unsafe if left alone.

Analysis: In this case, appropriate interventions include but are not limited to the following: contacting a family member or friend to make arrangements to stay with the client; placing an emergency HHA immediately in the home to assist the client; or having the client transported back to the hospital until a more appropriate discharge plan can be arranged. This situation requires immediate intervention as the nurse cannot leave the client until arrangements are made. It is most important to ensure Mr. Fields' safety. In this particular case, the family could not be located and the client was sent back to the hospital until a more appropriate discharge plan could be arranged. The fact that Mr. Fields could not ambulate at all was the determining factor here. If left alone he would not be able to manage his own care and there was no doubt he was in an unsafe predicament without 24-hour direct assistance. The home care services were not enough to meet Mr. Fields' needs to ensure his safety.

Likewise, the discharge plans from the hospital need to be re-evaluated. If Mr. Fields is to be sent home, he needs an appropriate level of assistance until he regains strength and the ability to manage alone. This might mean arranging for the services of a 24-hour private aide or companion, or contacting the family for a commitment to stay with the client during the hours when a home health aide is not present. The family might consider bringing the client to their home and home care services be provided there. A referral to an agency that serves that community can be made for them. If Mr. Fields cannot pay for the level of care required to ensure a safe home environment, applying for Medicaid might be an option. The home health agency can authorize a social work visit to help the client and family apply for Medicaid in order to facilitate this process, or to discuss what plans can be made in Mr. Fields' best interest.

Safety risks are increased if a client's functional status includes any alteration in weight bearing ability (none or partial), need for assistance or use of an assistive device in ambulation or transfer activities, or weakness due to lack of activity or exercise. As clients age, they may encounter sensory limitations. Any limited vision (especially at night), blindness, hearing problems, or slowed reaction times also increase the risk to safety.

Medications (the action and interaction of medications, or a medication regime), particularly those that cause orthostatic changes, alter heart rate and blood pressure, or cause diuresis or sedation, must be considered as potential safety hazards.

A client history of drug or alcohol abuse can be a major cause of accidents and may be difficult to detect. The home care nurse needs to observe for any changes in the client's behavior, such as poor personal hygiene, poor diet and nutritional status, tremors, and repeated history of falls. Lonely elders who are not coping effectively with the loss of a loved one or with personal health changes may be substituting alcohol for food and putting themselves at risk for nutritional and safety related health problems.

Clients who have one or any combination of the above conditions are at risk for falls, burns, and other life-threatening occurrences. In addition, if clients have any of these health problems, their ability to independently perform activities of daily living (ADL) and instrumental activities of daily living (IADL) is compromised, which also puts them in a risk-for-falls category.

The initial clinical assessment of the client's health status and functional ability is very important, but it does not give the whole picture. The client's home environment and lifestyle also contribute to risk for falls and injury, and this requires an ongoing safety assessment. As the client's health status stabilizes, improves, or deteriorates, the plan of care must be revised to address the current needs of the client, including safety needs.

ENVIRONMENTAL ASSESSMENT

The nurse's assessment of the client's environment begins before meeting the client. As the nurse approaches the client's dwelling, the following questions should run through the nurse's mind:

- What is the neighborhood and building like? Are they safe?

- Are there stores nearby? Is public transportation nearby?
- Is the client's home in decent repair and the entrance to the dwelling physically accessible to the client?
- How many steps are there and will the client be able to manage without too much difficulty?
- Is there a working elevator the client can operate?
- Does the doorbell work and can the client hear the bell?
- How long does it take the client to answer the door?
- Can the sound of a cane or walker, clicking across the floor as the client approaches the door, be heard?
- Can the client open the door, or is it blocked by the assistive device the client is using?

The home safety assessment is a continuous process that extends beyond the initial visit. The initial visit, however, is a crucial time for assessment because obvious risk factors need to be identified. There are potential risk factors in every environment, and the challenge is to alert clients to those factors in their own environment that put them at risk for potential injury.

There are many factors to consider when determining environmental hazards and situations that pose a threat to the client's safety. Evaluating the home to identify safety risks entails a room-by-room assessment, and this must be done in the most nonjudgmental and respectful manner.

A good safety assessment includes questioning the client about safety risks encountered since arriving home, if the client was just discharged from the hospital. Negotiating a cluttered hallway may not be the first big risk identified by the client. An inability to reach the phone located in another room may be a far riskier situation to the client and can cause greater stress than risk factors identified by the nurse.

The nurse must always obtain permission from the client or family to look around the home. If the nurse explains why a home assessment is necessary, this can alleviate clients' worries that the nurse is "checking up on them" or is just "nosy." These issues are also addressed in Chapter 3.

It is now standard practice for most home care agencies to require the nurse to assess for the following safety conditions in the home on the initial visit and to record data on an assessment form provided with the paperwork when beginning home care services to a client. The assessment parameters are usually presented in a checklist format (see Figure 4-1, Home Safety Checklist).

HOME SAFETY CHECKLIST

ASSESSMENT PARAMETERS:
EXTERNAL CONDITIONS LEADING TO RISK OF FALLS AND OTHER INJURIES

	YES	NO
Are lamps, extension cords, and telephone cords placed out of the flow of traffic?	☐	☐
Are cords out from beneath furniture and rugs or carpeting?	☐	☐
Are cords attached to the walls or baseboards with nails or staples?	☐	☐
Are electrical cords in good condition and not frayed or cracked?	☐	☐
Do extension cords carry more than their proper load, as indicated by the ratings labeled on the cord and the appliance?	☐	☐
Are all small rugs and runners slip-resistant?	☐	☐
Are emergency numbers posted on or near the phone?	☐	☐
Is there access to a phone in case of a fall that limits reaching a wall phone?	☐	☐
Is there at least one smoke detector on every floor of the house?	☐	☐
Are the smoke detectors properly working and tested regularly?	☐	☐
Can lights be turned on without first having to walk through a dark area?	☐	☐
If fuses are used, are they the correct size for the circuit?	☐	☐
Are volatile liquids tightly capped and stored away from ignition sources?	☐	☐
Are any outlets or switches unusually warm or hot to the touch?	☐	☐
Do all outlets and switches have cover plates, so that no wiring is exposed?	☐	☐
Are light bulbs the appropriate size and type for the lamp or fixture?	☐	☐
Are appliances or heaters with three-prong plugs being properly used in three-hole outlets or with proper adapters?	☐	☐
Are small stoves, space heaters, and other heating sources away from flammable materials such as curtains or rugs?	☐	☐

FIGURE 4-1 • Home Safety Checklist *(continued on the next two pages)*

HOME SAFETY CHECKLIST (continued)

	YES	NO
Is wood-burning equipment installed properly?	☐	☐
Is there an emergency exit plan and an alternate emergency exit plan in case of fire?	☐	☐
Are towels, curtains, and other flammable materials located away from the range?	☐	☐
Is clothing with short or close-fitting sleeves worn while cooking?	☐	☐
Are lamps or light switches within reach of each bed?	☐	☐
Are smoking materials located far away from beds and bedding?	☐	☐
Is anything covering an electric blanket when in use?	☐	☐
Are the sides or ends of an electric blanket "tucked in"?	☐	☐
Does anyone go to sleep with a heating pad that is turned on?	☐	☐
Is there a telephone close to the bed?	☐	☐
Are kitchen ventilation systems or range exhausts functioning properly and are they in use while cooking?	☐	☐
Are all extension cords and appliance cords located away from the sink or range areas?	☐	☐
Does good, even lighting exist over the stove, sink, and counter-top work areas—especially where food is sliced or cut?	☐	☐
Is there a step stool that is stable and in good repair?	☐	☐
Are chimneys clear from accumulations of leaves or other debris that can clog them?	☐	☐
Have the chimneys been cleaned within the past year?	☐	☐
Are hallways, passageways between rooms, and other heavy traffic areas well lit?	☐	☐
Are exits and passageways kept clear?	☐	☐
Are bathtubs and showers equipped with nonskid mats, abrasive strips, or surfaces that are not slippery?	☐	☐
Do bathtubs and showers have at least one (preferably two) grab bar?	☐	☐
Is the water heater temperature set at 120 degrees or lower?	☐	☐
Is a light switch located near the entrance to the bathroom?	☐	☐
Are small electrical appliances, such as hair dryers, shavers, and curling irons, unplugged when not in use?	☐	☐

FIGURE 4-1 • Continued

HOME SAFETY CHECKLIST (continued)

	YES	NO
Are all medicines stored in the containers that they came in and are they clearly marked?	☐	☐
Are stairs well lighted?	☐	☐
Are light switches located at both the top and bottom of stairways inside the home?	☐	☐
Are sturdy handrails fastened securely on both sides of the stairway?	☐	☐
Do the handrails run continuously from the top to the bottom of the entire flight of stairs?	☐	☐
Do the steps allow secure footing?	☐	☐
Are steps even and of the same size and height?	☐	☐
Are the coverings on the steps in good condition?	☐	☐
Are the edges of the steps clearly visible?	☐	☐
Is anything stored on the stairway, even temporarily?	☐	☐

ADDITIONAL ENVIRONMENTAL CHECKLIST ITEMS

	YES	NO
Functioning refrigerator	☐	☐
Proper food storage	☐	☐
Floor surface even, easy to clean, requiring no wax, free of deep-pile rugs	☐	☐
Doorways painted a contrasting color from wall	☐	☐
Windows screened and easy to reach and open	☐	☐
Ample number of safe electrical outlets, preferably three feet higher than level of floor for easy reach	☐	☐
Does not use burners on stove or the oven to supplement heat	☐	☐
Shelves within easy reach, sturdy	☐	☐
Faucet handles easy to operate, clearly marked hot and cold	☐	☐
Adequate resources in home to promote mental stimulation and fill time: e.g., television, radio, hobbies, books, magazines, newspapers	☐	☐
If driving, car in safe operating condition, license current, vision adequate for day and night driving, seat adjusted for postural changes	☐	☐
If not driving, adequate access to transportation for medical appointments, shopping, and other errands	☐	☐

FIGURE 4-1 • Continued

If the environment is unclean, unsanitary, or hazardous, the home care agency's social service staff should be immediately notified. Steps must be taken to make emergency improvements to the living conditions so that it is appropriate and safe for the client to receive home healthcare services or, if necessary, to transfer the client to a safer environment. This needs to be done tactfully as clients have the right to keep their environment to their liking.

The client's permission is needed before any alteration is made to the client's home. The nurse must always be aware of the tendency to want to fix or correct what does not appear to meet the nurse's own personal standards. Unless the home environment presents a safety hazard, the nurse should respect the client's preferences.

If there are obvious hazards in the environment that the client refuses to address, the nurse can request the assistance of the home care agency social worker. The social worker can further assess the client's reasons for not wanting to correct the situation and can determine if it is due to financial concerns, lack of understanding of the problem, or judgment or competency issues. If it is an issue of competency, then primary care provider notification and a referral to Adult Protective Services or a similar advocacy agency need to be made. If the cause is financial or it is a tenant/landlord situation, the social worker can assist in negotiating to help address and fix the situation. Many times a client has been in the unfortunate situation of not being able to manage household chores because of illness, and an unexpected hospitalization adds to housekeeping problems. The client's family may be willing to assist and prefer to manage without agency intervention. An understanding attitude can facilitate the client accepting the help needed to make the environment clean and safe. However, if conditions in the home imminently threaten the safety of the client or home care staff, or if the client's needs are beyond the scope of agency services required to ensure client safety, then the agency, on a case-by-case basis, will terminate the care and arrange for the safe transition of the client to a more protective environment or to an alternative healthcare provider.

The nurse performs a room-by-room assessment of the home, with special attention given to the rooms the client will be using most often. The nurse makes recommendations to the client and family about any changes required for the client's safety and convenience, as documented in the Home Safety Checklist (Figure 4-1). Items checked "no" need to be corrected for the client's safety, and plans for change should be incorporated into the individualized care plan.

Cooking and smoking accidents are major causes of fatal fires involving senior citizens. The following is a list of safety tips that the home health nurse can use and review with clients to help prevent fires and injuries occurring in the kitchen:

- Don't wear loose clothing or dangle dish towels near a hot stove.
- Don't hang towels, curtains, or other combustibles near the stove.
- Don't store flammable liquids or aerosol cans near the stove or oven.
- Don't store items above the range. You could get burned reaching for them.
- Don't use the stove (oven or burners) to heat the room.
- Don't leave food unattended on the stove. If you must leave the room, take a pot holder or a wooden spoon as a reminder.
- Don't let grease build up on the stove or oven.
- Don't extinguish a grease fire with anything but baking soda or a pot lid. Keep both items within reach of the stove, but not stored above it.
- Do check the kitchen before going to bed. Are the oven and burners off? Are the appliances and coffee pot off?
- Check monthly to see that smoke alarms and carbon monoxide detectors are present and working.

PRIMARY PREVENTION

The safety and risk assessment is an ongoing process that is revised as needed and evaluated regularly. The most reliable way to assess a client's ability to function within the home is through direct observation. Have the client ambulate and note the gait, balance, and endurance. If the client lives alone and is only able to ambulate a short distance without assistance, the nurse must determine if the client can manage safely with the amount of services authorized under the client's home care insurance benefit. The important point the nurse must always keep in mind is the client's ability to function alone when there is no one around to provide assistance.

Nursing interventions must be client-focused in order to be effective. It is important to ask clients what tasks they feel uncomfortable performing or if they have any fears related to falling. The nurse can review a list of general ADL and IADL and ask if the client feels confident to perform them alone or with some assistance. This information is used when developing a "home health aide activity sheet" for the home health aide (HHA) or when making recommendations to the family. The HHA activity sheet may include assistance with bathing or showering, dressing and undressing, cooking simple meals, household chores, shopping, walking out of doors, and ambulating at home.

Appropriate interventions and recommendations can then be made based on the client's confidence and perception of the ability to manage. The goal is to promote safety and to assist the client in maintaining or obtaining a maximum level of safe, independent living, regardless of whether the client lives alone or with family. The nurse, in addition to teaching, addresses any concerns related to the care plan or safety issues that the family or caregiver may have.

Teaching

After assessment skills, teaching is the next most important skill for home care nurses. All teaching is ultimately directed toward encouraging safe and healthy behaviors. The nurse's teaching goals include good nutrition and exercise and ensuring that the client understands the scheduling and proper doses of prescribed medications. Simple advice such as encouraging the client to wear well-fitting shoes, comply with therapy regimes, and use assistive devices are part of the nurse's teaching. Teaching also includes recommendations about eliminating obvious environmental dangers and unsafe behaviors, such as not climbing on chairs to reach items and immediately wiping up spills off the floor. For clients who are afraid to move for fear of falling, the dangers to their overall health by being immobile are also addressed.

If the client is dependent on others for ADL and IADL, the nurse observes the family's and caregivers' ability to provide care and supervision. When teaching a client, family member, or aide, a return demonstration of the skill or procedure being taught assures the nurse that the skills are performed correctly. Reinforcing safety occurs on each home visit. As the home health nurse observes the client, suggestions and recommendations are made both verbally and in writing so that clients and their caregivers can refer to the instructions when the nurse is not present.

Assistive Devices

The nurse may determine that the client can benefit from the use of an assistive device, such as a walker or cane, after completing an environmental safety assessment. The nurse first consults with the primary care provider. If the primary care provider agrees, orders must be obtained and a durable medical equipment (DME) company notified to order the equipment. A referral for physical or occupational therapy may be considered to fit the device to the client's height, to teach proper use of the device, or to teach exercises to increase strength and mobility.

If the client is using assistive devices, the nurse must assess on each visit that they are in good working condition and that the correct device is being used based on the client's needs and the doctor's order. The nurse should reinforce instruction on the proper use of the assistive device and have the client, family member, or aide demonstrate proper use. It is important to note whether the client is compliant with the use of the equipment.

If the client has additional assistive equipment in the home, such as a bath seat, bedside commode, or mechanical lift, the nurse must ensure the equipment is being used safely and is in good working order. At times, suggesting the need for the use of a bedside commode, bedpan, or urinal at night, instead of ambulating to the bathroom, may be an additional safety measure.

Safe Administration of Oxygen

If oxygen therapy is ordered, it is essential to assess that the environment is safe for its use and that the client and family are instructed in the safe use of oxygen. Teach about the obvious dangers of smoking or having a lighted flame, candle, or electrical appliance in the same room. The electrical outlets should be checked to make sure they are not overloaded.

Oxygen tanks or oxygen concentrators need to be placed so that the client and others will not trip and fall over the length of oxygen tubing or electrical cords. A "No Smoking—Oxygen in Use" sign should be placed on the front door and another on the door of the room where the oxygen tank/concentrator is located. For additional compromised respiratory status concerns, see Chapter 17.

Safety in the Community

Clients who are able to go outdoors are encouraged to keep safety in mind. Suggestions might include always using the assistive device when outdoors. It is surprising how many clients don't want to be seen "with a cane!" Having an aide or friend accompany them on walks is a good idea. Encourage clients to slowly increase their endurance by adding a block or half a block at a time to their walking regime. Pacing their walking distance and turning around before they get too fatigued is also important. There may be community agencies or senior groups that sponsor transportation for shopping trips that clients can be referred to for assistance.

In icy conditions or extreme heat temperatures, caution should be taken when being out of doors. For most elders, it is advised not to be outside when environmental conditions may adversely affect health status, unless the reason is extremely important and it is done with safety in mind. This includes wearing proper, warm attire and footgear in cold, wet, or icy weather and using sunscreen and shade in the heat of the summer.

Some people have a hard time accepting or asking for help, and this behavior could result in injury. Encourage clients to let neighbors help with snow shoveling and errands. Acknowledging dependence can be difficult for some, so explain that allowing assistance helps them to keep their independence. Acceptance of limitations is a big step in ensuring safety.

SECONDARY PREVENTION

However diligently the home care nurse works to prevent injuries and ensure safety, a client may still experience a fall or injury. If this happens, the nurse must respond according to safe effective nursing practice and follow the home care agency's protocols regarding notification, documentation, and follow-up care.

Unless the nurse actually witnesses a client fall or get injured, the only way it comes to the nurse's attention is if the client, family, or aide reports it. The nurse routinely inquires about any injuries that may have happened, notes any bruising or other injuries during the physical assessment, and documents all findings. Surprisingly, elderly clients are often reluctant to report what they consider to be minor injuries, or they minimize the extent to which they were injured. The clients' reasons for this are many but are often based on fear of losing their independence. Clients fear that someone will decide they are unable to remain at home and need to move to a more restrictive environment, such as an assisted living center or skilled nursing facility.

When a client reports a fall that the nurse did not witness, a thorough physical examination is required to assess for injury, with the following points in mind:

- If a client reports a head injury, assess and monitor vital signs and neurological symptoms for signs and symptoms of subdural hematoma.
- If a client reports injury to the chest, consider the possibility of fractured ribs.
- If a client complains of stiffness or decreased mobility of the lower extremities, suspect an injury to the hip.

After completing a physical examination and determining that there are injuries requiring treatment, the home care nurse contacts the primary care provider and home care agency via a report. If the client requires immediate medical attention, 911 or an ambulance service is called. The nurse or home care agency calls the client's family to advise them of the incident and make arrangements for follow-up care.

After completing a physical examination and detecting no injuries requiring treatment, the nurse arranges for follow-up care with the client's primary care provider and assesses the environment for a possible cause of the accident. Interventions and client teaching are initiated or reinforced to minimize or correct the situation. For example, if the client fell after rising from a sitting position and experienced dizziness or weakness prior to the fall, remind the client about rising slowly from a seated to standing position to minimize orthostatic changes.

If the nurse witnesses a fall or accident, the same steps would be taken as above. Assess for injuries, administer standard first aid, and, if needed, access emergency care and transport the client to the hospital as quickly as possible. The primary care provider, home care agency, and family are notified.

Incident Reports

When completing an incident report, it is important to include all information. The information usually requested includes the name of the client, the names of anyone else involved, the date and time of the incident, and where the incident occurred.

A complete description of the incident is required, including all dates and specific events and actions taken. It must be clear who performed what action. For example, if the home health nurse (HHN) called emergency medical services (EMS) for assistance, document "HHN called EMS." Do not simply write "EMS was called," because that does not provide the specifics of "who did what."

Document any medical follow-up for which the client received medical assistance and any outcome of the medical follow-up. If safety instructions were given, document what was taught to the client at the time of the incident and the client's response to the teaching. Document all phone calls and reports given to the home care agency. Sign name and title on the report.

The incident report is kept in the agency and does not become a part of the client's chart. In the client's chart, the incident, steps taken, and so on are documented. No mention of completing an incident report is made. The incident report file system is a confidential record of incidents involving clients being served. It is used internally by agency management to conduct risk assessments, develop in-service programs, and to work with individual caregivers—HHNs, HHAs, and others—to improve client caregiving techniques.

Personal Emergency Response Systems

Renting a personal emergency response system may make some clients feel safer. This system operates via a remote calling device. The client wears the device, which is similar to a necklace. It has a button that can be pushed to activate the system if the client is in some kind of distress and can't get help through other means. When the client activates the system, an operator or a designated responder calls the client via the phone. If the client is unable to communicate or does not answer the phone, the system responder calls 911 or contacts someone who has access to the client's home to see if the client is in need. This system is very helpful for those who live alone because it provides reassurance that help is always available even if they can't get to the phone.

USE OF RESTRAINTS IN HOME CARE

Ensuring safety for elderly home care clients also includes a careful evaluation of medical symptoms and situations that might require the use of a restraint in order to protect the client from possible injury or harm. Home care agencies incorporate in their policy and procedure manuals, specific policies that guide the use of restraints in the home. The nurse must always be aware and alert to the potential harm that can be caused by the use of restraints. Restraints can cause both physical and psychological harm, including loss of dignity. They violate an individual's rights and can even cause death. Through teaching and demonstration of alternative interventions, nurses can support and encourage strategies to promote restraint-free environments.

The Joint Commission on Accreditation of Healthcare Organization (JCAHO) Standards (JCAHO, 1996) defines "a restraint" as "any method (chemical or physical) of restricting a client's freedom of movement, physical activity, or normal access to the body." The JCAHO mandates that "because the use of restraint can also be an intentional component of abuse and neglect, the home care provider has a responsibility to report suspected abuse according to applicable law and regulation [JCAHO, 1997]."

In using the term *restraint,* the nurse needs to consider the following three categories of restraints:

Physical restraint. Any manual method, physical or mechanical device, or material or equipment attached or adjacent to the client's body that the client cannot use easily and that restricts freedom of movement or normal access to the body.

Examples of physical restraints are leg restraints, arm restraints, hand mitts, soft ties or vests, and lap cushions or trays the client cannot remove. Other examples include using bed rails to keep the client from voluntarily getting out of bed as opposed to enhancing mobility while in bed; the practice of tucking in a sheet so tightly that the bed-bound client cannot move; using wheelchair safety bars to prevent the client from moving; or placing the client in a chair to keep the client from rising. Note that bed rails may be used to assist in the client's mobility and transfer; their use is prohibited if they are not medically necessary.

Chemical restraint. Any psychopharmacologic drug that is used for discipline or convenience and not required to treat medical symptoms.

Seclusion. Involuntary confinement of a person alone in a room where the person is physically prevented from leaving. The use of seclusion is never justified or supported in home care.

Before a restraint is used on a client in the home situation, the agency must demonstrate that (1) a medical symptom requires the use of a restraint; (2) the use would treat the cause of the symptom; and (3) the use will assist the client in reaching his or her highest level of physical and psychosocial well-being. Individualizing care plans and ongoing evaluations provide necessary treatment options that reduce or eliminate the need for restraints.

When it is determined that the use of a restraint is appropriate, the nurse and home care agency should consider the following elements:

1. The client's rights, dignity, and well-being are protected and preserved during restraint use.
2. The use of a restraint is based only on the client's assessed needs.
3. Decisions are made considering the use of the least restrictive methods first.
4. Safe application and removal of restraints by competent staff is assured.
5. The client is monitored and reassessed during use.
6. The restraints meet the client's needs during use.
7. A primary care provider's medical order is obtained for the use of the restraint on the client.
8. The medical order is time-limited.
9. The use and method of restraint is documented according to agency protocol in the client's medical record.

JCAHO standards mandate that when any restraint is used, the home care agency is obliged to educate the client and family/caregivers with individualized teaching plans that will instruct them in:

- the safe and effective use of medications in accordance with legal requirements and client needs.
- The appropriate use of restraints and alternatives to the use of restraints, including:
  —the correct application of the restraint.
  —attention to the needs of the client while the client is in the restraint.

Alternatives to the use of restraints include but are not limited to exploration of ambulation, positioning, active listening, exercise, appropriate lighting, and placing clients with a higher risk of falling near the center of activity within the home for closer supervision by the family or caregiver.

In addition to instructing the family, the nurse must instruct aides assigned to care for the client in the safe use of restraints. All teaching and response to teaching must be documented in the client's chart.

When a family requests the use of a restraint, it is necessary to determine what the behavior of the client is that the family feels necessitates the use of a restraint. There are other options to consider before using restraints. For example, have someone with the client at all times. This can be accomplished by enlisting family members to schedule themselves for time spent just sitting with the client or having an aide sit with the client if the cost of this fits with the client's and family's finances. The client should always be spoken to in a calm and reassuring manner and reoriented as needed. If the client is bed-bound and pulling at tubes, instead of restraining wrists or hands, have a person sit with the client to remind the client not to do so or move the tubes to a less obvious position. Keep the environment calm, quiet, and free of sudden and loud noises.

If the client is getting up at night and falling, the family may request restraints to keep the client safe. It may be that the client is getting up to use the bathroom. In this case, it would be helpful to provide a urinal or bedside commode or to have a family member set an alarm and get up to assist the client to the toilet according to the client's routine waking times. In this way, the family can plan to respond to the client's needs and possibly eliminate the behavior that they felt warranted a restraint.

There are situations in which the use of a restraint is a necessary safety measure to prevent injury and provide protection to the client. A mitten restraint prevents clients from scratching or digging at their bodies. Teaching for this includes instructing the caregiver to wash and dry the client's hand, put a rolled washcloth or gauze pad in the client's hand, and apply the mitt over that. It is important to check the circulation regularly and to remove the mitt to exercise the hand on a regular basis.

Safety vests and safety belts help prevent a client from falling out of a chair or bed. Teaching includes making sure the vest is applied correctly. Always crisscross the flaps in the front to prevent accidental choking if the client is restless and the vest rides up. The vest is always applied over clothing to prevent skin irritation from rubbing. It should be applied loose enough that a hand can be slipped between the vest and the client's abdomen.

Basic safety measures for all restraints include regular checks on circulation, skin integrity, and joint mobility. Clients can hurt themselves trying to get out of a restraint and should not be left unattended in a restraint. Explain to the client why a restraint is needed, such as "to keep you from falling out of the chair if you lean too far over." Toilet the client as needed and provide good personal care if the client is incontinent. Always use a knot or bow to secure the restraint so that it can be opened easily in an emergency.

SUMMARY

Care of the elderly client at home requires sensitivity to the issues of independence and dependency. Ensuring safety can be a crucial intervention for elderly clients struggling with the goal of remaining safe and independent in their own homes and communities. A thorough safety assessment is good, preventative, cost-effective nursing care! When possible the nurse attempts to approach safety through primary prevention techniques. These include assessment, teaching, and the proper use of equipment, oxygen, and assistive devices. At times, incidents cannot be prevented at the primary level and are first encountered at the secondary level of prevention. In this case, the nurse institutes proper emergency responses, which include documentation in the client's record and an incident report. The use of restraints in home care is a situation that requires close monitoring. Restraints are used only when all other options have been explored.

REFERENCES

JCAHO. (1996). Standards and intents. *Joint Commission Perspectives, 1996,* Jan/Feb.

JCAHO. (1997). *Comprehensive Accreditation Manual for Home Care.* Oakbrook, IL: Author.

5

PROMOTING AND MAINTAINING MOBILITY IN THE HOMEBOUND ELDERLY CLIENT

Dianna D'Amico-Panomeritakis
Joan Kurtz Sommer

◆ ◆ ◆

Health Changes and Aging
Activities of Daily Living
Impact of Functional Limitations
Promoting Activity Using the Nursing Process
Selecting Appropriate Mobility Devices
The Nurse's Role in Rehabilitation
Client and Caregiver Education
Summary

Maintaining mobility and function in the elderly is an important aspect of their being healthy. The potential impact of immobility on the elderly population can greatly alter the quality and length of life. The home care nurse is in a key position to assess the impact of acute and chronic conditions on the level of function, mobility, and quality of life among older adults. With knowledge, skill, and confidence, the home care nurse can frequently interrupt the downhill spiral of functional changes that often occur with older adults after a health crisis, new diagnosis, or hospitalization.

The process of rehabilitation or restorative nursing is meant to address these functional issues. Rehabilitation of the elderly focuses on mobilization in their own environment, safely using appropriate equipment and modifying the environment to facilitate independence. To do this, the home care nurse needs to become familiar with specific rehabilitation skills and techniques. The nurse begins the rehabilitation process with a functional safety assessment of the client as addressed in Chapter 4. The impact of limited mobility is considered in depth in this chapter, with a focus on increasing the nurse's rehabilitative/restorative role in promoting mobility in elders.

HEALTH CHANGES AND AGING

Three factors can affect a client's well-being: normal aging, a primary diagnosis, and existing secondary conditions. Each factor needs to be considered when a plan of care is being developed for the home care client.

Normal aging brings a gradual change in muscle strength and mass, flexibility, and the lubrication of joints, all of which affect range of motion and overall endurance. Additional changes in vision, hearing, center of gravity, and the sleep/wake cycle may further impact safe mobilization and the ability to care for oneself. These predictable changes are experienced by most people as they age, but at varying intensity. Aging does not necessarily mean limitations. Experienced over time, physical changes are readily compensated for by gradual changes in the way one does things. The home care nurse begins a functional assessment with knowledge of the normal aging process and the client's prior status on this continuum. What exactly the client was capable of before this spell of illness is an important piece of information to determine.

The client's *primary diagnosis* is often the first clue to assessing potential functional/mobility losses. The primary diagnosis is the current condition for which the client is being referred. Orthopedic and neurologic conditions are the most common primary diagnoses with an obvious impact on function. These include fractures, arthritis, joint replacements, degenerative joint disease, cardiovascular accident (CVA), Parkinson's disease, multiple sclerosis (MS), spinal cord impairment, and peripheral neuropathy. Table 5-1 lists activities that are most commonly affected by specific diagnoses. Whatever the diagnosis, the nurse must focus on the actual or potential loss of function incurred, always keeping in mind how the condition affects the client's ability to manage care. For example, an 84-year-old diabetic with generalized arthritis falls and fractures her right humerus. She is fitted with a cast and immobilized for six weeks. How will she bathe with one arm? Can she open cans and packages and prepare food with one hand? How will she cleanse herself after toileting? Can she maintain her balance safely for ambulation? How will she dress herself? Will she be able to manage her insulin injections? What was she capable of prior to this and how has that changed? In order for this client to manage safely, solutions to these dilemmas need to be reached.

Rarely is a referral for home care services void of multiple secondary diagnoses. *Secondary diagnoses* are all the other conditions that the client has. These may be long-standing (such as diabetes, cardiac disease, or respiratory compromise), or they may be a result of the primary diagnosis (e.g., surgery, pain, fatigue, or poor nutritional status). Additionally, the client may be experiencing debilitation from a previous hospitalization, cognitive changes from anesthesia or a change in environment, medication side effects, or depression as a result of trying to cope with a major change. The secondary diagnoses category often represents subtle issues that go unnoticed, yet dramatically impact functional ability. They tend to interact with and aggravate the current primary diagnosis. A thorough assessment of secondary diagnoses and their impact on functioning must be part of the home care nurse's plan of care.

After assessing the effects of the aging process and the primary and secondary diagnoses, the home care nurse explores their potential combined impact on the client's functional ability. The nurse must always consider how to address mobility issues and prevent debilitation. This includes considering the type of equipment or assistance that may help function as impaired abilities coexist.

ACTIVITIES OF DAILY LIVING

Activities of daily living (ADL) are the basic tasks a client needs to perform to minimally function on a day-to-day basis. Assessing a client's mobility answers such questions as how long, how much, and under what circumstances the client is able to perform ADL. In addition to ADL, there are instrumental activities of daily living (IADL), which

TABLE 5-1 • COMMON DIAGNOSES THAT IMPACT FUNCTION

Orthopedic Conditions	Potential Functional Issues
Fracture of the upper extremity	Dressing, grooming, bathing, feeding, toileting, bed mobility, meal preparation, ambulation
Fracture of the lower extremity	Dressing, toileting, bed mobility, positioning, transferring, sitting, ambulation
Arthritis, rheumatoid	Virtually all functions may be affected depending on joints involved or degree of flare up
Arthritis, osteo	Issues may vary depending on joints involved
Joint replacement, hip and knee	Bathing, dressing, toileting, bed mobility, transferring, sitting, ambulation
Degenerative joint disease Osteoporosis	Issues may vary with location. For example, if the spine is involved: grooming, feeding, toileting, positioning, bed mobility, transferring, sitting, ambulation

Neurological Conditions	Potential Functional Issues
Cerebral vascular accident Transient ischemic attack Hemiplegia—total loss of control Hemiparesis—partial loss of control	Dressing, grooming, bathing, feeding, toileting, positioning, bed mobility, transferring, sitting, ambulation, communication, vision Affect may vary depending on type of change
Parkinson's disease	Dressing, grooming, bathing, feeding, toileting, positioning, bed mobility, transferring, sitting, ambulation, cognition, communication
Spinal cord impairment Multiple sclerosis Spinal cord injury	Virtually all activities affected dependent on the level of impairment. The higher the injury, the more limitations.

include progressively independent functioning. Boxes 5-1 and 5-2 delineate types of activities in each category and presents them in question form to assist the home health nurse in the assessment process.

The home health nurse may notice that due to limitations in ADL and IADL, clients may modify how they perform these tasks. A client reports that she "can cook a meal," when what she is able to do is heat a frozen dinner in the microwave oven versus using the physical and cognitive skills it takes to prepare a meal from original ingredients.

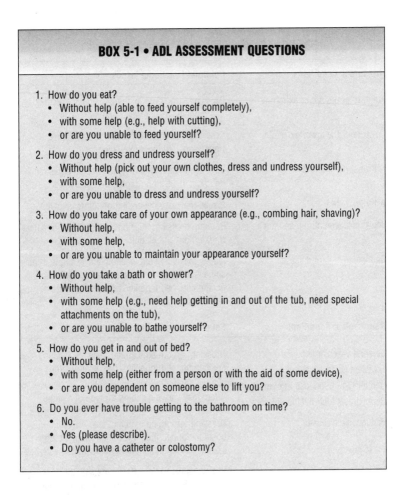

BOX 5-1 • ADL ASSESSMENT QUESTIONS

1. How do you eat?
   - Without help (able to feed yourself completely),
   - with some help (e.g., help with cutting),
   - or are you unable to feed yourself?

2. How do you dress and undress yourself?
   - Without help (pick out your own clothes, dress and undress yourself),
   - with some help,
   - or are you unable to dress and undress yourself?

3. How do you take care of your own appearance (e.g., combing hair, shaving)?
   - Without help,
   - with some help,
   - or are you unable to maintain your appearance yourself?

4. How do you take a bath or shower?
   - Without help,
   - with some help (e.g., need help getting in and out of the tub, need special attachments on the tub),
   - or are you unable to bathe yourself?

5. How do you get in and out of bed?
   - Without help,
   - with some help (either from a person or with the aid of some device),
   - or are you dependent on someone else to lift you?

6. Do you ever have trouble getting to the bathroom on time?
   - No.
   - Yes (please describe).
   - Do you have a catheter or colostomy?

Another client takes sponge baths only because he is afraid he will fall if he stands in the tub to shower and he won't bathe because he cannot climb in or out of the tub safely. Exploring client responses and not assuming to know the client's meaning is a responsibility of the home health nurse.

IMPACT OF FUNCTIONAL LIMITATIONS

When the elderly are hospitalized for any medical or surgical problem, they are usually immobilized, on bed rest, or have restricted mobility

BOX 5-2 • IADL ASSESSMENT QUESTIONS

1. Are you able to use the telephone?
   - Without help, including looking up numbers and dialing,
   - with some help (can answer phone or dial operator in an emergency, but need a special phone or help in getting the number or dialing),
   - or are you unable to use a telephone?

2. How do you get to places out of walking distance?
   - Without help (can travel alone on buses or taxis or can drive),
   - with some help (need someone to help or go with you when traveling),
   - or are you unable to travel unless emergency arrangements are made for a specialized vehicle, such as an ambulance?

3. Can you go shopping for groceries or clothes (assuming you have transportation)?
   - Without help (taking care of all shopping needs yourself),
   - with some help (need someone to go with you on all shopping trips),
   - or are you completely unable to do any shopping?

4. How do you prepare your own meals?
   - Without help (plan and cook full meals yourself),
   - with some help (can prepare some things but unable to cook full meals yourself),
   - or are you unable to prepare any meals?

5. How do you manage your housework?
   - Without help (can scrub floors and so on),
   - with some help (can do light housework but need help with heavy work),
   - or are you unable to do any housework?

6. Are you able to take your own medicine?
   - Without help (in the right doses at the right time),
   - with some help (able to take medicine if someone prepares it for you and reminds you to take it),
   - or are you unable to take your medicine?

7. Do you manage your own money?
   - Without help (write checks, pay bills, and so on),
   - with some help (manage day-to-day buying but need help with managing your checkbook and paying your bills),
   - or are you unable to handle money?

8. Do you do your own laundry?
   - Without help (get to machines or Laundromat, sort, wash, dry, and put clothes away),
   - with some help (transporting, carrying, managing the washing and ironing processes or putting clothes away),
   - or are you dependent on someone else for your laundry?

BOX 5-3 • MR. PETERS, PART I

Mr. Peters is 80 years old and has been discharged from the hospital after a three-day stay. He was admitted with complaints of shortness of breath and diagnosed with an acute exacerbation of congestive heart failure. While hospitalized, he was treated with IV Lasix. Presently, he is taking Lasix by mouth. During hospitalization, the client complained of shortness of breath and increased fatigue. He remained on bed rest.

Mr. Peters lives with his elderly wife on the second floor of their private house. Prior to admission, they were an active couple who liked to shop, walk, and visit friends. On the home care nurse's initial visit, Mr. Peters was in bed, where he has remained since discharge. He reports feeling lonely, having poor endurance and weakness, and can only walk to the bathroom with his wife's help.

For the nurse working in home care, Mr. Peters presents as a typical client. Presently he has decreased endurance and mobility and requires assistance with self-care. If Mr. Peters' prognosis is good, these limits will be temporary and long-term consequences minimal. However, if an elderly client's limitations are not identified, addressed, and intervened upon, complications can be expected. The nurse assesses the potential physical consequences of Mr. Peters' immobility. If he remains in bed for several days, he may potentially have complications with the cardiovascular, musculoskeletal, respiratory, integumentary, and gastrointestinal systems. He is already noting increased weakness of lower extremities and complains of constipation. Early mobilization for Mr. Peters can readily reverse these problems and prevent others.

---

due to pain or fatigue. Once home, they often continue to rest or find themselves in a deconditioned or debilitated state. This makes movement difficult, fatiguing, and, for some, a safety issue. The younger hospitalized client returning from a state of extended rest can easily compensate. For elderly clients, the return to a state of mobility or independence may be slow, labored, and frustrating.

To develop a plan to maintain or maximize mobility, the home care nurse needs a clear understanding of the potential complications. The impact of immobility on the elderly has consequences in physical, social, and psychological domains, as is best illustrated in the case study in Box 5-3.

In this case, the home care nurse instructs the client and caregiver of the need to: change positions frequently when in bed to prevent tightening of muscles, sit out of bed for meals, do strengthening exercises, walk to the bathroom, and assist with self-care. A walker may be recommended for temporary balance problems and assistance. Energy con-

---

BOX 5-4 • MR. PETERS, PART II

Mr. Peters has always been able to go with his wife shopping and visiting. He was the chauffeur for his wife and friends whenever they went out. He took care of all the bills and household chores. He now believes he is unable to participate in these activities and is beginning to feel "isolated" and "worthless."

---

servation techniques will also be included. Remember, the elderly may be experiencing limitations from normal aging, so even small changes in mobility can lead to unexpected complications. These activities encourage the client's mobility and function.

Social problems occur due to a client's inability to participate in activities outside the bedroom or home. The elderly person who is non-ambulatory or limited in mobility may find that most time is spent in bed or in the bedroom. A client may feel alienated from family activities, visiting with neighbors, and socializing at church or the senior center. The client may also find that roles within the family have changed.

Some potential social concerns related to decreased mobility include: a lack of stimulation, a lack of recreation and leisure, family separation, isolation from friends, a change of roles, loss of independence, and changes in quality of life (see Box 5-4).

By assessing the client's prior level of functioning and types of leisure activities, it gives the nurse a better understanding of the depth of impact the functional limits are having on lifestyle. The nurse may suggest encouraging friends to visit, sitting at the table for meals with family, making phone calls, and involvement in a hobby. These interventions encourage physical as well as mental activity.

The *psychological* consequences of limited function can occur at any time. The negative feelings that go with limited functioning are depression, poor self-esteem, withdrawal, loss of control, and helplessness.

The elderly often mention these feelings when recounting their diagnoses. Hospitalization may trigger feelings of being out of control and excluded from decisions. As the nurse entering a client's home to provide care, it is important to remember to include the client in all decisions, support the client's wishes when possible, and plan interventions jointly. Clients who are unable to control their slowing bodies, even from the aging process, need to believe some order can be brought to their lives (see Box 5-5).

BOX 5-5 • MR. PETERS, PART III

The nurse must include Mr. Peter in decisions, ask him for suggestions to decrease his isolation, and discuss with his wife some tasks he can still perform in household management (e.g, paying the bills). He should also be encouraged to participate in areas of his treatment plan, such as scheduling appointments.

Physical and mental interaction and stimulation are important ingredients to ward off isolation. Maximizing a client's potential for mobility and self-care will minimize the complications of prolonged limitations and maximize feelings of self-worth. The home care nurse is in the best position to facilitate a client to be a decision maker rather than a decision taker.

PROMOTING ACTIVITY USING THE NURSING PROCESS

The nursing process is a useful framework in which nurses formulate their caregiving activities. It provides the structure needed to work effectively with clients. The five steps in the nursing process help to guide caregiving in a systematic manner.

Assessment

In this first step, all the data that can be gathered through observation, other objective data, and subjective information are used. The five areas of cognition, range of motion, muscle strength, balance, and endurance are the focus of the nurse's functional mobility assessment. First, one needs to be cognizant of what one is doing and where one is. Second, one needs range of motion in hips, knees, elbows, neck, and shoulders in order to turn, extend, sit, and stand. Muscle strength is necessary to push, lean, sit, stand, and walk. Without a sense of balance, one would have great difficulty sitting on the edge of the bed, standing, and walking. A degree of endurance—the ability to maintain an activity long enough to accomplish a task—is essential to maintain independence safely.

There are two approaches to assessing these five functions. One is subjective, or what the client reports. It can be elicited by having the client answer questions about mobility capabilities. The answers give the nurse the client's perception of the client's abilities and limitations. At times, the client's report may be contrary to what the nurse actually observes. The nurse's observation is called objective measurement. It entails asking the client to perform specific tasks and assessing for function and limitation. This is a hands-on approach. Together, a subjective and objective assessment provide a more accurate picture of the client's current function. Table 5-2 gives assessment areas and examples of subjective and objective data. A comprehensive collection of data includes the client's primary and secondary diagnoses, functional limitations, family support system, and environmental barriers.

The skilled home care nurse will very quickly learn to incorporate observations and questions into the overall assessment, diminishing the time constraints often faced. The following is an example of gathering data efficiently: the nurse observes the client sitting on the edge of his bed, leaning to answer the phone, and picking up his shoes. The nurse can quickly move past the issues of balance, bed mobility, sitting, and range of motion to these joints and focus attention on standing and walking. The nurse weaves this information into what is already known about normal aging and the client's primary and secondary diagnoses.

Nursing Diagnosis

Having completed the assessment, the home care nurse is ready for the second step, formulating a nursing diagnosis. A nursing diagnosis is created by analyzing the assessment data and arranging the information into patterns with scientific bases, and it concludes with an identification of a standard nursing diagnosis. Standard nursing diagnoses were developed by the 10th Conference on Nursing Diagnoses (NANDA) in 1992. Each home care agency uses these or a list of diagnoses widely used in the agency's community. Client's with mobility needs may have nursing diagnoses such as: a knowledge deficit related to —, at high risk for injury related to —, pain (acute or chronic), impaired physical mobility related to —, self-care deficit (feeding, bathing, hygiene, dressing, grooming, toileting), self-esteem disturbance, skin integrity impaired, impaired social interaction, social isolation, and at high risk for trauma.

Plan of Care

Step three is the development of the care plan. This requires the home health nurse to identify the present limitations and develop appropriate

TABLE 5-2 • OBTAINING INFORMATION FROM THE CLIENT

Assessment of:	Subjective Approach	Objective Approach
Cognition	Do you have complaints of forgetfulness, difficulty concentrating, or poor memory? Do you have problems with vision or hearing?	Check ability to follow commands, answer simple questions, and perform return demonstration. Is client aware of his own abilities and limitations? What types of medications does he take?
Range of motion	What position do you spend most of your time in? Are there any positions you are not able to maintain? Do you have any pain in any positions? Do you feel stiff anywhere?	Check all major joints. Check ability to lift arms and bend knees, hips, ankles, and neck. Ask client to perform a specific ADL (e.g., grooming, dressing, standing, walking). Check for contractures or joint limitations.
Muscle strength	What are you able to do for yourself? Do you have any weakness? Is there anything you can't do?	Check all four extremities. Check ability to reach, grip, push, lift. Check ability to do ADL: bathe, dress, eat, sit, stand, transfer, walk.
Balance	Can you sit on the edge of the bed alone? Can you sit/stand alone? Do you feel wobbly or dizzy when upright? Have you ever fallen? What caused it?	Check for ecchymotic areas. Observe sitting, standing, and gait. Check for head midline position during activities. Observe for leaning during activities.
Endurance	Do you feel fatigued? How much time do you sit out of bed? How far can you walk? Do you need to rest often?	Observe for shortness of breath, frequent changes in position, requests to rest, difficulty concentrating. Assess amount of energy to perform tasks: bed mobility, sit, stand, transfer, walk.

goals for the client. These goals must be specific, achievable, and mutually acceptable to both the client and nurse, and have measurable outcomes. Outcomes need to be divided into short-term and long-term goals. Usually, short-term goals are accomplished within four to six visits as the client progresses. Long-term goals are expected to be attained by the end of planned visits in the certification period.

Once a goal is identified, the home care nurse develops a plan to achieve the goal. An effective rehabilitation plan must include the components of an exercise program with progressive activity tolerance and progressive activity, environmental modification, and family/caregiver participation. The rigor of any plan is individualized within the limitations of the client's diagnoses and is modified as the client responds to the plan.

The establishment of a home exercise program (HEP) assists the client in increasing range of motion, strength, endurance, and balance needed to perform all activities. Remember, using activities that are functional, fun, and rewarding are the best form of exercise. For example, grooming, dressing, and moving in bed are the best forms of range of motion and more likely to be done by the client. Exercises should increase in duration, complexity, and exertion over time depending on the client's tolerance. The home care nurse instructs the client and caregiver in exercises to practice daily until the nurse's next visit. Written instruction may be helpful for further reinforcement. Performance of exercises may require supervision by caregivers until the client is independent.

Activity tolerance is defined as the client's ability to perform an activity without complaints or changes in the client's status. A client's ability to get out of bed and into a chair without complaints of dizziness, pain, or hypotension exemplifies this. The nurse works with the client on tolerating being out of bed for longer periods of time and more frequently throughout the day.

The concept of *progressive activities* is that one activity builds on another until independence is attained. A staircase is used to demonstrate the client's progression along this continuum:

PROGRESSIVE MOBILITY

STAIRS
WALKING
STANDING
TRANSFERRING
BED MOBILITY

The home care nurse may begin working with the bed-bound client on *bed-level activities,* which are turning, pulling up, lifting hips, rolling, sitting up on elbows, upper extremity lifting, dressing, bathing, grooming, eating, sitting on edge of bed, and balancing while sitting. Success at these tasks will allow the needed skills for the next step: transferring to a chair or wheelchair. *Transfer activities* are sitting balanced; trunk and abdominal muscle strengthening; hip, knee, and ankle flexion; bearing weight; dressing; reaching; pushing up in chair; sitting on edge of bed; and balancing with head at midline. For the client who is able to walk several steps, the intervention focuses on increasing the distance and safety in ambulation, then negotiating the stairs. *Ambulation activities* include marching in place, up and down transfers in chair, bridging (lifting hips off bed while lying), forward leaning while seated, standing in place, leg lifts, balancing on one leg, and weight bearing exercises.

The environment is another consideration in planning. Barriers to mobility and environmental changes needed are identified. Modifications to the environment need to occur early in the plan so they do not interfere with goals. Some environmental modifications may be as simple as removing a scatter rug, disposing of clutter, or changing dim light bulbs; others may require structural changes such as installing grab bars. The home care nurse discusses recommendations while being sensitive to the client's financial constraints, personal likes and beliefs, and realistic options.

Assisting clients in the exercise and activities program requires *family/caregiver participation*. Rehabilitation means repetition and reinforcement. The client and caregiver need instruction and clear expectations to continue practicing skills. The caregiver needs to assist the client to ensure safety and compliance in the treatment plan.

Implementation

Step four is implementing the plan. This includes conducting the actual activities needed to be completed in order to reach the goal or outcome. Rehabilitation interventions fall into three categories: prevention of further loss, complications, and injury; strengthening of abilities; and independence of activities.

As home health nurses proceed with interventions, they focus on the three categories. Prevention interventions include health and safety teaching, modifying the environment, and maintaining the client's current level of mobility. Strengthening interventions are woven into an active or passive exercise regimen, which may include family and caregivers. Strengthening activities are geared toward a progressive demonstration of ability, such as sitting versus lying, standing versus sitting, and walking versus sitting. The third intervention incorporates activities that will decrease the client's dependence. Incorporating more and more involvement in ADL and IADL, within the limitations of the client's diagnoses and prognosis, is key to success in this step.

Evaluation

Step five in the nursing process is evaluation. The client's response to interventions, progress toward goals, and need for modifications to the plan are measured. At this time, both the subjective and objective data are reviewed. The home care nurse needs to reevaluate the plan at each visit and change it appropriately. Some modifications may be temporary, as when a client complains of increased fatigue due to poor sleep resulting in an inability to practice stair climbing. Other changes may be permanent, such as cardiac or respiratory problems that make ambulation contraindicated, in which case the nurse can revise the goal to safe wheelchair transfers with the caregiver's assistance.

SELECTING APPROPRIATE MOBILITY DEVICES

Mobility devices serve as an adjunct in the rehabilitation process for many elderly clients. Devices may be recommended for a client's use for any of the following goals: to maximize mobility, ensure safety, or minimize workload.

An elderly client who has severe arthritis of both knees may be unsteady when walking and report a history of falls. The nurse may discuss the possibility of using a device for safer ambulation. There are numerous gait and mobility aids available. The home care nurse needs to be familiar with the options, purpose, and limitations of these devices. Table 5-3 presents some of the more common devices ranging from maximum support to minimum support. For a severely arthritic client, Table 5-3 indicates that a walker would be most appropriate for lower extremity weakness and balance problems. Good balance is necessary for using a cane or crutches.

When choosing the appropriate device for an elderly client, it is important for the nurse to know where the client needs the assistance and why it is needed, the client's ambulation ability, and the safest way for the client to be mobile. It is also important to be aware that the client can progress to different devices. The client may initially need the support of a walker, yet has a long-term goal of independent ambulation with a cane. Devices can be recommended on a temporary or permanent basis.

With all assistive devices instruction to the client and caregivers on equipment parts and safety is essential.

TABLE 5-3 • MOBILITY DEVICES AND OPTIONS

Mobility Device	Types of Option	May Use for Clients With These Problems	Potential Problems With This Device	Safety Tips for Using This Device
Walker	Standard Folding Rolling Junior Hemi-walker	Poor balance Lower extremity weakness No weight bearing on one leg Amputation	Narrow doorways and walkways are difficult Stair climbing Need use of bilateral upper extremities except with hemi-walker Obese clients require special equipment	Correct height is at client's wrist Step halfway into walker space Encourage leaning on walker for increased support Always place all four legs on floor at same time
Crutches	Lofstrand Axillary	No weight bearing on one lower extremity Partial weight bearing	Need good balance Need to be able to sequence steps Need good upper extremity strength	Place crutches with space wide enough for body Correct height, two fingers under armpit, slight bend to elbow Weight is on palms, not armpit Go upstairs with strongest leg first and come down with affected leg first

(continued)

TABLE 5-3 • Continued

Mobility Device	Types of Option	May Use for Clients With These Problems	Potential Problems With This Device	Safety Tips for Using This Device
Cane	Straight Narrow base Wide base Pyramid	Weakness of one lower extremity Weakness of both lower extremities Use of only one arm As a signal to others that assistance may be needed	Need good balance Cannot use if you need bilateral upper extremity support	Correct height is at client's wrist Longer legs of quad cane point away from body Keep within six inches of body Use on affected side if possible
Wheelchair	Standard Lightweight Junior Amputee One-arm drive	Poor endurance Paralysis or paresis Outside and distance mobility Poor balance	Need wide doorways and walkways Need upper body strength to self-propel Weight of wheelchair can be difficult if client has poor endurance Difficult to propel on carpeting	Remove foot rests and arms during transfers Check correct fit and height to avoid posture and skin problems Client can use feet to self-propel, remove foot pedals Lock and check brakes

THE NURSE'S ROLE IN REHABILITATION

Having completed a thorough assessment and identified a client's reha-
bilitative/restorative needs, such as mobility or ADL training, home care
nurses must also decide where their boundaries lie. What can home health
nurses accomplish and what requires another discipline's expertise? Long
before the 1990s, the home care nurse was a generalist, concerned with
and prepared to deal comprehensively with clients' needs. With increasing specialization in all aspects of healthcare, however, referring the client
became a common practice. Clients typically are seen by a nurse, assessed,
and then referred to a physical or occupational therapist for assistance
with mobility and ADL issues. Over time, some home care nurses have
lost confidence in their ambulation, exercise, positioning, and transfer
skills. Their teaching plans focused on medication, nutrition, and disease
management. Mobility and ADL activities lost priority as nurses grappled
with new and multiple client care problems.

Although the team approach to care is by far superior, its practical-
ity and cost in home care often becomes an issue. If the home care
agency has a physical therapist on staff, it is ideal to have the therapist
make an initial home visit at the time the nurse makes the first visit in
order for these two professionals to coordinate care. A problem occurs
for clients when their healthcare needs must wait for an outside professional to respond to a referral.

The future healthcare reimbursement climate will more than likely
make it more and more difficult to justify the use of many specialized
services. Home visits will be limited and based on diagnosis. Priori-
tizing client needs will be key, and nurses will be asked to address many
of the mobility and ADL issues. Making the most appropriate referrals
will become a focus of the managed care environment.

A clear example of the nurse's role in this method of caregiving
management is with an elderly client with a lower extremity fracture
who is non–weight bearing. The nurse is expected to prevent complications, maintain proper positioning, work on strengthening exercises,
assist with learning ADL, and teach safe transfers and wheelchair
mobility. The limited physical therapy visits are focused on ambulation
training and strengthening post–cast removal. The client will progress
more quickly if the nurse intervenes long before the cast is removed.
The nurse sees to it that the client works on upper body strength for
wheelchair and walker training and teaches safe transfers, wheelchair
mobility, and short distance ambulation with a walker, such as to the
bedside commode.

Documentation of goals and outcomes is not only necessary but mandatory for reimbursement. Restorative/rehabilitative nursing is a reimbursable service under Medicare. Sandwiched between several common nursing diagnoses, it reflects the nurse's ability to identify and intervene in common mobility and ADL issues.

With today's technology, there are many complex client care needs. Home care nurses must be able to assess, identify, and discern their role and intervene appropriately. There are many common mobility issues that can be readily managed by the nurse within the regular visit. Based on previous skills of progressive mobility, the home care nurse can identify safety issues related to mobility and institute an active plan of progressive mobility. Common mobility issues readily managed by the home care nurse include: loss of ambulation due to deconditioning, problems with ADL, post-hospitalization debilitation, mobility devices for lower extremity problems (foot sores, weakness), post–abdominal surgery pain, debilitation from cancer treatment, poor endurance, exacerbation of chronic disease, and weakness.

Rehabilitative/restorative nursing is based on possibilities and achievements, not limitations. With skill training, the home care nurse can assist in mobilizing the client and identify possibilities for the client. There will always be a clear need for therapist referral, particularly in orthopedic and neurologically impaired clients. However, virtually all clients will have some issues related to mobility or ADL. The nurse has many opportunities to intervene and can reinforce and review what physical and occupational therapy has recommended. Rehabilitative/restorative nursing is all about repetition and reinforcement, something nurses in all settings have always done.

CLIENT AND CAREGIVER EDUCATION

Working with elderly clients frequently involves elderly spousal caregivers. For them, remaining together and being independent is a priority. In other families, clients may be very old, in their late eighties and nineties, and cared for by older adult children who are in their sixties and seventies. The home care nurse needs to include these caregivers in the assessment of the client and environment. These caregivers know the client intimately and can provide detailed information if they are included in the assessment and care planning. Determining their physical and emotional capabilities in reinforcing the agreed upon plan may be critical to the recovery of the client. Do not underestimate their abilities, even if they appear frail. The years of commitment to their loved one, and perhaps months or years of caregiving, establishes their remarkable stamina. However, the nurse needs to assess caregivers for burnout and risk to their own health and well-being. They may very much need information about resources to assist them, such as home health aide and homemaker assistance, meals on wheels, and so on. Perhaps there is someone to provide direct care when needed, or supportive care so that caregivers can focus energy on their family members' needs, not household needs.

The home health aide and caregiver can unknowingly sabotage a rehabilitation plan if they are not included. If the home health nurse has taught the client to transfer to a chair by standing and pivoting, this can be sabotaged by a home health aide who lifts the client quickly into the chair. The client is up but has lost the benefit of learning balance, weight bearing, and range of motion.

There are many ways to accomplish a goal. Caregivers are usually anxious to learn, and at times the nurse can learn from caregivers. When the nurse teaches about moving in bed, body mechanics, transfers, and ambulation, it frequently applies to caregivers as well. The following guidelines are helpful when teaching elderly clients and caregivers at home.

The approach:

- Keep a positive attitude that is focused on abilities, not limitations.
- Keep safety at the forefront of all interventions.
- Include all family members and caregivers in the plan.
- Choose an area to teach first that the client is motivated to learn.

Things to include:

- Provide tips on energy conservation.
- Include how to manage and maintain equipment.
- Provide resources for support, information, equipment, and assistance.
- Include information on respite services if appropriate.
- Help the family develop a home emergency escape plan.

Home health nurses who help to rehabilitate clients are always thinking what they can teach their clients to do for self-care. Time and effort, however, must not be wasted on tasks that have no functional value for the elderly. A focus must be maintained on function. Independence and being able to function in life is what everyone wants no matter their age and what gives quality to the years.

SUMMARY

Everyone has a perception of what it means to grow old and age. For some, it is a time of slowing down, reminiscing, and peace. Others may see it as a time of sickness, the unknown, waiting for "the other shoe to drop," or letting go and giving up on things. Still for others, it is a period free of many responsibilities where time allows new adventures, hobbies, and fun. Seniors often take up tennis, travel, bowling, or skiing. It is paramount that home care nurses be aware of their own attitudes about aging and then put them aside to focus on the client's perceptions and meaning to this life issue. All too often, the elderly are hindered by caregivers' and other's attitudes toward them. It is important to be careful and look beyond the client's current health crisis and debilitation and see the potential that exists. Growing old is a natural, expected process all people experience. It should not mean an inability move, sit, walk, or manage care. A rehabilitation perspective, therefore, serves the elderly well because it focuses on ability not disability.

A home care nurse who focuses on rehabilitative/restorative nursing seizes this challenge, finds a way, coaches and supports, repeats and reinforces. The home care nurse sees the uniqueness of each elderly client and provides dignity and respect for their long journey on life's continuum.

6

MAINTAINING OPTIMUM NUTRITION AMONG ELDERLY CLIENTS AT HOME

Vilma Baltazar
Olivia Babol Ibe
Judith A. Allender

◆ ◆ ◆

The Importance of a Healthy Diet Among Elders
Accessibility of Food
Special Dietary Considerations
Adaptive Feeding Mechanisms
Summary

Dietary decisions impact health and functional capacity. Likewise, eating is a social activity. In fact, in the United States, most social gatherings focus on food. Whether people are happy or sad, celebrate or grieve, food is central in the get-together as emotions are expressed. People meet friends and family in restaurants, eat out as often as they cook meals at home, and most cannot see a movie without a bucket of popcorn and large soda. With such a cultural emphasis on food, it should be easy for the home health nurse to recognize the need to assess clients for the ability to eat and the adequacy of food and food storage and to make appropriate recommendations and referrals as needed.

This chapter focuses on promoting healthy dietary practices in the elderly home care population. By conducting a nutritional assessment of the elderly client, the home care nurse can determine the client's strengths and deficits, from which a care plan can be developed. This should lead to teaching healthy dietary changes that incorporate the client's budget, cultural differences, medical or surgical limitations, and interest in eating. Since home care nurses are privileged to enter the client's environment, they are in an ideal position to provide this valuable resource to clients, family members, and caregivers.

THE IMPORTANCE OF A HEALTHY DIET AMONG ELDERS

Eating properly at any age is important. However, elders generally consume fewer calories, so those calories should be of higher quality to ensure an adequate intake of nutrients. An adequate diet provides the body with nutrients to defend against disease, maintain structural normality, and provide the energy needed to engage in everyday activities of living.

Maintaining optimum nutrition is a continuous process and an important one. Any deviation from the normal nutritional intake can facilitate development of other health conditions. The home care nurse must help clients maximize their quality of life in the home care setting, especially their level of independence in eating and choosing their foods. The nurse must have nutritional information and resources to help clients and families broaden their knowledge on the different aspects of nutrition.

Frequently, clients have alterations in nutrition that were identified or incurred during hospitalization. With these clients, the nurse is aware that a focus of the caregiving involves dietary assessment, management, and modification as described in the referral and carried out in the plan of care. Other clients, however, may have diagnoses with which dietary concerns are not as obvious. Such diagnoses as stasis ulcers of the lower extremities, fractured hip or wrist, mastectomy, or hernia repair are not diagnoses where a nutritional assessment appears as being of primary importance. The information on healthy diets in this chapter is shared especially with those clients in mind, since their dietary needs may be seen as secondary to other health concerns.

BOX 6-1 • THE NUTRITIONAL ASSESSMENT

HISTORY

- Review health history and medical records for evidence of diagnoses or conditions that can alter the purchase, preparation, ingestion, digestion, absorption, or excretion of foods.
- Review medications for those that can affect appetite and nutritional state.
- Consider the client's description of diet, meal patterns, food preferences, cultural and religious influences on food choices, and dietary restrictions.

PHYSICAL EXAMINATION

- Inspect hair. Hair loss or brittleness can be associated with malnutrition.
- Inspect skin. Note persistent "goose bumps" (vitamin B_6 deficiency), pallor (anemia), purpura (vitamin C deficiency), brownish pigmentation (niacin deficiency), red scaly areas in folds around eyes and between nose and corner of mouth (riboflavin deficiency), dermatitis (zinc deficiency), or fungus infections (hyperglycemia).
- Test skin turgor. Skin turgor, although poor in many elders, tends to be best in the areas over the forehead and sternum; therefore, these are preferred areas to test.
- Note muscle tone, strength, and movement. Muscle weakness can be associated with vitamin and mineral deficiencies.
- Inspect eyes. Ask about changes in vision and night vision problems (vitamin A deficiency).

BIOCHEMICAL ASSESSMENT

- Obtain blood samples for screening of total iron binding capacity, transferrin saturation, protein, albumin, hemoglobin, hematocrit, electrolytes, vitamins, and prothrombin time.
- Obtain urine sample for screening of specific gravity.
- Inspect oral cavity. Note dryness (dehydration), lesions, condition of tongue, breath odor, and condition of teeth or dentures.
- Ask about signs and symptoms: sore tongue, indigestion, diarrhea, constipation, food distaste, weakness, muscle cramps, burning sensations, dizziness, drowsiness, bone pain, sore joints, recurrent boils, dyspnea, anorexia, and appetite changes.

COGNITION AND MOOD

- Test cognitive function.
- Note alterations in mood, behavior, cognition, and level of consciousness. Be alert to signs of depression (which can be associated with deficiencies of vitamin B_6, magnesium, or niacin).
- Ask about changes in mood or cognition.   *(continued)*

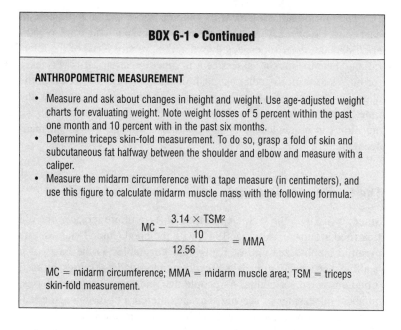

BOX 6-1 • Continued

ANTHROPOMETRIC MEASUREMENT

- Measure and ask about changes in height and weight. Use age-adjusted weight charts for evaluating weight. Note weight losses of 5 percent within the past one month and 10 percent with in the past six months.
- Determine triceps skin-fold measurement. To do so, grasp a fold of skin and subcutaneous fat halfway between the shoulder and elbow and measure with a caliper.
- Measure the midarm circumference with a tape measure (in centimeters), and use this figure to calculate midarm muscle mass with the following formula:

$$\frac{MC - \dfrac{3.14 \times TSM^2}{10}}{12.56} = MMA$$

MC = midarm circumference; MMA = midarm muscle area; TSM = triceps skin-fold measurement.

The Nutritional Assessment

A complete nutritional assessment has several components: a history, physical examination, biochemical evaluation, assessment of cognition and mood, and anthropometric measurement (see Box 6-1). The client history gives the home care nurse information about the client's perception of dietary practices, medications that affect appetite, and actual foods and amounts consumed during a typical week. Physical examination of skin, hair, eyes, and muscle tone give information about overall nutritional status. A biochemical evaluation is more invasive and may include obtaining blood and urine samples for screening. The home care nurse may see the need for such an evaluation and discuss the need with the client's primary care provider. The remaining parts of the biochemical assessment are inspecting the oral cavity and inquiring about untoward gastrointestinal signs and symptoms. Cognition and mood affect appetite and eating, so their assessment is vital. A final component is determining anthropometric measurements, such as height and weight, determining triceps skin-fold measurement, and measuring the midarm circumference. The home care nurse should keep a standard height and weight chart among the materials brought into the home during visits. Such charts can be gotten from life insurance companies.

The nutritional assessment is comprehensive and takes time, with data collected over several home visits. It is wise not to attempt to gather all data on one visit, especially when the primary focus of the referral may take the nursing assessment in other directions. It is very easy for nurses to want to gather as much data as possible to best assist the client. In the enthusiasm to be complete, the nurse may overlook the time this consumes and the burden it places on the client. In contrast, nutrition can be neglected as an important component of client management.

The Food Guide Pyramid

Since April 1992, the U.S. Department of Agriculture replaced the old four food groups, in use since 1946, with the Food Guide Pyramid. The pyramid emphasizes grains, fruits, and vegetables as the basis of a healthy diet (see Figure 6-1). Recommended daily servings in each group are noted for adults. As people age and require fewer calories, numbers of servings or serving sizes are altered. For instance, the recommended daily allowance (RDA) for calorie intake in a male adult aged 25 to 65 is 2,800 kcal. Among male elders aged 65 to 75, the RDA is reduced to 2,300 kcal, and for those over age 75, it is decreased to 2,050 kcal. The figures are about 600 to 800 kcal less at each age for females. A balanced diet with high-quality calories is still needed for all elders, but it becomes harder to get the nutrients in as the calories are reduced. Frequently, vitamin and mineral supplements are recommended to maintain the appropriate levels of important vitamins and minerals.

Seven guidelines developed by the U.S. Department of Agriculture and the Department of Health and Human Services can be shared with elderly clients. The home care nurse should include the following instructions when teaching clients:

1. Eat a variety of foods.
2. Maintain a healthy weight.
3. Choose a diet low in fat, especially saturated fat and cholesterol. (The American Heart Association recommends a diet with less than 30 percent of calories from fat.)
4. Choose a diet with calories primarily from the bottom of the Food Guide Pyramid (plenty of vegetables, fruits, and grain products).

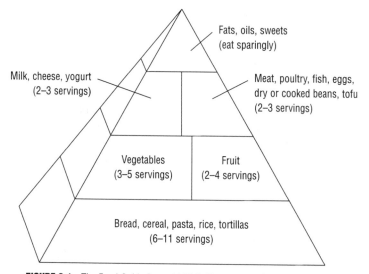

FIGURE 6-1 • The Food Guide Pyramid (U.S. Department of Agriculture, 1992).

5. Use sugar sparingly.
6. Use salt and sodium in moderation.
7. Drink alcoholic beverages in moderation.

Dietary Recommendations

The eating habits of older adults have taken a lifetime to develop and are not easily changed. This is important for the home care nurse to remember when making dietary recommendations on behalf of clients.

Mealtime is usually very important for the client. Elders may have a standard time for breakfast, lunch, and dinner; or drink coffee all day and eat just one meal late in the day; or nibble all day on cookies and candies, washed down with white wine. Eating three well-balanced meals a day may not be the norm for the client. Clients may eat in a pattern that served them well when they were working, caring for a family, and generally more active. Now they may neglect eating any nutritional foods. The following are helpful suggestions for the nurse to consider when making dietary recommendations:

• Remember this adage, "Eat like a king at breakfast, a prince at lunch, and a pauper at dinner." Namely, elders are better off if they eat a hearty, well-balanced breakfast, a moderate-sized midday meal, and have just a snack-sized meal at dinner. This way, they will have more energy earlier in the day and can digest food throughout the day, and indigestion will not disturb their night's rest.

- For some elders, "grazing" is a perfectly healthy way to eat. This consists of eating 5–7 small meals all day long. Here is what one 75-year-old "grazing" grandmother had to eat one day: 7:00 a.m.—a glass of orange juice and a piece of toast (while she reads the newspaper); 10:00 a.m.—a container of yogurt and a handful of raisins (while watching her favorite talk show); 1:00 p.m.—half of her 2-year-old granddaughter's McDonald's Happy Meal (her daughter and granddaughter visited); 4:00 p.m.—a banana and a piece of chocolate (while folding laundry); 7:00 p.m.—a bowl of vegetable soup and peanut butter on crackers (before settling in to watch evening television); 10:00 p.m.—a cup of warm milk and two cookies (warm milk always helps her sleep better). Her intake was perhaps not perfectly balanced, but it was nutritious and filling. The home care nurse critiquing this day's meal pattern might suggest whole grain crackers or breads, adding a salad with the soup, having low fat yogurt and milk products, and making sure water intake meets fluid needs.

- Incorporating fluid needs in dietary teaching includes reminding clients who have no fluid restrictions to consume eight eight-ounce glasses of fluids (other than milk) each day. This may need to be started gradually if the client is not used to drinking that much. Many elders restrict fluids thinking they won't have urinary accidents or frequent trips to the bathroom at night. This is where additional information about urinary health and toileting habits can be included (see Chapter 11 for more information).

- Food choices within the Food Guide Pyramid should reflect the client's food preferences and meet any dietary restrictions (medical, cultural, or religious).

- Style of food preparation only needs modification if it increases "empty" calorie intake, such as frying foods and using lard or oil. If individual eating habits do not affect the quality of the diet, they should be ignored. For example, an elderly client may eat all foods at room temperature, a habit developed when he had to feed his wife before she died and he got so used to eating his food cold that he prefers it this way now. Others may desire combinations of food that bring back memories of another time. Beans on pancakes, catsup on everything, or eating raw cookie dough may sound strange to some people but not to others.

- Eating as a social activity with family and friends should be respected and encouraged. Elderly clients benefit by having a friendly social atmosphere at mealtime. They may eat poorly if they eat alone. Holidays are more meaningful to clients when they can share in lifelong family traditions of cooking and eating favorite family foods. The home care nurse can encourage modification of some recipes so the client can enjoy desired food and not have to pass it up or eat it and have it affect comfort or health status.
- The religious practice and cultural background of the client may be the basis for food preferences. A knowledge of certain religious holidays and beliefs and religious or cultural dietary restrictions is beneficial to the home care nurse.
- The home care nurse should develop an individualized plan of care to meet a client's nutritional needs and have the client share views and preferences. The family and primary caregivers are also reliable sources in giving input about the client's dietary practices, and the home health nurse should involve them in the planning and implementation of care.

ACCESSIBILITY OF FOOD

The home care nurse who is new to home care may neglect to consider the accessibility of food. When clients are in inpatient settings, food is always available. This is not the case for many clients, especially elderly clients. Accessibility can be affected by many factors. Shopping and getting foods into the home takes money, transportation, physical endurance, and cognitive ability. The loss of any one of these will alter the availability of foods in the home.

Consider the case of one home health nurse who visited a client to fill insulin syringes for the client's use during the week. The nurse found milk in the refrigerator that had an expiration date of two months previous to the current date, no running hot water, spoiled meat in the refrigerator, sweet rolls on the counter, and no indoor toilet facilities. This type of information is important in determining if the client can safely remain in the home or if education and intervention can correct the situation.

Food Costs

Food and medication costs are of concern to elders on fixed incomes. Elders often try to manage their budget by skimping on food purchases and skipping medications. Housing costs remain fixed so adjustments there are impossible. This leaves food, medicines, and other necessities as costs they can control. Sadly, it is too frequently reported that an elder is found dead in a home because the heat was turned off to save on fuel costs. The home care nurse must make an assessment of resources to buy food and determine eligibility for programs to help seniors "stretch" their food dollars.

There are several programs that help clients reduce food costs. The Food Stamp Program is a federal program based on income and assets and is available to eligible people regardless of age. Commodities programs distribute surplus foods (such as cheese, peanut butter, and rice) to senior centers. Subsidized home meal delivery programs, such as Meals on Wheels, deliver hot foods daily at midday with a sandwich for evening or they bring frozen dinners weekly to clients with microwave ovens. Many of these programs ask for a suggested donation but will deliver meals whether the client pays or not.

Physical Accessibility

Clients who have become homebound because of health deterioration or a lack of transportation can benefit from a meal delivery program such as Meals on Wheels. In addition, the nurse can intervene by locating a grocery store (and pharmacy) that delivers and setting up a regular delivery service based on the client's food preferences and needs.

If the client is not able to leave the home and get food because of a decline in cognitive skills, a volunteer, friend, family member, or hired in-home assistant is needed in order for the client to remain at home safely. While the client is receiving skilled nursing services, a home

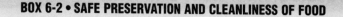

BOX 6-2 • SAFE PRESERVATION AND CLEANLINESS OF FOOD

BEFORE HANDLING FOOD

- Wash hands and all food preparation surfaces and utensils thoroughly with soap and water.

WHEN PREPARING FOOD

- Wash foods that are to be eaten raw and uncooked thoroughly in clean water. This includes foods that are to be peeled that grow in the ground or come in contact with soil.
- Cook all meat products thoroughly.
- Do not allow cooked meat and other food to come in contact with dishes, utensils, or containers that were used with the meat when it was raw and uncooked.

WHEN STORING LEFTOVER FOODS

- Cool cooked foods quickly; store under refrigeration in clean, covered containers.

WHEN REHEATING LEFTOVER FOODS

- Heat foods thoroughly. Bacteria that contaminate food grow and multiply in a temperature range between 39 and 140 degrees Fahrenheit.

Spradley, B. W., & Allender, J. A. Community health nursing: Concepts and practice. Philadelphia: Lippincott–Raven, 1996, p. 509.

---

health aide can visit daily and may help with food preparation for the client. Since this is a form of temporary assistance, it is the responsibility of the home care nurse to put into place a permanent solution to this ongoing problem for the client.

Food Safety

Another area of concern is the safe storage and preparation of foods. If the client is suffering from memory loss or a decline in visual acuity, safety at home in general is of concern, especially with stove top cooking and using the oven. In addition, the home care nurse needs to be familiar with the increased emphasis on food safety and the development of safety guidelines in order to share this information with clients. Some of the specific food safety concerns are listed in Box 6-2.

SPECIAL DIETARY CONSIDERATIONS

Not all elders can eat what they want, when they want, in the same way that they did when they were younger. Many older people have a poor dental history and eat foods that are more easily chewed. Others have difficulty with swallowing and tend to eat foods pureed or liquified. Some clients have specific dietary modifications based on medical or surgical conditions that require alterations in food types, amounts, or timing of when they are ingested. Common adaptive nursing, safety, and dietary considerations are shared here.

The Normal Swallow

A common problem that the elderly client may experience is a change in the ability to swallow. This, together with other age-related changes, causes clients to have a hard time ingesting adequate amounts of nutrients to maintain their weight and stay healthy. The home care nurse needs to be able to differentiate between a normal swallow and dysphagia. Information on dysphagia, especially common symptoms, should be discussed with elderly clients and their families. The home care nurse should be sensitive to these manifestations so that appropriate caregiving, including the initiation of a referral, can be implemented.

The normal swallow of an individual consists of three phases:

The oral phase consists of chewing food, mixing it with saliva, and moving the bolus of food backward toward the base of the tongue. This phase is under voluntary control of the 5th, 7th, and 12th cranial nerves.

The pharyngeal phase begins when the bolus of food reaches the base of the tongue. The swallow reflex is triggered, which involves the upward and forward movement of the larynx, the closure of the epiglottis, and the closure of the vocal cord to protect the airway. Pharyngeal peristalsis moves the bolus into the esophagus through the relaxed cricopharyngeal sphincter (upper esophageal sphincter). This phase is involuntary and is totally reflexive depending on the intact 9th, 10th, and 12th cranial nerves.

Finally, the esophageal phase begins with the lowering of the larynx and closing of the upper esophageal sphincter so that food will not be regurgitated into the respiratory system. Peristalsis moves the food down the esophagus through the lower esophageal sphincter into the stomach.

Dysphagia

The frail elderly are prone to dysphagia, an inability to swallow properly. The three phases of the normal swallow are interrupted, and the client's safety while eating is compromised. Examples of clients who are at risk are clients who cough when they eat or drink, hold food in their mouth for an extended time, have excessive drooling, or have frequent choking.

Common symptoms of dysphagia that require a swallow evaluation include: unexplained weight loss, the client refusing food, dehydration, accelerated breathing while eating, pocketing or holding food in the mouth, food residue in the mouth after swallowing, unexplained pneumonia, coughing out food after a swallow, spitting out food, drooling, decreased food intake, and discomfort while swallowing. When the swallow is altered, mechanical dietary modifications are needed to ensure client safety and adequate nutritional intake.

Nursing Management

If the home care nurse identifies a problem with swallowing or taking in food, the nurse needs to discuss the findings with the client's primary care provider because further evaluation may be needed. The nurse needs to make an individualized plan, based on the finding, that involves the client, family, and primary care provider. The first step is to have the client or family monitor the food and fluid intake for three days. They are asked to complete a very detailed three-day food and fluid intake list for the home care nurse. The list should include what the client eats and drinks and the exact amounts. The amount of food and fluid intake should be very specific: 25 percent of a piece of bread, two ounces of juice, and so on. The client's weight should be monitored closely; weigh the client at the same time of day on the same scale.

Types of Dietary Modifications Needed

The home care nurse needs to know how to assist the client and family in understanding how to prepare modified diets. Diets with modified consistencies are prepared because of a client's dental status, maxilla-facial problems, swallowing difficulties, or general weakness (too weak to chew and caloric intake is needed).

Mechanical soft diet. This diet is designed to minimize the amount of chewing necessary for the ingestion of food and is given in conjunction with a specific diet. Most foods are of a chopped consistency and used with client's who have dry mouth, ulceration of the mouth or gums, gastrointestinal disorders, missing teeth, ill-fitting dentures, oral surgery, or a broken jaw. Home care nursing responsibilities include:

1. Evaluating each client for appropriate size of chopped pieces of food for safety and adequate intake.
2. Assessing clients for ability to advance to their regular eating habits or regressing to need a pureed diet.
3. Instruction on adding small amounts of liquid (broth, gravy, or milk) to achieve appropriate consistency.
4. Instruction on proper positioning during eating (sitting at a 90-degree angle to prevent choking).

Pureed #1 soft diet. This is a diet wherein foods can be swallowed with no chewing involved. It is used with client conditions as in the mechanical soft diet. It can be used in conjunction with any type of diet. Home care nursing responsibilities include:

1. Evaluating each client for the appropriate soft or pureed consistency (for a thinner or thicker consistency).
2. Assessing those who may aspirate liquids and recommending the use of a commercial product such as Thickit.
3. Monitoring bowel function. As soft or pureed diets lack fiber, supplements with fiber can be included.
4. Giving oral supplements to assure adequate nutrition.
5. Instruction on adding small amounts of liquid (broth, gravy, or milk) to achieve appropriate consistency.
6. Reinforcing safety; the client needs to sit at a 90-degree angle to prevent choking.

Pureed #2 soft diet. This is a diet for clients with dysphagia who need a pureed consistency that is thinner than the regular pureed #1 consistency. This can be used in conjunction with a specific diet. Home care nursing responsibilities include:

1. Making sure a swallowing evaluation has been done.
2. Checking the client's gag reflex.
3. Recommending oral supplements to ensure adequate nutrition.
4. Monitoring bowel function as this diet lacks fiber.
5. Instruction on proper positioning during eating (90-degree angle to prevent choking).

Regular no-concentrated sweets diet. This is a diet that places the client on an unmeasured or free diet, restricting only sugar and foods high in concentrated sweets. This diet represents a liberal approach for the treatment of diabetes (see Chapter 15 for more information on diabetes), and it can be adapted to other diets. Home care nursing responsibilities include:

1. Checking with the client to ensure that sugar and foods high in concentrated sweets are not included in the diet. Ask to take a look at the client's kitchen. Are cookies, sweet rolls, and the like on the counter? Is ice cream in the freezer? Are chips and snack foods out? The client may not understand what foods to avoid.
2. Checking the clients blood glucose level if indicated.
3. Monitoring the client's weight.

Foods to avoid on a regular no-concentrated sweets diet include canned, frozen, or dried fruit to which sugar has been added; sweetened fruit juice; any processed or prepared meat, fish, or poultry to which sugar has been added; candied sweet potatoes; all candies and other sweets made with sugar, jelly, honey, and syrup.

Diagnosis-Specific Dietary Changes

In this section, dietary changes are discussed based on specific medical diagnoses commonly seen among elderly home health clients. Clients should become familiar with the new nutrition labels on all foods made in the United States. They give information about nutrients in the product, including calories, fiber, and fat grams, all based on a standard portion size noted on the label.

Caloric restricted diet. This diet puts emphasis on the total calories rather than the components of carbohydrates, protein, and fat (e.g., a 1,200 calorie diet). Such a diet is indicated for weight reduction, weight maintenance, and in diabetes. The home care nurse's responsibilities include:

1. Monitoring the client's blood glucose level.
2. Monitoring the client's dietary adherence.
3. Monitoring the client's weight.
4. Teaching the client, family, or caregivers to recognize signs of hypo- or hyperglycemia.

Sodium restricted diet. this is a normal diet that restricts the sodium intake to a certain specific level. With this diet, foods are always prepared without added salt. This diet is indicated for clients with hypertension, impaired liver function, cardiovascular disease, renal disease or chronic failure, edema, or ascites. The home care nurse's responsibilities include:

1. Monitoring the client for any edema.
2. Identifying foods the client prefers that are high in natural sodium content and should be used in limited quantities.
3. Instructing the client in the use of a salt substitute.
4. Monitoring the client's blood pressure and weight.
5. Instructing on the client's use of ordered medications, such as diuretics and potassium supplements.

Foods to avoid on a sodium restricted diet include commercial salad dressings, canned vegetables, cold cuts, herring, smoked fish, salted cheese, regular canned tuna or salmon, potato chips, salted popcorn, pretzels, corn chips, bouillon, commercially prepared soups, catsup, olives, Worcestershire sauce, meat tenderizers, salted nuts, and prepared mustard.

Fat restricted diet. This diet has no more than 40–45 grams of fat and is not modified in the ratio of saturated to polyunsaturated fat. It is used for clients who have diseases of the liver or gallbladder or disturbances of digestion and absorption, and for clients who are following the American Heart Association recommendations regarding fat restriction or who want to decrease their intake of fats. The home care nurse's responsibilities include:

1. Assisting a client's adherence to the specific diet.
2. Suggesting ways to modify favorite foods to obtain a lower fat content.

Foods to avoid include all foods made with cream or eggs, ice cream, chocolate milk, whole milk, evaporated milk, buttered popcorn, quick breads, muffins, biscuits, popovers, snack crackers, sweet rolls, doughnuts, griddle cakes, waffles, commercial stuffing, french toast, granola-type cereals made with fat, coconut, nuts, and whole milk yogurt. Today there are many products on grocery shelves that say "low in fat" or "fat free." Consumers must be enlightened shoppers to know what they are really getting when these words are used on packaging. To be sure, fat free products are the best to buy. If there are less than three grams of fat in one serving of a product, it should fit into a diet low in fat.

Renal diet. This is a diet for clients whose kidneys have limited function. This diet provides controlled amounts of protein, sodium, and potassium. A fluid restriction may also be indicated. This type of diet is indicated in acute renal failure, proteolysis (hemodialysis or peritoneal), or a kidney transplant. The home care nurse's responsibilities include:

1. Collaborating with primary care provider or dietician for safe home management of the renal client, especially in regards to diet. The client should have printed material indicating the number of servings of food groups and fluids allowed. These instructions may need to be interpreted or reinforced by the home care nurse.
2. Monitoring dietary compliance. Instruct the client to use a scale to weigh meat if protein is severely restricted.
3. Monitoring intake and output, blood pressure, and weight. Instruct the client to use measuring devices to measure fluids.
4. Assessing for early signs and symptoms of complications.

High protein, high caloric diet. This diet is high in protein and high in calories. It is indicated in hyperthyroidism, metabolic increase colitis, decubitus healing, wound healing, AIDS, cancer, and in the prevention of skin breakdown. The home care nurse's responsibilities include:

1. Monitoring the client's intake of calories and protein.
2. Teaching clients and family members (especially the primary shopper and cook for the client) that an increased caloric diet is utilized to meet the increased metabolic needs of the body.

There is usually an increase in protein and vitamins when increased calories are needed.

3. Encouraging the client to eat high protein foods such as fish, fowl, meat, and dairy products, since a high protein diet is necessary for tissue building.

As a note, it is important to keep fat grams under control when loading a client with extra protein and calories. The fat in foods will make the client feel full and will limit the amount of other foods the client should eat, so lean meats and low fat dairy products are best. Adding dry nonfat milk to soups or evaporated skim milk to beverages adds calories and protein without added fat. Occasionally, a client is so cachectic that any foods the client will tolerate are encouraged; this is not a time to count fat grams.

ADAPTIVE FEEDING MECHANISMS

Because of illness or injury, some clients have difficulty feeding themselves independently and need to have an adaptive environment in order to ingest an adequate amount of nutrients. These mechanisms include positioning, mechanical food changes (mentioned earlier), and adaptive devices designed to administer nutrients passively to medically debilitated clients. Even the totally dependent client can be nutritionally managed at home with an informed and educated caregiver. Active feeding assistance includes physical assistive devices that help the client or caregiver with oral ingestion of foods specifically prepared for the client. Passive feeding assistance includes enteral and parenteral feeding mechanisms.

The following are two common examples of nursing responsibilities for clients who need active feeding assistance. For clients with a cerebrovascular accident (CVA), the home care nurse can best be of assistance by:

1. Encouraging self-feeding with assistive devices as needed.
2. Instructing client/family to place food in the unaffected side of the client's mouth.
3. Ensuring that the client sits at a 90-degree angle when eating.

For clients with Parkinson's disease, the home care nurse can best be of assistance by:

1. Encouraging self-feeding as much as possible, using assistive devices.
2. Encouraging rhythmic patterns to attain timing and allow rest periods for the client.
3. Ensuring that the client sits at a 90-degree angle when eating.

Adaptive Devices

The use of adaptive feeding devices are considered for clients whose loss of body function affects specific parts of the body involved with the eating process, such as the hands, wrists, or arms. Equipment usually can be changed or made to meet a person's needs.

The home care nurse needs to know the proper referral and follow-through for clients needing an evaluation for an adaptive device. Collaboration with the primary care provider, occupational therapist, client, family, caregivers, and other appropriate others is essential. In other instances, clients may already have been given an adaptive device when they were admitted to the hospital or nursing home for short-term rehabilitation, or clients may come home from the acute care setting with the device.

Eating utensils that are commonly used for clients with special needs include:

1. Cuffed fork, which fits over the client's hand.
2. Rounded plate that helps keep food on the plate.
3. Special plate grips and swivel handles.
4. Glass or cup holders for clients who have difficulty grasping.
5. Plate guards to help stabilize the plate, keeping food in place.
6. Knives with rounded blades, which are rocked back and forth to cut food.

The home care nurse needs to respect the client's frustration, and at times discouragement, at trying to eat independently while using assistive devices. The nurse should be sensitive enough to understand that the progress may be slow or some efforts unsuccessful. Empathy also needs to be conveyed to the primary caregivers (who are with the client up to 24 hours a day).

A demonstration and return demonstration of storage, care, and use of devices are good teaching techniques to use with caregivers as they develop strategies to work with the client and assistive devices. The home care nurse needs to ensure proper application of the adaptive device and that the adaptive device is used as instructed. The client's progress on the use of the device is coordinated with the occupational therapist. Successful use of the device may be documented by regular client weights, if maintaining or gaining weight is a client goal. A reevaluation of the adaptive feeding device should be done as indicated. If a client is not productive in using a particular device, a reassessment is indicated.

Enteral Feedings

A client who has a functioning GI tract but who is not able to orally ingest enough nutrients to meet nutritional needs is a candidate for tube feeding. The client may have chewing or swallowing problems, have poor food and fluid intake, be in a coma or semicomatose state, or have very high nutrient requirements.

Enteral feedings, via gastrostomy tube or nasogastric tube, are administered to a client after a complete medical and GI evaluation. Balanced liquified feedings are administered at room temperature through a tube inserted into the stomach or duodenum via gastrostomy tube or nasogastric tube to meet the nutritional needs of the client.

The nurse needs to evaluate clients for enteral feedings, especially those clients who are unable to take adequate nutrition orally. The nurse should assess the overall client nutritional status, including:

1. Evaluating oral intake—adequate, moderate, or altered.
2. Assessing nutritional requirements—are they being met?
3. Assessing the status of the GI tract—is it functional?
4. Assessing the client's capacity to swallow.
5. Checking for presence of a gag reflex.
6. Evaluating the client's respiratory condition.
7. Checking for renal complications.
8. Checking for vomiting and diarrhea.

After the assessment process, the home care nurse needs to discuss the findings with the client, family, and primary care provider. It may be the client's wish not to have life prolonged through the use of artificial nutritional supplements. If the client has completed advance directives, the client's wishes must be considered at this time. The primary care provider needs to discuss possible options with the client and family.

If the client chooses to have enteral feedings, the primary care provider orders them after all alternatives have been considered. In most

BOX 6-3 • TEACHING GUIDELINES FOR NASOGASTRIC TUBE FEEDINGS

1. Wash hands before and after handling instruments.

2. Keep all equipment in one place. Wash all reusable equipment in warm, soapy water.

3. Keep these orders and instructions within view:
   - The amount of water to be given before and after.
   - The amount and type of feeding to be given, with the specific time schedules.
   - Instructions for giving medications. Make sure instructions are followed and that medications are finely crushed to avoid blockage.

4. Care of the mouth:
   - Clean the mouth with water (especially if lips are dry).
   - Apply mouthwash and use a cotton swab to clean area around mouth if client is unable to do oral care.
   - Brush the teeth, gums, and tongue at least twice a day with a regular toothbrush and toothpaste.

5. Care of the nose (nasogastric or nasointestinal):
   - Gently clean inside the nostrils with a cotton swab moistened with warm water.
   - Check that nostrils are patent.
   - Clean the edges of both nostrils daily.
   - Use a water soluble lubricant on the nostril edges.
   - Check for signs of redness, bleeding, or numbness in nose.

6. Taping the tube:
   - Change the tape holding the tube.
   - Make sure tape has been cut and is ready prior to changing.
   - Remove the tape slowly from nostrils while holding the tube securely in place.
   - Clean the area with soap and warm water.
   - If taping the tube to the cheek, do not allow the tube to kink.
   - Do not allow the tube to obstruct the nose.
   - The tube should not pull or rub the side of the nose or mouth.
   - Make sure the tape holds the tube securely.
   - Rotate site where the tube is taped on the skin.
   - If taping tube to the nose:
     — Cut a tape about three inches long.
     — Cut the piece of tape halfway down the center.
     — Place the wide part over the bridge of the nose.
     — Wrap the two thinner pieces around the tube.
     — Be careful that the tube does not rub against the side of the nose.

BOX 6-4 • DRESSING A GASTROSTOMY SITE

PREPARATION

Note: Wash hands before changing the dressing, wear gloves, and wash hands after changing the dressing!

- Place client in a supine position.
- Gently remove the old dressing.
- Clean the area around the site with water to eliminate any discharge or drainage.
- Inspect for evidence of leakage or infection, such as erythema, purulent drainage, edema, or tenderness.
- Use cotton-tipped applicators or 4 × 4 gauze to wash the surrounding skin with soap and warm water. Start from the insertion site of the stoma and work out using a rotary motion. Rinse with water.
- Clean encrusted secretions from the tube with a cotton-tipped applicator
- Rinse site with 4 × 4 gauze and warm water. Pat dry.
- Apply a skin protectant as ordered by the primary care provider.
- Apply 4 × 4 gauze, slit to center, around the feeding tube.

EQUIPMENT

- Irrigation set/syringe.
- Prefilled container and tubing.
- Prescribed formula.
- Stethoscope.

- Emesis basin.
- Tap water
- Infusion pump.
- IV pole.

(continued)

---

cases, the home care nurse is the liaison between the primary care provider and family members in discussing the need for enteral feeding. The primary care provider has to order enteral feeding that will provide the client with nutrients to sustain a normal diet and fluid and electrolyte balance. Four areas that should be considered when choosing a tube feeding formula are digestive and absorptive function, placement of the tube, nutrient requirements, and individual tolerances and allergies.

Clients who need tube feeding often have not been eating for a period of time and may have a difficult time tolerating a large volume of concentrated nutrients. When a tube feeding is first started, water may be added to the formula to dilute it to one-third or one-half strength at a slow rate. The need to dilute the formula is eliminated if isotonic feedings are used.

BOX 6-4 • Continued

PROCEDURE

- Wash hands.
- Use measuring cup to measure the amount of formula needed. Keep unused formula in the refrigerator.
- If using a prepared formula, turn container upside down and shake vigorously.
- Measure tap water and pour into container.
- Gather all equipment and follow the directions for feeding administration and pump, if used.
- Check for patency and position:
  — Insert the tip of the syringe into the feeding tube.
  — Open the clamp on the feeding tube.
  — Place stethoscope over the stomach area with earpiece in your ear. Inject 10–20 cc air and listen for a whooshing sound.
  — Repeat the above steps if you do not hear a whooshing sound.
  — If you still do not hear the sound, *do not* give the feeding. Call the primary care provider.
- Aspirating stomach content also confirms that the tube is patent and properly positioned:
  — Attach syringe to feeding tube.
  — Draw back the syringe plunger to withdraw stomach contents (called gastric residual).
  — Read the amount of gastric residual.
  — Gently push the contents back into the stomach with the syringe.
  — It may be necessary to call the client's primary care provider if the gastric residual is greater than a predetermined number of milliliters.

There are two ways that a client is fed via the GI system. The first option is with a nasogastric tube, where the tube is introduced through the right or left nares, through the esophagus, and into the stomach. The other option is with the creation of a gastrostomy. An opening (ostomy) is surgically created in the stomach (gastro). This feeding method is indicated when food cannot pass normally from the mouth to the esophagus and into the stomach.

Once the preferred formula is ordered and equipment delivered to the client's home, the client and family must be taught how to administer the feedings safely (see Box 6-3 for guidelines).

If the client has a gastrostomy tube for enteral feedings, the guidelines include additional considerations. A dressing is usually in place over the site where the gastrostomy tube enters the stomach. See Box 6-4 for

BOX 6-5 • NASOGASTRIC AND GASTROSTOMY FEEDING METHODS

ONE DOSE OR INTERMITTENT FEEDING (Using a Syringe)

- Pinch proximal end of feeding tube.
- Attach syringe to the end of the tube and elevate 18 inches above the client's head.
- Fill syringe to empty gradually, refilling until prescribed amount has been delivered to the client.
- If gavage bag is used, attach the bag to the feeding tube and raise bag 18 inches above client's head. Fill bag with prescribed amount of the formula, allow bag to empty gradually over 30 minutes. When all of the formula has been given, pour the tap water into the syringe. When water has been flushed through, close clamp and detach syringe.

CONTINUOUS DRIP METHOD (Manual or Using a Pump)

- Hang feeding bag to IV pole or a wall hook about 2 feet above the head of a standing person.
- Squeeze the drip chamber until it is about one-third to one-half full of formula.
- Open the flow regulator clamp and fill the tube with formula, then close the clamp.
- Attach the tip of the tube to the feeding tube.
- For gravity drip feeding, open the flow regulator clamp and adjust the flow rate. The formula should run freely.
- In feedings administered by a pump, follow the manufacturer's instructions for setting the flow rate.
- When all of the formula has been given, close the flow regulator clamp. Close the clamp before the drip chamber is empty. If a pump is being used, turn it off.
- Observe the client during and after feedings for any problems that may result from feeding, such as reflux, nausea, diarrhea, and abdominal cramping.
- Pour the premeasured tap water into the container. Open the clamp (remove the tube from the pump if one is being used for this phase of the feeding).
- When the water has run in, close the clamp.
- Clamp the feeding tube and detach the administration set from the feeding tube.

additional guidelines in the care of the gastrostomy site, equipment needed, and preparing the equipment.

When teaching the client and caregivers about administering feedings, note that there are positioning guidelines for client comfort and safety that need to be followed. The client needs to sit upright during the feeding and for 30 to 60 minutes after the feeding. Positioning clients in a high- or semi-Fowler's position prevents the possibility of gastric reflux and aspiration. With bed-bound semicomatose or comatose clients, this is best accomplished by using an electric hospital bed to raise the client to a sitting position. Do not have the client lie flat, as this may cause nausea and vomiting.

There are two ways to feed clients through nasogastric or gastrostomy tubes and these methods are outlined in Box 6-5: the one dose or intermittent feeding method (where a syringe is used) and the continuous drip method (often using a pump).

SUMMARY

Healthy older adults are not much different than the rest of the healthy adult population, especially when it comes to nutrition. All people have specific nutritional needs that must be met in order to remain at or regain a healthy state. However, some elders have special nutritional needs because of chronic illness or damage to the body. Some effects of illness or injury alters what the client can eat, how the client eats, or the client's ability to eat independently.

This chapter focused on three aspects of maintaining nutrition in elders. The first focused on meeting the nutritional needs of the elder who has no dietary restrictions. Ways to assess nutritional status and introduce principles of nutrition using the Food Guide Pyramid were presented. The second part outlined common diets used with clients who have chronic illnesses. The types of modifications needed were outlined. The final section focused on assistive devices used when clients cannot meet dietary needs independently. Active assistive devices help clients with self-feeding. Passive assistive devices are used when clients are unable to chew and swallow on their own. Guidelines for safe administration of nasogastric and gastrostomy tube feedings complete the chapter, covering the possible nutritional issues that the home health nurse encounters.

7

ENHANCING INTIMACY AND SEXUAL HEALTH

Mary Ellen McCann

◆ ◆ ◆

We must learn not to ignore the disquieting sexual aspects of a patient's humanity, nor should we overtly or covertly stigmatize him or her. We are healthcare providers, not theologians, law enforcement officers, or moralists. We cannot be committed to total patient care without considering the patient as a sexual being.

Marianne Zalar, RN

Intimacy and sexuality are important aspects of one's overall well-being. Nursing professionals are intellectually aware of this, yet, when it comes to caring for clients, especially the elderly, nurses can easily focus on the referral, home safety, and medications. Enhancement of the client's sexual health is not often addressed. Perhaps this is because the nurse is inexperienced and uncomfortable with discussing the subject. If this is true, this chapter gives home care nurses the needed knowledge and confidence to discuss this important subject with their clients.

DEFINITION OF SEXUALITY

Sexuality is integral to both person and personality in all age groups, yet it is overlooked or avoided by nurses during nursing assessment and interaction, especially with the elderly. A holistic view of sexuality focuses on human qualities and intimate feelings and does not reduce sexuality solely to genital contact and function. It includes all the biological, psychological, emotional, social, cultural, and spiritual qualities that make a person who she or he is. Sexuality incorporates masculine and feminine traits into a self-concept, which is enhanced in the elderly client by the wisdom of a long life. A person is a sexual being from birth—and maybe before—until death, and perhaps beyond it (McCann, 1989).

Webster's Ninth New Collegiate Dictionary (1990) defines sexuality mechanistically as the quality of being sexual, the condition of having sex, sexual activity, and expression of sexual receptivity or interest, *especially when excessive* (author's italics). The World Health Organization (WHO) views sexual health as the integration of the somatic, emotional, intellectual, and social traits in ways that are enriching to personality, communication, and love, which corresponds to nursing philosophy.

SEXUALITY SELF-ASSESSMENT

Sexuality is more than what kind of sexual activity a person chooses. Sexuality is a life force, a way to express self and emotion to the world that affects mood, health, wellness, and intimacy. Sexuality and intimacy can be a look, a glance, a touch, desire, sharing of thoughts and feelings, or any manifestation of warmth and love. Sexual life experience ranges from celibacy (living without sexual activity), to masturbation (experience with oneself), to activity with one partner or more at a different or the same time; whereas sexual preference may be heterosexual (with a partner of the other sex), homosexual (with a partner of the same sex), or bisexual (with a partner of either sex). A basic rule in nursing assessment of sexuality in home care is for the nurse to let go of any preconceptions about what a client chooses sexually. This is particularly true with the elderly, whom too many view unfairly as asexual.

A nurse gives permission for free-flowing discussion of sexuality by assuming that everyone does everything (Fontaine, 1991). Everyone, including nurses and clients, has preconceptions, values, and biases about sexuality. No one is value free, but an important first step for nurses in self-assessment is to view themselves as sexual beings (Poorman, 1987). A nurse must first reach a healthy attitude toward his or her own sexuality. Such self-understanding helps nurses to develop an atmosphere of acceptance and respect for the sexual beliefs and practices of older adults (Burke & Walsh, 1997).

WAYS TO ADDRESS SEXUALITY

The best principle for any nurse to enact when discussing sexuality is to be as real as possible. Authenticity promotes ease of communication and connection with a client of any age, but a sense of connection is particularly soothing to the elderly. Being authentic or real takes practice and usually involves trial and error. Humor is a powerful icebreaker and eases discussion of any topic that is potentially embarrassing, as long as the humor is well chosen. Any humor that shows ambivalence about sexual activity in the elderly is not the wisest choice, but laughter or joking about any anxiety or uneasiness felt by the nurse or client may lessen the tension.

The renowned geriatrician Robert Butler and his associate Myrna Lewis (1976) have long recognized the importance of sexuality as a life force in the elderly, and they, along with others, provide some helpful views for the home care nurse:

- Sex is one of the great free and renewable pleasures of life.
- Sexual play can generate pleasure, exhilaration, release of tension, a sense of well-being, and provide mild exercise benefits.
- There is little reason for the elderly to abstain from sex, except by choice or circumstance, and many reasons to engage in it.

- Aging does not exclude growing wise sexually, nor does it destroy sexual desire.
- There is no known age limit to sexual activity, and there is nothing in the biology of aging that automatically shuts down sexual function (Burke & Walsh, 1997).
- Age is not a barrier to satisfying expression of sexuality and fulfillment of sexual needs.
- The best predictor of sexual activity and interest in old age is sexual activity and interest at a younger age (Burke & Walsh, 1997).
- Loss of sexuality is not an inevitable aspect of aging, and the majority of healthy people remain sexually active on a regular basis until advanced old age (Kaplan, 1990).
- The primary reason given for cessation of sexual intercourse in older adults is the physical illness of one or both partners, or the unavailability of any partner.
- Depression may be a cause of lessened sexual interest, as well as a consequence (Burke & Walsh, 1997).

Johnson (1996) studied a community-based sample of 69 men and 92 women who were over the age of 55, living independently in the community, and able to read and write English. She found that:

- Women are more interested, active, and satisfied with relational and nongenital activities.
- Men are more responsive visually to stimuli and are more interested, active, and satisfied with genital sexual behaviors.
- Men and women have similar scores for the activities of sitting and holding hands, having a sexual conversation, and hugging and kissing.
- Men and women have lower interest in masturbation and oral sex.

These are important findings for home care nurses to apply when assessing any elderly client because it is estimated that 75 percent of nursing practice involves therapeutic relationships with people over the age of 65, both individuals and couples (Johnson, 1996). Because Johnson's sample is community-based, the research alerts home care nurses to what they may expect to hear about sexual desires in the elderly. It is helpful to be prepared with specific information for ready response; forewarned is forearmed.

Sexuality is expressed in hairstyle, makeup, moustache, beard, dress, hopes, dreams, fantasies, writing, art, music, and within all relationships. Intimacy fulfills needs of love and belonging and can be expressed by emotional or physical means (Needham, 1993). Nurses can use personal photographs to discuss significant relationships in the life of the elderly client. This may create a natural progression to talk about preserving intimate relationships and sexuality.

WHAT TO DO WHEN EMBARRASSMENT OCCURS

It is all right to be embarrassed, as long as there is no pretense about it. Embarrassment occurs as a natural consequence of sexual health assessment. Home care nurses are in a unique position to address sexuality because such discussion frees older clients to talk about intimate realities of their life, regardless of whether they are sexually active. Home care nurses can use the familiar and known environment of the home to advantage, because it is likely to be the most comfortable space for private talk.

Trust is built on authenticity of response, which means that words match feelings. Home care nurses do not have to be sexual experts, but they do need to be open-minded about whatever a client entrusts them to hear. It is natural to be embarrassed, uneasy, or anxious at times about what a client reveals, as long as the nurse manifests a nonverbal response that corresponds to the emotion. A client is less likely to trust a nurse who smiles when there are nonverbal indicators of uneasiness.

Openings to discussion of sexuality can take many forms, direct and indirect. An elderly woman may reminisce about her childbirth experiences, what it was like to go through menopause, or how difficult it is to be alone. A woman might also talk about her sexuality if she has just experienced a mastectomy, hysterectomy, or colostomy, or if she is infected with HIV. A man may discuss his sexuality in relation to any prostate or urinary changes, after coronary artery bypass graft or after a heart attack, or if he notices change in erectile function that he suspects is related to illness such as diabetes or a medication side effect. There is overlay of some clinical implications for either sex.

The nurse can use the aforementioned cues for smoother entry to sexual topics. Nurses are often daunted at the prospect of broaching the topic of sexuality. This is a common, real, authentic, and human response, since many people perceive it as embarrassing and intrusive, even unmentionable. There is a misconception within nursing that nurses must "know it all." What is important is that home care nurses know available resources, maintain confidence in what knowledge they have, and have a realistic view of their limitations (Poorman, 1987).

Home care nurses routinely encounter intimate, joyous occasions such as recovery and progression of activity, and at other times witness the sad, physical and emotional intimacies of loss, death, grief, nakedness, bodily invasion, excretion, and elimination. Seeing sexuality as a similar entity can ease a nurse's comfort in assessing it. It may reassure the home care nurse to keep in mind that the client may experience embarrassment equal to or surpassing that of the nurse during sexual discussion. Such moments of humanity provide a means to connect and to enhance trust in the client-nurse relationship.

HOW TO PROMOTE INTIMACY

Loneliness and social isolation are a common reality among the elderly, a dismal consequence of loss, and a mirror of societal attitudes. Home care nurses create connections to alleviate isolation by developing a sense of therapeutic trust and appropriate touching in their interactions with clients. Sometimes, the nurse is the sole contact an elderly client has with the outside world. Touch promotes intimacy and conveys comfort, reassurance, support, and consolation (Fontaine, 1991). Nurses can help the elderly relearn or reactivate vital sensual pleasure.

Older adults may cling to possessions and memories to keep loved ones alive to preserve a sense of security and connection. This can overcome the shadow of loss and nearness of death. Friends, spouses, lovers, acquaintances, and children move away or die. Reminiscence and dialogue about memories of pleasurable times keep the elderly grounded in reality and create powerful bonds within the therapeutic relationship. Reminiscence is especially therapeutic for demented or confused elderly. It is comforting to competent elders, as well as for those who prefer to live in nostalgia for what they see as the "rose-colored," seemingly more desirable past. The story telling in reminiscence is also therapeutic and revelatory. Stories provide much information about the lived experience of any individual, and even more so with the elderly.

Nursing the older adult means recognizing who that person was, is, and hopes to be and preserving a sense of belonging. Intimacy, whether interpersonal or sexual, is a universal need, and the nurse can help the elderly person to discover or renew its joys.

Common barriers to joyful intimacy are monotony of a repetitious, staid, rigid sexual interaction; mental, emotional, or physical fatigue; breathlessness; overindulgence in food or drink; physical or emotional infirmity; generalized anxiety or fear; and performance anxiety. Butler (1976) recommends that the elderly try a warm bath or shower, exchange massage, turn the lights low, or listen to music to unwind. The home care nurse can give specific suggestions about these sensual modes of intimacy, as well as help the elderly experience the calm of meditation; the sensuality of massage; the relaxation of deep breathing, visualization, and yoga; and the invigorating effects of exercise, activity, and good nutrition. Each cultivates a healthy sense of self, intimacy, and sexuality. (Box 7-1 provides an example of an exercise to help the elderly learn creative visualization for coping with stress or for enhancing sexual fantasy.)

WHAT TERMS TO USE

One way to get comfortable with addressing sexual topics is to include sexual history questions in each nursing assessment. This becomes routine and less threatening with practice. Getting comfortable with asking about or discussing a particular sexual behavior or choice does not require or indicate approval of it (Beresford, 1988). There is no need to change beliefs and attitudes, but it is necessary to suspend them to spare the client any overt or covert judgment. Judgment damages intimacy and deadens dialogue. It is helpful for nurses in home care to analyze what inhibits their competence or comfort with sexual counseling, since nurses usually reach a comfort level when faced with other physical and emotional intrusions inherent in nursing practice. Nurses often cope with or avoid sexuality assessment by clinging to the prevalent perception that a client is asexual, a label that is too often attached to the elderly and the infirmed. This undermines the therapeutic relationship because it is based on a false premise. Use of terms such as "usual," "common," and "typical" are less threatening than "normal." "Normal" implies judgment, as if there is a standard to meet. It is advisable to assume engagement in sexual activity be-

BOX 7-1 • SAMPLE VISUALIZATION EXERCISE I

- Close your eyes.
- Take a few deep breaths.
- Imagine yourself in your favorite hideaway.
- You feel very relaxed in this place.
- See yourself in your chosen place of privacy, calm, and comfort.
- Imagine yourself alone or with a partner, whichever you prefer.
- Enjoy the comfort your special place gives you.
- You want to give and receive pleasure.
- Feel the delight of sensual touch.
- Enjoy an imaginary massage, or begin to massage yourself.
- Revel in the fantasy of the erotic joy of whatever sensual or sexual pleasure you desire, whether you see yourself alone or with a partner.
- Connect with your loving feelings.
- Let your imagination help you feel pleasure.
- Let go of any pressure to perform.
- Inhale the pleasant and earthy aromas within your special place.
- Hear your favorite music.
- Allow yourself as much time as you want to spend in this reverie or fantasy.
- Feel capable and powerful.
- Let your capacity for sexual intimacy feel limitless.
- Take a few more deep breaths whenever you feel ready.
- Remember that you can try this sensual and sexual escape whenever you want.
- Open your eyes, whenever you feel ready.

cause it generally frees an elderly client to tell the truth and give a complete reply.

An aware nurse listens for the sexual terms used by the elderly so that the dialogue stays at their comfort level and in their language, whether delicately formal or shocking street slang. The home care nurse should clarify meaning; for instance: "When you say make love I assume you mean sexual intercourse. Am I understanding you correctly?" Such confirmation is important to effective assessment, because without checking, the nurse could later find out that the older adult equates making love with cuddling. Similarly, if an elderly client uses a term that induces embarrassment, awkwardness, or uneasiness in the nurse, the nurse can respond, "When you use that word, I hear 'sexual intercourse,' and I feel more comfortable saying that [Beresford, 1988]." This relieves any discomfort the nurse feels without tainting the relationship with judgment.

QUESTIONS TO INCLUDE IN A SEXUAL ASSESSMENT

Progress in the realm of nursing and sexual health is often incremental because it is still a relatively uncharted area, despite the alleged sexual revolution. Nurses in home care can develop and incorporate questions about sexuality into a nursing history. This can be tried bit by bit, and as the nurse's comfort grows, the nursing assessment will become more comprehensive and complete. Trust and privacy elicit more information about personal and intimate experience than any number of questions. Nurses in home care should start with the least sensitive and move toward more sensitive topics when taking a sexual history. A broad question about relationships and significant others is safer than starting with more threatening topics, such as erectile function or vaginal lubrication (Johnson, 1995).

Certain questions create a sense of permission and openness to nurture intimate exchange of information. Open-ended questions allow elderly clients to answer in any way they choose. These questions do not set up an expectation of a correct answer, and they free the interaction from any sense of judgment about what might be labeled as right or wrong. There is an intimacy to this approach, which avoids the "yes" or "no" responses usually elicited predictably by a closed-question format. Open questions and comments have a number of other potential benefits. Openness develops the nurse-client relationship and allows for many possibilities of answers. These unpredictable and unexpected responses make the relationship more authentic. Examples of open-ended questions or statements that can be used by the nurse are:

- What intimate or close relationships do you have?
- What do you do to nurture these relationships?
- How do you keep intimacy or closeness alive in your life?
- What problems or obstacles are there to intimacy?
- How do you think you contribute to any problems?
- What do you think you can do to enhance or renew intimacy?
- What has worked for you in the past?
- What is (was) your illness like for you?
- Can you tell me what changes it causes (caused) in your life?
- How do you think I can best help you?

The nurse can help elderly clients learn to use similar questions to safeguard intimacy within their personal network. They can be eye and ear openers if asked within the family unit, or between person and partner, friend, or significant other.

The home care nurse assesses a client based on a comprehensive health history, which includes capability with activities of daily living and any physical or emotional obstacles to sensual and sexual health. Questions that the nurse can include in a sexual history are:

- How often do you engage in sexual activity?
- What kinds of sexual activities?
- Are your partners men, women, or both?
- What difficulties do you have with sexual interaction? (These can be physical, emotional, psychological, spiritual, or situational.)
- What sexual activities do you enjoy?
- What gives you pleasure or joy?
- With whom do you share your feelings, whether happy or sad?
- What helps you to lubricate vaginally? (The home care nurse can recommend use of a water soluble lubricant, hormone cream, or saliva to improve or supplant lubrication. The nurse should advise against any vaseline-based product because it obstructs lubrication.)
- What helps you to have an erection? (This assumes that a man is capable of erection, and it also allows a man to discuss any difficulty with erection. The term impotence should be avoided; inability to have an erection interferes with intercourse but does not disempower a man and partner from other gratifying sexual play.)

The nurse can comfort the client by noting that if, during sexual activity, a man experiences erectile limitation (or a woman does not lubricate vaginally) and intercourse is not possible, there is always another time (McCann, 1989). This is also an opportune time to remind the client about other ways to enjoy sex. Nurses should avoid putting sexual activity in context because it is judgmental and limits discussion. For example, a question to avoid would be: "Are you able to have an erection during sex with your wife?" This is a closed format and may yield only a "yes" or "no" reply. Moreover, it conveys that heterosexual sex with a spouse is deemed the only acceptable option, which could impede discussion of erectile difficulty (Beresford, 1988). The open format yields information about fantasy, masturbation, erotic literature or movies, sex with a nonspouse, or sex with someone of the same sex. A home care nurse has to grow in ability to address sexual matters, if only because of the safe sex learning the nurse must foster to safeguard clients from contacting or spreading the human immunodeficiency virus (HIV). Since HIV/AIDS does not bypass the elderly, nurses can build on this reality.

Reflection helps clients acknowledge feelings and allows nurses to check the accuracy of their listening ability and empathy. Questioning is effective, as long as over-questioning is avoided. Over-questioning often happens when the nurse feels embarrassed or uncomfortable with the content of the discussion or tries to overcome any uneasiness with silence (Beresford, 1988). Silence is a way to create an open atmosphere and promote reflection. It communicates acceptance and permission for the client to continue with his or her story. Allowing silence is active listening, not passive ignoring. Silence is a difficult strategy because it often causes stress.

"Focusing" examines more closely any expressed concern: "Tell me more about your concern about your erection." One element of authenticity is for the nurse to admit distraction, such as when the mind wanders. This humanizes the nurse in the eyes of the client. The nurse can say something like, "Would you mind running that by me again? I got a bit distracted" (Beresford, 1988). Such an admission prevents distortion of information or missing an important piece of data.

Retirement, illness, injury, or loss of a significant other may cause an older adult to feel less attractive or compromise self-esteem. Men may see inability to achieve erection as a loss of manhood, and fear of repeated failure of erection may lead to less frequent sexual activity or a repeated cycle of inability to achieve or maintain an erection (Johnson, 1995). Isolation, anxiety, or depression lessen sexual desire and expression. The home care nurse has time to develop a therapeutic relationship with the client, and the experience of such closeness often reassures the client about his or her capability with personal intimacy, and this restores self-confidence.

The nurse creates an atmosphere that encourages dialogue and sharing. Home care nurses can facilitate interaction in group settings. Such a forum helps men and women learn about the sexuality of peers, what factors affect sexuality, and ways to enhance sexual interest, activity, and satisfaction. This can be an option in support groups and in community senior centers (Johnson, 1995). Confidentiality is crucial to rapport and is integral to professional and therapeutic relationships. A breach of confidentiality violates trust within any nurse-client interaction. This means that private matters are kept private.

SAFE SEXUAL CHOICES

Sexuality is a significant part of health, whether the client is sexually active solo or with a partner. Even if sexuality in an elderly client takes place only in the realm of fantasy, and desire in friendly banter, this empowers intimacy and sexuality. Activation of sexuality can override the bodily betrayal an elderly client experiences. At times the client may feel trapped in a physical body that is undependable. Home care nurses assist recovery by helping older clients reclaim faith in their capability as they progress in endurance and performance of activities of daily living (ADLs).

Talking and listening secure intimacy. Although this is a simple concept, it is much easier to say than do. Many attempts at talking end up with people talking at each other rather than talking with and listening to each other. There is an adage that says people have one mouth and two ears for a purpose. There are ways to help an older client learn how to start intimate dialogue. The client can take time to imagine what is going on in the life of his or her partner, much like the Native American metaphor of walking in another's moccasins. One partner can ask the other to visualize a personal experience and talk about what was imagined. This often stimulates two-way talk and eliminates hidden or personal agendas that restrict intimacy. These strategies can start simple discussions about the course of one's day or ease complex talk about the more personal experiences of aging, frailty, illness, and sexuality. The imagination can prompt more vivid interaction concerning each other's hopes, desires, joys, needs, fears, and disappointments. Other suggestions for the nurse to help catalyze "real" dialogue are questions like:

- What do you talk about to your partner?
- What limits communication with your partner?
- What can you change to improve communication?
- What qualities in your partner evoke affection?
- How do you express affection?
- What do you reminisce about?
- What do you love about yourself?

- What do you love about your partner?
- What opportunities do you and your partner make for contact? talking? comforting? sensual play? sexual play?
- Who is the matter with you? (This often seems like a silly question, until a nurse tries it a few times. It can elicit a wealth of information about personal relationships.)
- How do you share what pleases/displeases you with your partner? What pleases/displeases you sexually?

These questions are posed in a way that the older adult can use for improving intimacy. They can be modified for use between partners, friends, and significant others.

Writing questions and answers provides another entry to intimacy or connecting talk. Sometimes, writing fosters openness and honesty. Partners can create and write dialogue between the heart, mind, or sexual organs as ways to discover renewed attachment and pleasure.

It helps to remember that the skin is the largest sexual organ, and that the mind is the most powerful. This expands sensual and sexual horizons. Sexuality and illness share a fierce unpredictability that defies any illusion of control. They also share an unhealthy stigma and shame, something that home care nurses help dispel.

Masturbation is one of the most common sexual expressions, while at the same time one of the least acknowledged and guilt ridden (Fontaine, 1991). If an older client is comfortable with masturbation, which Butler (1976) refers to as "solo sex," the nurse can tell the client that it is an optimal and safe choice of sexual self-care. It gives one responsibility for one's own sensual and sexual pleasure and is a viable choice with or without a partner, and it frees one from dealing with a partner's pleasure needs or fears. "Solo sex" permits self-pacing, so one can test endurance, confidence, and capability safely (McCann, 1989). This is particularly beneficial for elderly patients who have fears about how safe sex is in the face of heart disease, pulmonary deficits, or profound fatigue. Masturbation also provides gratification and release for people who are without partners. The nurse in home care can remind elderly clients to enjoy whatever sensual or sexual pleasure they can and let go of performance pressure.

Specific and safe sexual information that can be given to clients who have heart disease include:

- Touching, cuddling, hugging, kissing, and sensual play are safe.

- Sex is safe six to eight weeks after a heart attack and sometimes sooner.
- Sex is very unlikely to trigger a heart attack (about 20 chances in a million [DeBusk, 1996]).
- The physical energy expended during sexual intercourse is equivalent to climbing two flights of stairs, or walking one block briskly.
- Sexual activity is optimal in a room or environment that is not too hot or cold.
- Heavy meals and drinking should be avoided prior to sexual activity, and it is a good idea to wait three to four hours after eating to allow time for the heart to recover from the work of digestion.
- It is a good idea to rest prior to sexual intercourse.
- Any activity, sexual or otherwise, should be stopped immediately, if there is any shortness of breath or chest pressure/pain.
- Prophylactic nitroglycerin, if prescribed, is helpful before sexual activity.
- Anal penetration may not be safe because it can slow heart rate.
- Oral sex is a safe and pleasurable option.
- It helps to remember that there is always another time.
- Viagra should not be taken if nitrates are prescribed.

Although these tips relate to clients who have heart illness, they are practical suggestions for anyone who may be symptom-limited in activity due to pulmonary disease, fatigue, and so on. Most of it is common sense, but clients are comforted by specifics. Nevertheless, the most common medical advice about sexual safety is the vague phrase "take it easy." Clients can derive encouragement from equating energy used during sexual intercourse with activities like climbing stairs or walking. A meaningful translation of some of the above suggestions is to recommend that clients consider changing sexual activity from the evening to the morning, after a good night's sleep—or from the dessert to the appetizer (McCann, 1989).

FACTORS THAT LIMIT SEXUAL RECOVERY

Most medical data on healthy sexuality are limited to the physical realm. This essentially likens intimacy with physical contact, usually vaginal intercourse. Intimacy goes beyond physical boundaries, and

---

BOX 7-2 • SAMPLE VISUALIZATION EXERCISE II

- Picture in your mind your personal experience of sexuality.
- Focus on the physical, emotional, mental, and spiritual energy that you expend when you participate in sexual activity with yourself, or with a partner.
- Visualize in your mind another activity in which you engage that uses a similar amount of your energy.

---

sexuality is expressed in contexts other than heterosexual marriage and in contact other than genital. The nurse can suggest a visualization activity and encourage the elderly patient to see what it is like (see Box 7-2).

Use of a visualization exercise provides an opportune way for the nurse to discuss endurance, breathlessness, fatigue, isolation, fear, joy, thrill, and so on, and how each translates or adapts practically to safe, healthful sexuality. Nurses also have the opportunity to provide many older people with affirmation of their sexuality by making a positive comment about a good-looking tie or a new hairstyle or reaching out to touch the elder's hand (Burke & Walsh, 1997). These are small acts with major impact—affirming an older adult's sexuality is a gift of enormous dimension. Intimate contact is preserved through talk and touch, which helps recovery and instills hope in the elderly.

Failure of erection may lead to less frequent or avoidance of sexual activity, or it may initiate a repeated cycle of inability to achieve or maintain an erection. This can happen due to side effects of medical therapy; the home care nurse can inquire about erectile ability when helping the client learn about the side effects of any suspected drug.

Illness affects sexuality because the body uses energy to recover, and little energy may be left for sexual activity (Johnson, 1995). Factors that limit or deter healthy sexuality in the elderly include age-related dryness and fragility of the vaginal canal; vaginal infection; erectile problems; sexually transmitted disease; cardiovascular, pulmonary, and neurological illness; diabetes mellitus; decreased production of hormones; arthritis; pain; prostate problems; cystocele; rectocele; effect of medications; obesity; fatigue; over-imbibing of alcohol or use of other mind-altering drugs; anxiety; fear; lack of a partner; unwilling or unable partner; widowhood; guilt; depression; stress; lack of privacy; religious conflict; altered appearance; and negative self-concept (Eliopoulos, 1993).

A client's illness can be used to introduce the sexual history to the nursing assessment. For example, 60 percent of men who have diabetes experience erectile dysfunction (Burke & Walsh, 1997). The home care nurse can relate sexual questions to discussion of other complications of diabetes, or whatever chronic condition, if the nurse feels more at ease with such a strategy. Chronic illness, which is common in the elderly and a reality amongst the home care population, tends to develop slowly over time. Resultant changes in sexual functioning may develop insidiously and may be mistakenly attributed to aging rather than to the chronic disease process (Burke & Walsh, 1997). Effective nursing assessment differentiates the two.

PHARMACOLOGIC EFFECTS ON SEXUAL CAPABILITY

Medications prescribed for the elderly affect potency, libido, orgasm, and ejaculation. Some of these drugs include but are not limited to: beta-blockers, clonidine, guanethidine, haloperidol, phenothiazines, reserpine, sedatives, thiazide diuretics, tranquilizers, and tricyclic antidepressants. For a review of pharmacologic effects of medications on an elder's well-being, see Chapter 8.

It is important for the home care nurse to prepare older people for the potential changes in sexual function that drugs can produce (Eliopoulos, 1993). Some nurses avoid telling clients about the side effects of drugs, especially if it affects erection, because of concern about the "self-fulfilling prophecy," yet it is probably more reassuring to a man to attribute erectile difficulty to a drug than to a sense of sexual inadequacy (McCann, 1989). Moreover, it is helpful for the man or woman to know that trying another drug therapy may reverse the problem. Change in sexual function caused by use of drugs is reversible; the dose can be reduced or another drug substituted (Johnson, 1995).

INSTILLING HOPE

Sexuality is rarely the primary reason for intervention by a home care nurse, but sexual intervention is essential to comprehensive nursing. The home environment provides a wealth of data about emotional and social support and the tapestry of intimate connections within the client's world. Nurses are intuitive, sensitive, and subtle caregivers. Nursing focuses on the client's response to wellness and illness, promotes health, and restores self-care capability. Home care nurses assess an elderly client's strength and recovery potential, link a client to community resources, and enhance coping strategies to overcome anxiety and stress. Sexuality and intimacy thrive in such nurturing.

Nurses are wellsprings of hope, and instilling hope is essential to nursing care. Hope is often defined in relation to hopelessness or despair; when hope is lost, one becomes despondent and loses energy necessary for hopefulness (Morgante, 1997). Although hope is often seen as the absence of hopelessness, no experience is static. It is just the language that limits our vision to an either/or experience. One can move from hope to hopelessness from moment to moment. Recognition of this ever-changing process can inspire hope even in moments of despair. Hope is the smallest or largest expression of the spirit of optimism. Hope and sexuality share a dynamism that manifests in a song, poem, painting, flower arrangement, or a smile (Morgante and McCann, 1992). Life is also dynamic, and if home care nurses nurture a forward, futuristic outlook toward vital intimacy and sexuality in the elderly, they promote hope, preserve health, and enliven spirit.

SUMMARY

Home care nurses are in a unique position to assess the lived experience of illness in the familiar environment of the client's home. The comfort of this setting is likely to promote intimate therapeutic interaction between the home care nurse and the client. The therapeutic relationship becomes a model for healthy human connection and can enhance a client's capability of interacting with intimate partners, family, and friends. Intimacy and sexuality are linked, and intimacy can be enhanced in the elderly if they perceive that their feelings matter and think that their words are heard.

Many nurses feel embarrassed about discussing sexuality. This is common, and it is fine as long as it is acknowledged. Attempts to hide discomfort interfere with authenticity in the nurse-client relationship. It helps to remember that nurses ask many other kinds of "intrusive" questions and participate in many intimate life events. Clients are not neuter, whether sick or well.

Home care nurses can give permission to clients to discuss sexual concerns. Broaching the topic with a simple inquiry such as "What sexual concerns do you have?" often relieves the client of uneasiness about sexuality. This is therapeutic, even if this is as much as the nurse is able to do at the moment. If the nurse lacks knowledge, the nurse can always consult a colleague for answers.

A comprehensive nursing assessment should include questions about sexuality, yet this is still relatively uncommon, even though the twenty-first century is nigh. The nurse should instruct all clients about safe sex in respect to HIV transmission; otherwise, the nurse is contributing to risk of transmission. It is ageist to think that the elderly are asexual.

It is also important to remember that the elderly have intimacy needs and sexual desires. Compliments and contact can do much to preserve their self-esteem and overcome any sense of isolation. These needs are real, whether or not a person is sexually active.

This chapter contains suggestions to help the client grow in intimacy and to guide the nurse in ways to address sexuality. This is often a process of trial and error but one that can enrich and reward the home care nurse and client. In essence, it is life.

REFERENCES

Beresford, T. (1988). *Short-term sexual counseling*. Baltimore: Planned Parenthood of Maryland.

Burke, M. M., & Walsh, M. B. (1997). *Gerontological nursing: Wholistic care of the older adult*. St. Louis: Mosby–Yearbook.

Butler, R., & Lewis, M. (1976). *Sex after sixty*. New York: Harper & Row.

DeBusk, R. F. (1996). Sexual activity triggering myocardial infarction: One less thing to worry about. *Journal of the American Medical Association, 275,* 1447–1448.

Eliopoulos, C. (1993). *Gerontological nursing*. Philadelphia: J. B. Lippincott.

Fontaine, K. L. (1991). Unlocking sexual issues: Counseling strategies for nurses. *Nursing Clinics of North America, 26,* 737–743.

Johnson, B., Stanley, M., & Beare, P. G. (eds.) (1995). *Sexuality and aging: Gerontological nursing* (pp. 426–438). Philadelphia: F. A. Davis.

Johnson, B. (1996). Older adults and sexuality: A multidimensional perspective. *Journal of Gerontologic Nursing, 22,* 7–15.

Kaplan, H. S.(1990). Sex, intimacy, and the aging process. *Journal of the American Academy of Psychoanalysis, 18*(2), 187.

McCann, M. E. (1989). Sexual healing after heart attack. *American Journal of Nursing, 89,* 1133–1138.

Morgante, L. (1997). Hope: A unifying concept for nursing care in multiple sclerosis. In J. Halper & N. J. Holland (Eds.), *Comprehensive nursing care in multiple sclerosis* (pp. 189–201). New York: Demos Vermande.

Morgante, L., & McCann, M. E. (1992). *The energy and power of hope*. Unpublished manuscript.

Needham, J. F. (1993). Exercise and activity. In J. F. Needham (Ed.), *Gerontological nursing: A restorative approach* (pp. 43–102). Albany, NY: Delmar.

Poorman, S. G. (1987). *Human sexuality and the nursing process*. Connecticut: Appleton & Lange.

HOME CARE MANAGEMENT OF ISSUES COMMON TO ELDERLY CLIENTS

his unit's five chapters address common issues found in the older home care population. The chapters focus on medication usage, coping effectively with hearing and vision problems, dealing with physical and verbal abuse, managing urinary and bowel changes, and maintaining skin integrity and caring for compromised skin. With this unit, we begin concentrating on secondary prevention—the early diagnosis and treatment of health problems.

As much as all nurses would like to spend most of their time teaching and helping older adults in maintaining a wellness state, this is only a part of the nursing care given. Unfortunately, for many elders, the accumulation of years of wear and tear, bodily use and misuse, and exposure to disease-causing agents results in negative changes in various systems. On a positive note, as one author once said, "considering the alternative, old age is not so bad." Home care nurses should be as optimistic as that author when dealing with elders who are coping with age-related changes. Hopefully, thoughts shared in this unit will help the home care nurse work effectively with older clients.

The first chapter in this unit, Chapter 8, provides the home care nurse with up-to-date, important information about the use, side effects, and possible deleterious effects of polypharmacy. In Chapter 9, the reader is exposed to the frustrations hearing- and vision-impaired clients may feel. These changes are common in elders, and it behooves the nurse to be able to maximize the client's potential to improve the quality of life. Chapter 10 prepares the home care nurse to effectively manage a client's or caregiver's inappropriate or abusive behavior. Chapter 11 takes a proactive approach in managing urinary and bowel problems. The final chapter in this unit, Chapter 12, focuses first on maintaining intact and healthy skin and second on promoting wound healing in clients whose skin has been compromised.

Since these issues may be common to many elders, regardless of medical diagnoses, they are presented prior to specific medical and surgical concerns, which are addressed in Unit IV. This unit builds on the foundational home care information presented in Unit I and health promotion strategies found in Unit II and leads into the chronic and acute healthcare issues covered in the final chapters.

8

MANAGING MEDICATION REGIMENS IN ELDERLY CLIENTS

Henry Cohen

◆ ◆ ◆

Medication management in the elderly is complex and presents a challenge to the home care nurse. The home care nurse must consider and minimize medication compliance barriers. The expert nurse consults with the primary care provider if any problems are found, as the provider may need to tailor medication regimens to incorporate age-related changes affecting drug pharmacokinetics and pharmacodynamics. Collaboration among healthcare professionals, specifically the primary care provider, pharmacist, and nurse is paramount. It is the responsibility of the home care nurse to ensure that all clients are well-educated regarding their medications and possible adverse reactions and that clients become as independent as possible with their medication management.

Medication use in the elderly continues to be associated with significant morbidity and mortality—the etiology is multifactorial. An overt lack of medication knowledge may lead to inappropriate use of medications and subsequent drug misadventures. Drug misadventures involve a drug's failure to accomplish its intended purpose due to inappropriate prescribing, lack of compliance, or adverse drug reaction. An adverse drug reaction is described as a response to a drug that is harmful and unintended, one which requires discontinuing a drug, modifying a dose, prolonging hospitalization, or administering supportive care. Examples of adverse drug reactions include: diphenhydramine-induced drowsiness, dizziness resulting in a traumatic fall, prazosin-induced orthostatic hypotension, and ibuprofen-induced asthma—all are unintended responses to a drug and may require dose adjustment, discontinuation, prolonged hospitalization, or supportive care. Expenditures incurred by society for adverse drug reaction-induced morbidity and mortality exceed billions of dollars annually.

Medication use and polypharmacy are commonplace among the older adult population and account for the extraordinary high rate of adverse drug reactions. Polypharmacy is described as the use of multiple prescription and over-the-counter medications by one person. The elderly, while comprising approximately 12 percent of the entire general population, consume greater than 40 percent of all prescription drugs. Over 40 percent of home-dwelling elders take five or more drugs daily, and 20 percent take seven or more drugs daily. In the United States, over nine million adverse drug reactions occur annually in clients over 65 years old. Adverse drug reactions account for over 30 percent of all hospital admissions by elders. Drug misadventures are directly attributed to a client's lack of medication compliance. Medication compliance in the elderly is affected by many factors, including impaired cognition and diminished vision, hearing, and strength (Darnell, 1986; Fowles, 1991; Lamy, 1985; National Center for Health Statistics, 1994).

COGNITION AND COMPLIANCE

Cognition—defined as the mental activities associated with thinking, learning, and memory—is often impaired in elderly clients and becomes progressively worse with aging. Clients often forget or misunderstand medication-related instructions. Therefore, it is paramount to keep the home care client's medication regimen as simple as possible. Dosing schedules incorporating once- and twice-daily regimens are preferred and afford 90 percent and 80 percent compliance, respectively. Dosing schedules with three and four times daily administration are associated with lower compliance rates of 60 percent and 40 percent, respectively. Efforts should be made to use longer acting or sustained release once- or twice-daily medications whenever possible.

Many drugs are available in transdermal (skin patch) systems that allow for daily to weekly administration, and these should be considered. Transdermal systems are applied to a hairless portion of the skin, generally the upper torso or chest area; however, application site is dependent on the individual drug. Agents available in transdermal dosage forms include nitroglycerin, clonidine, fentanyl, and estrogen. The primary care provider should be made aware of any compliance problems, as long acting or sustained release preparations of a drug or a pharmacologically similar long-acting agent may be needed.

Fixed drug products (a combination of more than one medication in a dosage form), unit-of-use packaging, and unit-dose blister packaging will all aid in reducing the complexity of a client's medication regimen. Commonly prescribed fixed drug products include the combination of antihypertensives, such as Capozide (captopril and hydrochlorothiazide), Inderide (propranolol and hydrochlorothiazide), Combipres (clonidine and chlorthalidone), and Vaseretic (enalapril and hydrochlorothiazide). Two examples of manufacturer-prepared unit-of-use packaging are Medrol Dosepak-21 and Helidac. Medrol Dosepak-21 contains individualized doses of methylprednisolone titrated from high to low dose. Helidac, indicated for the treatment of an active duodenal ulcer associated with H. pylori infection, contains individualized daily doses of bismuth subsalicylate, metronidazole, and tetracycline.

All drugs are generally available in unit-dose blister packs, which may facilitate compliance since the client can easily inspect the package visually and determine if the medication was administered. Checking for compliance of medications stored in vials would require remembering a daily count and removing the drug from the vial in order to determine the count, which could lead to drug spillage and is error prone. Some pharmacies possess the mechanical technology to place drugs in unit-dose blister packs. Additionally, readily available plastic blister packs compartmentalized to the days in a week can be purchased in the pharmacy.

When compatible, the administration of medications after a meal is preferred. An after-meal regimen will serve as a compliance reminder and may aid in minimizing drug-induced gastrointestinal side effects.

TABLE 8-1 • ANTICHOLINERGIC OPHTHALMIC AGENTS	
Generic Name	**Brand Name**
Atropine	Isopto Atropine
Homatropine	Isopto Homatropine
Cyclopentolate	Cyclogyl, Pentolair
Scopolamine	Isopto Hyoscine
Tropicamide	Mydriacyl, Opticyl, Tropicacyl

PHYSICAL STRENGTH, MANUAL DEXTERITY, AND COMPLIANCE

Diminished strength and limited physical and manual dexterity may lead to a lack of compliance and may preclude the use of self-administered ear and eye drops, injectables, and inhalers. For example, a client with debilitating rheumatoid arthritis and limited manual dexterity may not be able to open prescription vials or administer eye and ear drops, injectables, and inhalers.

In most states, pharmacists are required to dispense medications in difficult-to-open child safety vials. The elderly client should always request nonsafety capped vials from the pharmacist, except when there are children in the house. Nonsafety capped vials generally require a gentle twist-off or push-open motion.

Administration of Ophthalmic Preparations

In elders with peripheral vascular disease or diabetes mellitus, the administration of eye drops can be a difficult and hazardous task. These clients may not be able to feel the number of drops they are self-administering to the eye and inadvertently may instill multiple drops. Most eye drops are potent drugs in a concentrated solution. Even when ophthalmic preparations are administered appropriately and at recommended doses, they may have systemic effects.

Anticholinergic ophthalmic preparations (e.g., atropine, homatropine [see Table 8-1]) indicated for cycloplegic refraction and for pupil dilation in inflammatory conditions of the iris and uveal tract are associated with many toxic, systemic adverse events. These agents can cause significant systemic anticholinergic effects, including constipation, urinary retention, dry mouth, hyperpyrexia, blurred vision, hallucinations, bizarre

TABLE 8-2 • OPHTHALMIC BETA-ADRENERGIC BLOCKING AGENTS

Generic Name	Brand Name
Betaxolol	Betoptic
Carteolol	Ocupress
Levobunolol	AKBeta, Betagan
Metipranolol	Optipranolol
Timolol	Timoptic

behavior, drowsiness, confusion, tachyarrhythmias, hypotension, and respiratory depression.

Ophthalmic beta-blockers indicated for glaucoma (e.g., timolol, betaxolol [see Table 8-2]) possess the same systemic effects as the oral products. Systemic toxicities include bradyarrhythmias, hypotension, cardiac failure, bronchospasm, dyspnea, wheezing, and asthma exacerbation.

Apraclonidine (Iopidine), an alpha-1 agonist indicated for elevated intraocular pressure, has been associated with anticholinergic-like effects and depression. Pilocarpine, a cholinergic direct-acting miotic indicated for the management of glaucoma, may have the propensity to cause bradyarrhythmias, hypotension, headaches, salivation, diarrhea, gastrointestinal spasms, urinary incontinence, and asthma.

In order to prevent excessive administration of eye drops, many products are now available in unit-of-use containers. These products contain calibrated droppers that can dispense precisely one drop per instillation. Alternatively, chilling eye drops in the refrigerator prior to administration will allow for a cold sensation, thereby alerting the client to the number of drops administered.

Compression of the lacrimal sac for three to five minutes after instillation of eye drops will aid in minimizing systemic absorption of ophthalmic drops and should be employed in all clients. Compression of the lacrimal sac will retard the passage of drops via the nasolacrimal duct into areas of potential drug absorption, such as the nasal and pharyngeal mucosa.

Administration of Metered Dose Inhalers

Clients utilizing metered dose inhalers (MDIs) require manual dexterity and good hand-lung coordination in order to master appropriate administration technique, maximize drug delivery, and minimize adverse drug events. Poor technique may lead to excessive oropharyngeal deposition, swallowing of drug, and gastrointestinal absorption and may increase the prevalence of systemic adverse events. For example, oropharyngeal deposition of corticosteroid inhalers may cause the development of oral thrush. Excessive gastrointestinal absorption of corticosteroids may cause osteoporosis, myopathy, fluid retention, hypertension, heart failure, glaucoma, cataracts, gastropathy, hypokalemia, hyperglycemia, and immunosuppression. Excessive gastrointestinal absorption of beta$_2$-receptor agonists (e.g., albuterol, metaproterenol) may cause tremors, headaches, dizziness, irritability, and palpitations.

The home care nurse should watch the client use an MDI to ensure the client can administer it properly. Up to 30 percent of clients cannot master the use of an MDI, but alternatives are available (Kamada, 1994). Alternatives include spacers, breath-actuated MDIs, and jet nebulizers. Spacers allow evaporation of the drug propellant prior to inhalation. Spacers do not require significant hand-lung coordination. When used with an MDI, spacers decrease oropharyngeal deposition and enhance lung delivery. Breath-actuated MDIs significantly reduce the need for hand-lung coordination; however, they cannot be used with a spacer. Jet nebulizers do not require significant client coordination or cooperation other than breathing. Jet nebulizers produce an aerosol from a liquid solution placed in a cup: A tube connected to a stream of compressed air or oxygen flows up through the bottom and draws the liquid up an adjacent open-ended tube. The air and liquid strike a baffle creating a droplet cloud that is then inhaled.

DOSAGE FORM, COUNSELING, AND COMPLIANCE

Dosage form preference may play a major role in maximizing medication compliance. Older clients may have difficulty swallowing large tablets or capsules. Studies have demonstrated that capsules are the preferred dosage form for most clients. Capsules, unlike tablets, are easier to swallow and rarely give the client a bad taste.

Clients who are unable to swallow tablets and capsules should have all their medications prepared in a liquid dosage form. Many medications are readily available from the manufacturer in a liquid dosage form. When liquid medications are not available from the manufacturer, the pharmacist is usually able to extemporaneously prepare a liquid dosage form. When a liquid preparation is not available and cannot be prepared by the pharmacist, the nurse can instruct the client or caregiver to crush the drug with a mortar and pestle, mix it in a cup with 5 to 10 mL of water, administer the mixture, rinse the cup with 5 to 10 mL of water, and immediately administer the rinse. Rinsing the cup will eliminate any drug residual adhered to the cup, thereby ensuring complete drug delivery. Most sustained release medications cannot be crushed. The home care nurse should always consult the pharmacist for information regarding medication crushing. Table 8-3 lists selected medications that should not be crushed.

It is important to administer all liquid medications individually, since some combinations may produce in-vitro incompatibilities. Liquid preparations can usually be stored in the refrigerator, maximizing stability and palatability. Pharmacists are now able to prepare almost any liquid medication in an assortment of flavors (e.g., strawberry, orange, pineapple/ banana). All dosage forms should be swallowed while sitting or standing and followed with a glass of water, unless otherwise instructed. This information is important to share with the client, involved family members, and other caregivers responsible for medication administration.

Written Counseling

Many pharmacists will offer, in addition to verbal counseling, written information on medication use. Written drug instruction usually contains information regarding indications and contraindications for use, adverse events, drug-drug and drug-nutrient interactions, and appropriate dosing schedules and administration techniques. By the year 2000, the FDA will require all pharmacists to supply written medication information to all clients for each individual drug dispensed. In order for written drug information to be effective, the home care nurse must evaluate the client's ability to read and comprehend the data. The home care nurse should review all drug information with the client, highlighting the most salient points to alleviate any reluctance or misunderstanding with compliance.

Vision Impairment

Vision impairment, especially with glare intolerance and loss of color discrimination, is the most common sensory deficit among elders and may hinder the use and efficiency of written drug information. Elders often have difficulty distinguishing among the different sizes, shapes, and colors of dosage forms. Distinguishing among colors, especially whites and yellows, or among different shades of a color is especially difficult.

TABLE 8-3 • SELECTED ORAL SOLID MEDICATIONS THAT SHOULD NOT BE CRUSHED

Medication	Manufacturer	Dosage Form
Bayer Extra Strength Enteric	Sterling Health	Slow release tablet
Bayer Adult Low Strength 81 mg	Sterling Health	Enteric coated tablet
Bayer Regular Strength Caplet	Sterling Health	Enteric coated tablet
Cardizem	Marion-Merrell Dow	Slow release tablet
Cardizem CD	Marion-Merrell Dow	Slow release capsule
Cardizem SR	Marion-Merrell Dow	Slow release capsule
Compazine Spansule	SmithKline Beecham	Slow release capsule
Depakote	Abbott	Enteric coated capsule
Diamox Sequels	Lederle	Slow release capsule
Dulcolax	Boehringer Ingelheim	Enteric coated tablet
Elixophyllin SR	Forest	Slow release capsule
Eryc	Parke-Davis	Enteric coated capsule
Erythromycin Stearate	Various	Enteric coated tablet
Erythromycin Base	Various	Enteric coated tablet
Feosol Spansule	SmithKline Beecham	Slow release capsule
Inderal LA	Wyeth-Ayerst	Slow release capsule
Inderide LA	Wyeth-Ayerst	Slow release capsule
Indocin SR	MSD	Slow release capsule
Ionamin	Fisons	Slow release capsule
Klotrix	Mead Johnson	Slow release tablet
Levsinex Timecaps	Schwarz Pharma	Slow release capsule
Lithobid	Ciba	Slow release capsule
Micro K	A. H. Robins	Slow release capsule
MS Contin	Purdue Frederick	Slow release tablet
Pancrease	McNeil	Enteric coated capsule
Prilosec	Astra Merck	Slow release capsule
Procan SR	Parke-Davis	Slow release tablet
Quinaglute Dura Tabs	Berlex	Slow release tablet
Ritalin SR	Ciba	Slow release tablet
Sinemet CR	DuPont Pharm	Slow release tablet
Slo-Bid Gyrocaps	Rhone-Poulenc Rorer	Slow release capsule
Slow-FE	Ciba Consumer	Slow release tablet
Slow-K	Summit	Slow release tablet
Slow-Mag	Searle	Slow release tablet
Theo-Dur	Key	Slow release tablet
Uniphyl	Purdue Frederick	Slow release tablet

All prescription drug labels should state the name of the medication, directions and indications for use, strength, and dosage form of the drug. Many pharmacists can print labels in large uppercase letters to enhance visualization. In addition, prescription labels and written information can often be printed in various languages. Pharmacists that are able to comply with these needs should be sought. Communication between the client, home care nurse, and pharmacist will maximize counseling information. For more information on visual acuity issues in elders, see Chapter 9.

Hearing Impairment

Presbycusis, the loss of auditory acuity, and hearing impairment are common in older adults. The home care nurse should be aware that 30 to 40 percent of people over age 65 have impaired hearing, and over 90 percent of people over age ninety suffer from a hearing handicap (Bess, 1989; Lichtenstein, 1988). Generally, men are more affected than women. The elderly often complain of difficulty understanding speech and, to a lesser extent, hearing sounds. Any type of hearing or speech impediment will interfere with client counseling. The home care nurse must speak slowly and clearly and reinforce oral communication with written information. For more information about hearing impairments, see Chapter 9.

Taste Impairment

Dysgeusia (taste disturbance) is also common in older adults. Dysgeusia may adversely affect compliance of a client's drug and nutrition regimen. Older adults develop a diminished ability to taste sweetness, sourness, and bitterness—saltiness is not affected. Taste disturbances may affect medication palatability and compliance. Certain drugs—including the angiotensin-converting enzyme inhibitors (ACEI) captopril, enalapril, lisinopril, and fosinopril—may cause dysgeusia in up to 10 percent of the population. Reports of ACEI-induced metallic taste and anorexia, as well as ACEI-induced sweetness and significant weight gain, have been reported. Other agents that may cause dysgeusia include metronidazole, ofloxacin, and clarithromycin.

MEDICATION STORAGE

Inappropriate storage of medication may lead to diminished drug stability, increased drug degradation, and lack of pharmacologic effect. Most clients store medications in the kitchen and bathroom. Both the kitchen and bathroom are hot and humid and are detrimental to heat-sensitive medications. All medications should be stored in a cool dry place, away from light. Most medications can be stored in pill boxes; however, they should not be exposed to extreme temperatures. Certain medications, such as nitroglycerin tablets, should never be removed from their original glass containers. All medications have specific storage requirements; these should be discussed with the pharmacist and strictly adhered to.

Medication storage is a common issue confronting home care nurses. It is not uncommon for older clients to have all of their medications out of the original containers and mixed together in one easy to open box or plastic container. Other clients keep all medication bottles (old and new) in a shoebox. At times, the home care nurse will notice prescribed generic and trade name medications and find that the client is taking both drugs, not knowing that they are the same medication. Observation, inquiry, and teaching are important nursing activities the home care nurse needs to engage in to promote medication safety among elders.

Hoarding Medications

Keeping medications for years and even decades is not an uncommon practice among elders. Some do this because they have learned that primary care providers often change medications and then reorder an old medication, so hoarding medications ensures they will not be wasted. Others hoard medications to extend the supply in order to stretch a limited income. A medication ordered for four times a day may be taken only twice a day so that the medication lasts twice as long; or a daily medication may be taken every other day or only when the client feels it is "needed." Elders on fixed incomes may take shortcuts with medications, food, and heating costs. It is imperative that home care nurses approach this subject and be ready to provide resources to eliminate this problem.

Most medications have less than a two- to three-year expiration date from the date of production in optimal storage conditions, and at best most homes do not provide this environment. Most states do not require pharmacists to place expiration dates on prescription labels, so the date the medication order was filled may be the nurse's or client's only clue as to the age of the medication. It is wise for the client to be a self-advocate and ask the pharmacist to place the expiration date on the label. If this is not possible, family members or the home care nurse should follow through.

The Pharmacist's Role

Pharmacists are the healthcare professionals most qualified to help consumers make the best use of medications. Pharmacists are experts on the thousands of medications available today, on how each one works in the body, and in the ways to use each one safely. The public should be aware that the pharmacist is obligated by law to provide pharmaceutical care. Pharmaceutical care requires the pharmacist to review the client's prescribed drug regimen, intervene and adjust medication regimens as necessary, and educate the client, hence maximizing the client's care to ensure a positive outcome. The pharmacist's role is vital to client care. It is paramount that the consumer seeks out an effective pharmacist willing to provide complete pharmaceutical care services.

Enacted into federal law in 1987, the Omnibus Budget Reconciliation Act (OBRA) requires pharmacists in all states to answer the following questions for every prescription filled: (1) Is the medication prescribed indicated? (2) Does the client have any contraindications to the medication prescribed? (3) Is the dosing schedule and administration route appropriate? (4) Are there existing or potential problems with drug side effects, drug-drug interactions, drug-nutrient interactions, or adverse drug reactions? (5) What recommendations can be made to minimize adverse effects while maximizing efficacy?

In order to maximize positive medication outcomes, the pharmacist must take a thorough history from the client—a good historian is crucial. The client must inform the pharmacist of all allergies, adverse events incurred, dietary regimens, vaccination schedules, and medications utilized, including over-the-counter drugs, homeopathic agents, and home remedies. Failure to utilize the pharmacist's services may be life-threatening. Having a prescription filled by a nonpharmacist health professional does away with the crucial quality checks that pharmacists provide in detecting and preventing harmful drug interactions or reactions and potential mistakes.

It is important for home care nurses to familiarize themselves with the client's prescribed regimen and to thoroughly review each drug's pharmacology. Additionally, clients must be encouraged to choose one pharmacy for all their medication needs. Since most clients will see several primary care providers concurrently, the risk of drug interactions and contraindications is high. Clients may have multiple medications from different providers and pharmacies, each not knowing the other is providing care and service. Choosing one pharmacy enables the pharmacist to maintain an accurate medication profile and detect any potentially harmful drug combinations. The home care nurse can help clients find a local pharmacist who delivers to the home and takes the client's medication insurance plan.

OVER-THE-COUNTER MEDICATIONS

With the plethora of over-the-counter agents and non-FDA regulated homeopathic and home remedies, as well as the continued conversion of prescription drugs to nonprescription status, the risk of drug interactions and adverse events has escalated dramatically. Elders routinely self-medicate without seeking professional advise. They will borrow and self-administer drugs from friends, based on anecdotal life experiences.

Most homeopathic remedies, like prescription medications, originate from natural sources, are pharmacologically active, and illicit side effects. For example, the popular mahuang plant used for weight reduction contains ephedrine and can cause hyperactivity, irritability, insomnia, elevations in blood pressure, tachyarrhythmias, and seizures. The home care nurse is responsible for obtaining a complete list of medications that the client takes. If the client uses homeopathic or home remedies, the primary care provider needs to be aware of this. The provider may or may not incorporate this into the client's plan of care.

Serotonin Syndrome

L-tryptophan, used for the management of depression and as a sedative hypnotic, is decarboxylated into serotonin, thereby increasing serotonin synthesis. When L-tryptophan is combined with serotonergic agents (see Box 8-1), an abnormally high concentration of serotonin in the central nervous system occurs, which subsequently can produce the serotonin syndrome.

The serotonin syndrome is a constellation of mental status changes and nervous system and neuromuscular effects that result from an excess of serotonin. Diagnosis of the serotonin syndrome may be made when three of the following develop: agitation, diaphoresis, diarrhea, fever, hyperreflexia, uncoordination, mental status changes, myoclonus, shivering, or tremor. Other manifestations include seizures and muscle rigidity. The onset of symptoms are usually within minutes to hours, as is the resolution. Combinations of meperidine and the popular cough suppressant dextromethorphan, both serotonin reuptake inhibitors, may significantly increase serotonin concentrations within the neuronal synapse, potentially yielding a severe serotonin syndrome that may be deadly. Any combination of serotonergic agents, or a high dose of an individual serotonergic agent, may predispose clients to the dangerous serotonin syndrome.

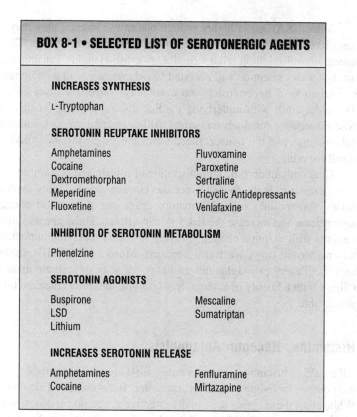

BOX 8-1 • SELECTED LIST OF SEROTONERGIC AGENTS

INCREASES SYNTHESIS

L-Tryptophan

SEROTONIN REUPTAKE INHIBITORS

Amphetamines	Fluvoxamine
Cocaine	Paroxetine
Dextromethorphan	Sertraline
Meperidine	Tricyclic Antidepressants
Fluoxetine	Venlafaxine

INHIBITOR OF SEROTONIN METABOLISM

Phenelzine

SEROTONIN AGONISTS

Buspirone	Mescaline
LSD	Sumatriptan
Lithium	

INCREASES SEROTONIN RELEASE

Amphetamines	Fenfluramine
Cocaine	Mirtazapine

Nonsteroidal Antiinflammatory Drugs

Nonsteroidal antiinflammatory drugs (NSAIDs) have many indications and are generally used for their antiinflammatory, analgesic, and antipyretic properties. Unfortunately, NSAIDs are associated with many significant adverse effects, especially peptic ulcer disease. It is important to note that only misoprostol (Cytotec) is effective in preventing NSAID-induced gastropathy. Antacids, sucralfate, and histamine$_2$-receptor antagonists (e.g., cimetidine, ranitidine) have not been consistently effective in reducing NSAID gastropathy. Aspirin, generally considered more toxic than the nonaspirin NSAIDs, may be found in products such as Pepto Bismol, Alka Seltzer, and Brioschi. Aspirin toxicity may present with dizziness, confusion, tinnitus, and headache. Tinnitus, a hallmark of aspirin toxicity, may often go unnoticed in the hearing impaired geriatric client.

Since NSAIDs are highly protein-bound to albumin, they may be associated with numerous protein displacement interactions. These agents may also inhibit renal vasodilatory prostaglandins, causing sodium and water retention and elevated blood pressure with a subsequent exacerbation of hypertension and eventually congestive heart failure. The older adult with underlying cardiac disease is most sensitive to NSAID-induced renal adverse effect. Although controversial, sulindac, nabumetone, and the nonacetylated salicylates (e.g., salsalate) may be renally sparing.

Concomitant chronic administration of aspirin and acetaminophen (e.g., Excedrin) is ill advised, since this combination is highly nephrotoxic. Nonsteroidal antiinflammatory drugs can also inhibit platelet aggregation and increase the risk for hemorrhage. These agents should be used with extreme caution, if ever, in clients receiving anticoagulation therapy (e.g., warfarin, heparin). Moreover, NSAIDs inhibit bronchodilatory prostaglandins and may cause or exacerbate asthma. Clients with a history of asthma, nasal polyps, and rhinorrhea are most susceptible.

Histamine$_2$-Receptor Antagonists

All available histamine$_2$-receptor antagonists are readily available over-the-counter, including cimetidine, ranitidine, famotidine, and nizatidine. While all of these agents are equally effective in equipotent doses, some agents are associated with significant drug-drug interactions. Cimetidine is a potent inhibitor of the hepatic cytochrome P-450 system and may decrease hepatic clearance and increase serum concentration of propranolol, diazepam, chlordiazepoxide, flurazepam, procainamide, quinidine, phenytoin, theophylline, and warfarin. Ranitidine has only mild effects on these agents; however, in some clients, a pronounced effect will occur. Both famotidine and nizatidine weakly bind to the hepatic cytochrome P-450 system and are not associated with any significant hepatic cytochrome P-450 drug interactions. Spacing medications is ineffective in preventing hepatic cytochrome P-450 interactions. Both cimetidine and ranitidine may significantly increase blood alcohol concentrations. Since histamine$_2$-receptor antagonists are primarily eliminated renally, dosage adjustment is mandatory. Excessive histamine$_2$-receptor antagonist concentrations will lead to a high prevalence of central nervous system toxicities, including confusion, lethargy, and headaches.

PHARMACOKINETIC AND PHARMACODYNAMIC CHANGES

The elderly have a greater propensity for adverse drug reactions because of the way their bodies handle drugs. Both pharmacokinetics (relating to the disposition of drugs in the body; i.e., absorption, distribution, metabolism, and elimination) and pharmacodynamics (relating to drug action in the body) are significantly altered in the elderly population. Significant interclient variability exists among these important factors. Each factor affects the manner in which an individual body handles drugs. When prescribing medications to the elderly, all factors must be weighed individually and collectively in order to decide on the most appropriate drug and dose. Conservative prescribing in the elderly—as stated in the old adage: "go low, go slow," meaning initiate therapy with very low doses and titrate upward slowly—is suggested and prudent.

Bioavailability

Bioavailability, defined as the rate and extent of drug absorption, is significantly affected by changes from aging. Normal gastrointestinal acid secretion declines with aging, and the resultant pH of the gastrointestinal tract may become alkaline. A lack of gastrointestinal acid can adversely affect the bioavailability of agents that require an acidic environment for absorption (e.g., iron, ketoconazole [see Table 8-4]). In such cases, these agents may have their absorption diminished to less than 1 percent, therefore losing their entire pharmacologic effect. To enhance bioavailability, acid-requiring agents may be administered with acidic supplements, such as orange juice, cranberry juice, glutamic acid tablets, and vitamin C.

As people age, they often develop diminished gastrointestinal motility, gastric emptying rate, and absorptive capacity. This may culminate in enhanced drug destruction in the stomach and lack of absorption in the small intestines. Anticholinergic drugs (e.g., propantheline, atropine), opiates (e.g., morphine, codeine), and other agents with anticholinergic-like effects (e.g., tricyclic antidepressants, neuroleptics, clonidine, methyldopa) may slow gastric motility. Conversely, elders with chronic diarrhea often display decreased drug bioavailability, since the drug will pass through the gastrointestinal tract before it can be absorbed. Agents that stimulate gastric motility include metoclopramide, cisapride, cholinergics (e.g., bethanechol, urecholine), reserpine, guanethidine, and guanadrel.

TABLE 8-4 • AGENTS REQUIRING ACIDIC GASTRIC MEDIA FOR ABSORPTION

Generic Name	Brand Name
Clorazepate Dipotassium	Tranxene
Enoxacin	Penetrex
Hydroxyzine Pamoate	Vistaril
Imipramine Pamoate	Tofranil-PM
Iron	Fergon, Feosol, Slow FE, Mol-Iron
Itraconazole	Sporanox
Ketoconazole	Nizoral

Distribution

Drug distribution is significantly altered in the older client. Elders have a decline in total body weight, lean body mass, and increased body fat. Total body fat content increases between ages 18 and 35 years from 18 to 35 percent in males and from 33 to 48 percent in females. Drugs that are distributed primarily in body water or lean body mass (e.g., lithium, digoxin, aminoglycosides [gentamicin, amikacin, streptomycin, tobramycin]) require lower doses than drugs that distribute primarily in fat. Additionally, when dosing a drug for the geriatric client, one must be cognizant that manufacturers' package insert recommendations are for young (20 years old), healthy, 70-kilogram adults with normal renal and hepatic function. Administration of full doses to an elderly client leads to an exaggerated drug response and adverse events. Therefore, based on weight, a 35-kilogram client should receive at most less than half the usual recommended dose.

Generally there is a decline in serum albumin either due to malabsorption/malnutrition syndromes or hepatic dysfunction. Drugs highly bound to serum albumin, approximately greater than 90 percent, will have a disproportionately higher free-drug concentration in the serum. Only the free drug traverses into cells to produce a pharmacologic effect. Drugs highly bound to serum albumin include weakly acidic drugs such as warfarin, aspirin, NSAIDs (e.g., ibuprofen, naproxen), phenytoin, valproic acid, carbamazepine, chlorpropamide, tolbutamide, and tolazamide. These agents may displace each other, based on the drug that has the highest intrinsic affinity for albumin. The displaced drug will initially exhibit an increased free concentration, resulting in an exaggerated pharmacologic response.

Metabolism

Hepatic metabolism, which is responsible for the majority of drug metabolism, decreases significantly with age. Hepatic mass and hepatic blood flow decrease over 45 percent between the ages of 25 and 65. Drugs that undergo phase-I metabolism in hepatic microsomes—often referred to as the mixed-function oxidase system (cytochrome P-450 system)—have decreased or unchanged clearance. Box 8-2 lists drugs that are hepatic enzyme inducers and inhibitors that undergo phase-I metabolism.

Drugs that induce the hepatic cytochrome P-450 system enhance the hepatic clearance of the substrate drug and decrease substrate drug serum concentration. For example, rifampin (a potent hepatic cytochrome P-450 microsomal enzyme inducer) will increase the hepatic metabolism and clearance of the estrogen component in an oral contraceptive (the substrate drug), resulting in decreased estrogenic concentrations and a possible subtherapeutic effect. Conversely, drugs that inhibit the hepatic cytochrome P-450 system decrease hepatic clearance of the substrate drug and increase substrate drug serum concentration. For example, erythromycin (a potent hepatic cytochrome P-450 microsomal enzyme inhibitor) will increase the hepatic metabolism and clearance of terfenadine (the substrate drug), resulting in increased terfenadine concentrations and possible toxicity.

Drugs that undergo phase-II metabolism, which involves conjugation, sulfonation, glucoronidation, and acetylation, do not require dosage adjustment since this metabolic method is not affected by age. Drugs that undergo phase-II metabolism include lorazepam and oxazepam. Unfortunately, hepatic function cannot be measured quantitatively, thus only empiric dosage adjustments can be made.

Elimination

Renal excretion declines progressively with age, approximately 1 percent annually beginning with the second decade of life. The decline in renal function may be attributable to a diminished number of functioning renal cells and absolute number of nephrons. Renal function may be measured by utilizing the serum creatinine. Serum creatinine is derived from creatine and phosphocreatine and is a major constituent of muscle. Creatinine is released from muscle into plasma and is excreted renally by glomerular filtration. A decrease or increase in the glomerular filtration rate of the kidneys result in a decrease or increase in the serum creatinine concentration, respectively.

BOX 8-2 • DRUGS THAT ARE HEPATIC ENZYME INDUCERS AND INHIBITORS

INHIBITORS

Alcohol (< 3 days use)
Allopurinol (daily dose > 300 mg)
Amiodarone
Chloramphenicol
Cimetidine
Ciprofloxacin
Clarithromycin
Diltiazem
Disulfiram
Enoxacin
Erythromycin
Fluconazole
Fluoxetine
Isoniazid
Itraconazole

Ketoconazole
Metronidazole
Miconazole
Phenelzine
Omeprazole
Propoxyphene
Quinidine
Quinine
Sertraline
Sulfinpyrazone
Sulfonamides
Trimethoprim/Sulfamethoxazole
Troleandomycin
Verapamil

INDUCERS

Alcohol (> 3 days use)
Aminoglutethimide
Carbamazepine
Cigarette smoking
Glutethimide
Griseofulvin

Marijuana smoking
Phenobarbital
Phenytoin
Primidone
Rifabutin
Rifampin

Generally, serum creatinine measurement allows for accurate determination of renal function. A normal serum creatinine is approximately 0.6–1.4 mg/dL. However, renal function should not be measured solely by using serum creatinine because this parameter also tends to decline with age due to diminished muscle mass and thus may not accurately represent renal function in the older client. To accurately assess renal function, creatinine clearance must factor in age, weight, and gender. The Cockroft and Gault Equation (Figure 8-1) is a simple equation that determines the creatinine clearance. The Cockroft and Gault Equation has been well studied and validated for accuracy. This equation will show that a 20-year-old client and a 70-year-old client may have the same serum creatinine (e.g., 1 mg/dL), but the 70 year old will have half the renal excretory capacity of the 20 year old. Hence, the 20 year old may have

Step 1: Calculate the patient's lean body weight (LBW)

   LBW for males in kg = 50 + (2.3) × (height in inches > 5 feet)

   LBW for females in kg = 45 + (2.3) × (height in inches > 5 feet)

Step 2: Calculate the patient's creatinine clearance (Clcr) from serum creatinine
   (Scr)

$$Clcr \ (mL/min) = \frac{140 - AGE \times (LBW)}{72 \ (Scr)^*} \quad \text{(Multiply by 0.85 for females)}$$

*If serum creatinine is less than 1, use 1; otherwise, use actual Scr.

FIGURE 8-1 • Calculation of Creatinine Clearance Using the Cockroft and Gault Formula

a calculated creatinine clearance of 100 mL/minute, compared to the 70 year old's calculated creatinine clearance of 50 mL/minute. Both are considered normal relative to age, yet the latter is obviously diminished.

If a drug is eliminated primarily via the renal route, decreased elimination will lead to accumulation and possible toxicity. For example, a standard dose of ampicillin 500 mg four times daily ordered for a 90 year old with a creatinine clearance of 15 mL/minute is excessive. Due to decreased renal function, ampicillin will accumulate in the body and may cause toxicity, manifesting with severe diarrhea and possibly seizures. Manufacturers' package inserts often contain dosing guidelines for clients with diminished renal function, based on the Cockroft and Gault Equation. Box 8-3 lists drugs that are significantly eliminated renally.

Pharmacodynamic Adverse Events

Pharmacodynamic changes involve concentration-response relationships and receptor sensitivity. The central nervous system exhibits a breakdown in its protective blood-brain barrier. The brain suffers atrophy and a reduction in cerebral blood flow and oxygen consumption. Inhibitory pathways (Gamma-aminobutyric acid [GABA], glycine) and excitatory pathways (acetylcholine, glutamate, and aspartate) are generally balanced to maintain cognition and behavior. This balance is altered in the elderly adult, evolving in altered cognition, anterograde (short-term memory) and retrograde (long-term memory) amnesia, confusion, hallucinations, and other mental status changes. Table 8-5 lists drugs that affect cognition and behavior in the older adult.

BOX 8-3 • SELECTED DRUGS THAT ARE SIGNIFICANTLY ELIMINATED RENALLY

Acetazolamide	Clonidine	Nadolol
Acyclovir	Diflunisal	Norfloxacin
Allopurinol	Digoxin	Phenazopyridine
Amantadine	Enalapril	Probenecid
Amiloride	Ethambutol	Procainamide
Aminoglycosides	Fluconazole	Ranitidine
Atenolol	Furosemide	Spironolactone
Aztreonam	Gabapentin	Sulfamethoxazole
Captopril	Lisinopril	Sulfinpyrazole
Cephalosporins (most)	Lithium	Thiazide Diuretics
Chlorpropamide	Methenamine	Trimethoprim
Cimetidine	Methotrexate	Vancomycin
Ciprofloxacin	Metoclopramide	

Extrapyramidal

Many elders are on neuroleptic agents, which are notorious for their extrapyramidal adverse effects. These adverse effects include dystonia, parkinsonism (akinesia), akathisia (motor restlessness), tardive dyskinesia, and neuroleptic malignant syndrome. Dystonia and tardive reactions predominate in the young; conversely, parkinsonian-like effects predominate in the old. The higher frequency of akinesia in the older population may be attributable to the age-related decline in the number of nigral cells, D2-dopamine receptors, and central dopamine concentrations. These factors enhance the dopamine receptor blockade of neuroleptics and predispose the elderly to a higher risk of drug-induced akinesia. Table 8-6 lists the offending neuroleptics. Metoclopramide is a non-neuroleptic with a high prevalence of extrapyramidal adverse effects.

Cardiovascular

In the myocardium, beta-receptor sensitivity declines with age, leading to a diminished effect of beta-blocker agents (e.g., propranolol). Elders tend not to respond to beta-blocker agents as well as young clients, yielding lower efficacy rates and necessitating higher doses. However, since these agents readily cross the blood-brain barrier, neurologic adverse ef-

TABLE 8-5 • SELECTED CATEGORIES OF ANTICHOLINERGIC DRUGS THAT AFFECT COGNITION AND BEHAVIOR

Therapeutic Class	Generic Name (Brand Name)
Antispasmodics	Belladonna Propantheline (Probanthine)
Antiparkinson	Benztropine (Cogentin) Trihexyphenidyl (Artane)
Antihistamine	Clemastine (Tavist) Brompheniramine (Dimetane) Chlorpheniramine (Chlortrimeton) Dexchlorpheniramine (Polaramine) Promethazine (Phenergan) Cyproheptadine (Periactin)
Antidepressant	Amitriptyline (Elavil) Clomipramine (Anafranil) Doxepin (Sinequan) Imipramine (Tofranil) Maprotiline (Ludiomil) Nortriptyline (Aventyl, Pamelor)
Antiarrhythmic	Disopyramide (Norpace) Procainamide (Procan, Pronestyl) Quinidine (Quinidex, Quinaglute)
Neuroleptic	Chlorpromazine (Thorazine) Clozapine (Clozaril) Mesoridazine (Serentil) Thioridazine (Mellaril)
Anxiolytic/Hypnotic	Hydroxyzine (Atarax, Vistaril)

fects with inherent neurotoxic beta-blockers such as propranolol, meto-prolol, labetalol, pindolol, and penbutolol may be exaggerated.

The elderly are highly susceptible to orthostatic hypotension due to diminished baroreceptor function and altered cerebral blood autoregulation. Orthostatic hypotension occurs in 20 percent of ambulatory clients over age 65, and in 30 percent over age 75 (Lipsitz, 1989). Clients with decreased cardiac output, clients receiving diuretics, and dehydrated clients are all at greater risk of orthostasis. Pharmacologic agents with a high propensity for orthostasis include potent vasodilators such as alcohol, nitroglycerin, isosorbide, prazosin, terazosin, doxazosin, guanethidine, guanadrel, minoxidil, hydralazine, angiotensin-converting

TABLE 8-6 • NEUROLEPTIC AGENTS AND RELATIVE INCIDENCE OF EXTRAPYRAMIDAL ADVERSE EFFECTS

Neuroleptic Agent (Brand Name)	Extrapyramidal Incidence
Chlorpromazine (Thorazine)	+++
Clozapine (Clozaril)	+
Fluphenazine (Permitil, Prolixin)	+++++
Haloperidol (Haldol)	+++++
Loxapine (Loxitane)	++++
Molindone (Moban)	+++
Perphenazine (Trilafon)	++++
Risperidone (Risperdal)	++
Thioridazine (Mellaril)	++
Trifluoperazine (Stelazine)	++++
Thiothixene (Navane)	++++

+ very low; ++ low; +++ moderate; ++++ high; +++++ very high.

enzyme inhibitors, tricyclic antidepressants, and neuroleptics. Of the tricyclic antidepressants, both desipramine and nortriptyline possess weak alpha$_1$ antagonist properties. Hence, they are least likely to induce orthostasis.

To minimize the risk of syncope and dangerous falls, clients should be instructed to dangle their feet for a few moments and to ambulate slowly from the supine or sitting to standing position. Avoidance of multiple orthostasis-inducing agents is suggested.

The renin-angiotensin-aldosterone system (RAAS), which preserves salt and water, becomes less efficient with age. When an elder is administered diuretics, the body attempts to maintain homeostasis by releasing renin and aldosterone, stimulating the RAAS system. Due to a diminished counter-regulatory RAAS, the older adult is at an enhanced risk of diuretic-induced dehydration and electrolyte disturbance. It was once thought that elders do not respond well to the effects of angiotensin-converting enzyme inhibitors (ACEIs)—perhaps due to a less efficient RAAS. However, recent data demonstrate equal efficacy for ACEIs among the young and old.

Endocrine

Many hypoglycemic elders will exhibit a diminished or nonexistent hypoglycemic symptom complex. Typical hypoglycemic symptomatology includes palpitations, tachycardia, tremor, and hunger, all of which are beta-adrenergic mediated. Elderly clients are often not aware that they are hypoglycemic until severe sequelae occurs, such as seizures, coma, and syncope. Tight control of hyperglycemia in the client with diabetes has become the standard of care; however, among elders, it may be associated with a significant risk of life-threatening hypoglycemia. Perhaps maintaining blood glucose at the upper limit of normal (100–125 mg/dL) or slightly above normal is preferable. Beta-blockers will blunt hypoglycemic symptoms and should be avoided in the diabetic older client when possible. Agents known to induce hypoglycemia include aspirin, pentamidine, disopyramide, quinidine, quinine, ACEIs, and high-dose sulfonamides.

Acute management of a hypoglycemic episode may include glucose tablets or gels, orange juice, or sugar water. Some clients keep a home supply of intramuscular glucagon for life-threatening hypoglycemia. The primary care provider needs to order this as part of the client's diabetic management. While glucagon is effective in the management of hypoglycemia, it has several limitations: (1) It requires adequate glycogen stores for gluconeogenesis—malnourished clients may be glycogen deficient. (2) It requires gluconeogenesis for activity; this delays its onset of activity, making it inherently slower than 50 percent dextrose in water. (3) Intramuscular injection requires adequate muscle mass for administration; older adults and people with diabetes often have poor muscle mass. See Chapter 15 for home care nursing management of diabetes.

Coagulation

Elders often require lower doses of the anticoagulation agent warfarin, due to enhanced intrinsic warfarin sensitivity. Additionally, less warfarin may be metabolized due to decreased hepatic clearance and more free drug may be available due to lower serum albumin concentrations. Moreover, warfarin is associated with many significant drug-drug interactions, specifically drug displacement and hepatic cytochrome P-450 inducer and inhibitor reactions. Malnutrition and malabsorption syndromes may lead to a decrease in vitamin K dietary supplementation, also culminating in a pronounced anticoagulant effect. Initial warfarin doses not exceeding 5 mg is recommended. Vigilant monitoring of the international normalization ratio is suggested and prudent. Clients may be sent home with a prescription for oral vitamin K, to be administered in the event of warfarin toxicity. Clients should be counseled to recognize the common signs and symptoms of bleeding, such as a general feeling of weakness, excessive gingival bleeding, epistaxis (nose bleeds), hematomas, hematuria, hemoptysis, hematemesis, and melena.

Clients who cannot tolerate oral anticoagulation agents may be placed on low-dose subcutaneous heparin (< 15,000 units daily in a 70-kilogram client). Low-dose heparin will not prolong the partial thromboplastin time; however, clients remain at risk for hemorrhage. Chronic heparin administration, even at low doses, has been associated with osteoporosis. To minimize the risk of osteoporosis, daily calcium with vitamin D supplementation is warranted.

Genitourinary

The genitourinary tract is adversely affected with aging in both women and men. In postmenopausal women, a decline in estrogen causes vaginal atrophy. Symptoms of atrophic vaginitis include burning, inflammation, pruritus, and occasionally bleeding. Estrogen replacement therapy effectively manages atrophic vaginitis.

Benign prostatic hyperplasia (BPH) is the most common cause of voiding dysfunction and one of the most frequent causes of disability in aging men. BPH is a nonmalignant neoplasm of prostatic epithelial and stromal tissue. BPH rarely occurs in men under 40 years of age. However, after age 40, the prevalence of BPH is age-dependent; approximately 50 percent of men over age 50 have moderate urinary difficulties due to BPH. By age 85, approximately 90 percent of men will have BPH (Brendler, 1994). Urinary symptoms of BPH may be irritative (e.g., dysuria, nocturia, urgency, frequency, burning) or obstructive (e.g., hesitancy, straining, dribbling, incomplete emptying). Many medications may exacerbate BPH and should be deleted from the client's medication regimen. Agents that exacerbate BPH include anticholinergics (e.g., disopyramide, tricyclic antidepressants, neuroleptics), alpha-adrenergic agonists, and calcium channel blockers (e.g., diltiazem, verapamil). General management of BPH includes alpha-adrenergic blockers, such as prazosin, doxazosin, and terazosin, and antiandrogens, such as finasteride.

In addition, there are many medications that inhibit libido and sexual functioning. These effects need to be discussed with the client, and the client must be given the opportunity to make an informed decision about the medication, substituting another if possible.

SUMMARY

This chapter gives the home care nurse invaluable information about common medication concerns with an aging population. The first concern deals with compliance and the client's cognitive and physical ability to administer medications safely.

Cost of medicines is a major dilemma for elders on fixed incomes, and drug effect and client health and safety may be compromised due to some behaviors initiated to stretch resources.

Many elders use over-the-counter medications, home remedies, and medications from other family members and friends. The safety of such practices needs to be monitored—the home care nurse being in an ideal position to effect safety changes as needed in these areas.

The final sections of this chapter give the home care nurse pharmacokinetic and pharmacodynamic information related to many common medications used by elders. It serves as an overview for the nurse who works with an ever-growing older population.

REFERENCES

Bess, F. H., et al. (1989). Hearing impairment as a determinant of function in the older patients. *Journal of the American Geriatric Society, 37,* 123.

Brendler, C. B. (1994). Disorders of the prostate. In W. R. Hazzard, E. L. Bierman, et al. (Eds.), *Principles of Geriatric Medicine and Gerontology* (3rd. ed., pp. 657–664). New York: McGraw-Hill.

Darnell, J. C., et al. (1986). Medication use by ambulatory older patients: an in-home survey. *Journal of American Geriatric Society, 34,* 1.

Fowles, D. G. (1991). *A Profile of Older Americans: 1991* (USDHHS AoA/AARP Publication No. PF3049). Washington, DC: U.S. Government Printing Office.

Kamada, A. K. (1994). Therapeutic controversies in the treatment of asthma. *Annals of Pharmacology 28,* 904–914.

Lamy, P. P. (1985). Patterns of prescribing and drug use. In R. N. Butler & A. G. Bearn (Eds.), *The Aging Process: Therapeutic Implications* (p. 53). New York: Raven.

Lichtenstein, M. J., et al. (1988). Validation of screening tools for identifying hearing impaired older patients in primary care. *JAMA, 259,* 2875.

Lipsitz, L. A. (1989). Orthostatic hypotension in older patients. *New England Journal of Medicine, 321,* 952.

National Center for Health Statistics. (1994). *Monthly Vital Statistics Report, 43*(6).

9

IMPROVING COMMUNICATION ABILITY OF OLDER ADULTS WITH HEARING AND VISION LOSS

Rae Lord Crowe

◆ ◆ ◆

Hearing and vision losses are common in older adults, increase in prevalence with longevity, and alter free-flowing communication. Some changes are a part of normal aging; others are related to diseases more prevalent in the later years, such as cataracts, diabetes, and strokes. These sensory deficits can affect the ability to perform many important daily activities, such as shopping, driving, and using the telephone. A loss of independence can lead to social withdrawal, depression, and cognitive impairment.

The home health nurse can prevent or postpone some conditions by teaching older adults ways to promote optimal hearing and vision. The nurse can identify community resources available to the client. In addition, screening to detect early hearing and vision loss followed by referral to the appropriate specialist can enhance treatment outcomes. The nurse can help older adults and their families understand the sensory changes associated with aging. With this knowledge, they can learn ways to compensate for these losses to optimize communication and independence.

◆ ◆ ◆

HEARING LOSS

Hearing loss is the most common sensory impairment in older adults, affecting half of all men and one third of all women over 65 years old (Eds. of Univ. of Calif. Wellness Letter, 1991). It is the third most prevalent chronic condition of the later years, surpassed only by arthritis and hypertension (USDHHS, 1991). Thirty percent of elderly adults living in the community self-report hearing problems, with 12 percent describing either unilateral or bilateral deafness (La Visso-Mourey & Siegler, 1992).

Studies suggest there is a 10 decibel (dB) reduction in hearing sensitivity per decade of life after age 60 (Heath & Waters, 1997). A decibel is a physical measurement that expresses the relative intensity of a sound. A whisper produces 20 dB, ordinary conversation is 60 dB, and potentially damaging sound, such as from a nearby revving motorcycle, is 85–90 dB (Eds. of Univ. of Calif. Wellness Letter, 1991).

IMPACT ON THE ELDER

Hearing loss is frequently an unaddressed problem for many older adults. Sixty-five percent of adults aged 85 and up report some hearing problem, but only 16 percent have a hearing aid or other assistive device and only 8 percent of these use their aid or device (Heath & Waters, 1997). Perhaps one reason so few elders seek hearing aids is that Medicare does not pay for these devices and the financial burden is on the client.

The major impact of a hearing deficit is the loss of free and easy communication. Socialization can become a chore. Trying to be attentive all the time can be very tiring for the person with a hearing loss. Hearing only parts of a conversation and knowing other parts are being missed can be frustrating and create tension. If listening is a continual struggle, hearing impaired people may choose to focus attention on only the parts of the conversation directed to them.

Hearing deficits irritate others because they impede communication. Having to repeat words or rephrase sentences hinders conversation and interrupts the speaker's train of thought. Frustration at being misunderstood can lead to shouting or to a minimal communication pattern of simple questions and answers.

The individual with hearing loss may feel lonely, depressed, and out of touch with others. Independence can be decreased as one struggles to carry out necessary daily activities, such as shopping and using the telephone. People may misinterpret the person's hearing loss as a cognitive or personality disorder.

A longitudinal research study examined the six-year impact of hearing impairment on psychosocial and physiological functions among adults age 65 and over (Wallhagen, 1996). Results suggest that these individuals had a significantly greater likelihood of depression and of perceiving their health as fair or poor when compared to those not hearing impaired. This is of concern as research suggests these indices are related to higher levels of morbidity and mortality. Thus, hearing loss may be indirectly associated with mortality. The hearing impaired also had a significantly greater likelihood of feeling left out, of just sitting and doing nothing and not enjoying their free time when compared to those not hearing impaired.

The home care nurse can use this information to educate the client, family, and caregivers. Understanding the psychosocial effects of hearing loss may eliminate unintentionally caused stress in a caregiving relationship and promote the quality of the client's life.

HEARING ASSESSMENT AND SCREENING

Responsibilities of the home health nurse include hearing assessment and screening, referral to a hearing specialist, and encouraging hearing rehabilitation for the hearing impaired older adult.

The home health nurse has the golden opportunity to see older persons in their home over a period of time. This can alert the nurse to cues suggestive of a hearing loss. These cues include failing to answer the doorbell or telephone, being late for appointments due to sleeping through the clock alarm, complaining that others always mumble, playing the radio or TV very loud, and avoiding social occasions such as parties and receptions where there is a lot of background noise.

The foundation of the hearing assessment is the client's health history, which includes specific questions about the client's health that may give some clues about the extent and perception of any hearing loss. Box 9-1 lists suggested questions to obtain a thorough hearing-specific health history and physical examination.

TYPES OF HEARING LOSS

Disorders in any part of the ear, the auditory nerve, or the brain can cause hearing loss. Hearing loss is often classified according to the component of the auditory system disrupted: conductive, sensorineural, or central.

Conductive Loss

In a conductive hearing loss, there is interference in the ear itself—a disruption in the transmission of sound in the external or middle ear to the internal ear. In pure conductive hearing loss, air conduction is worse than bone conduction on audiometric testing. Causes include otitis media, Paget's disease, damage to the tympanic membrane, cerumen impaction, and otosclerosis.

The most common cause of conductive loss in older adults is cerumen (earwax) impaction in the external ear canal. Cerumen is secreted by glands in the outer third of the ear canal. In non-Asians, the wax is a pale honey color, either dry or sticky; in Asians, it is usually gray, dry, and brittle. Clogged earwax is frequently overlooked, yet it is a reversible factor that occurs in 30 percent of older adults. The person with impacted cerumen may complain of tinnitus. Tinnitus is the hearing of sounds in one or both ears that are not occurring in the environment. Common descriptions of tinnitus are ringing, tinkling, bells whistling, and hissing. Management includes eardrops to loosen the earwax and, if indicated and if the tympanic membrane is intact, irrigation of the ear.

BOX 9-1 • HEARING-SPECIFIC HEALTH HISTORY AND PHYSICAL EXAMINATION

HEALTH HISTORY

Questions the home health nurse can ask:

1. Tell me about any disturbances in your hearing?
2. How do you rate your hearing: excellent, good, fair, or poor?
3. Do you hear better in one ear than the other?
4. Do you have problems hearing on the telephone, hearing soft voices, hearing children, or hearing in crowded restaurants and other noisy public places?
5. Do you have ear pain? Earaches? Infections? Discharge? History of recurring ear problems? Tinnitus? Vertigo? If the client answers yes to any of these questions, use symptom analysis to explore the problem and help the client describe the problem fully. Include:
   a. What causes the symptom? What makes it better or worse?
   b. What does it feel or sound like? How long does the experience last?
   c. Where is the symptom located?
   d. How bad is it? Is it getting better or worse?
   e. When did it begin? How often does it occur? Is it sudden or gradual?
6. What was your past and present exposure to excessive noise? Occupational noise? Noisy leisure activities?
7. Do you have a family history of hearing loss?
8. What is your medication profile—prescribed and over-the-counter drugs— (include dose, frequency, action, and effect)? If the client does not use over-the-counter drugs, evaluate further by asking specific questions:
   a. What do you do for a headache?
   b. What do you do for pain in your body?
   c. What do you do for a stomachache?
   d. What do you do for constipation? For diarrhea?
9. What is your medical history? What are your current medical problems?

The home care nurse should also assess the client's ability to perform instrumental activities of daily living (IADL), such as traveling, shopping, and telephoning. If family members, friends, or significant others are available, the nurse should ask if they have noticed any changes in the client's hearing ability.

(continued)

The most common cause of middle ear conductive loss is otosclerosis. Otosclerosis is caused by the formation of spongy bone, especially around the oval window, resulting in stiffening of the stapes, one of the three small bones of the middle ear. Symptoms include progressive

---

BOX 9-1 • Continued

PHYSICAL EXAMINATION

1. Inspect the ears for discharge, inflammation, and pain. If any are present, move auricle up and down, then press on tragus. Pain indicates acute external otitis. Pain behind the ear may indicate otitis media.
2. Conduct an otoscopic exam to inspect the external ear canal for discharge, inflammation, foreign bodies, and cerumen. Examine the integrity of the tympanic membrane. Normal color is pearl gray with a cone of light at 5 o'clock in the right ear, 7 o'clock in the left ear. A perforation appears as an oval hole with a shadow within.
3. A screening exam for hearing loss includes the whisper test. The whispered voice test is a fairly accurate, crude hearing test. However, it is insensitive to disorders of central auditory processing and speech understanding. To administer the whisper test, tell the client, "I am going to stand behind you. I will cover your left ear with my hand and whisper a word in your right ear. Please tell me what you hear." Standing behind the person, occlude the individual's left ear. At a distance of one to two feet from the person's right ear, breathe in and exhale completely to minimize voice intensity, then softly whisper a two-syllable word (e.g., baseball, nineteen, see-saw, postmark) or two numbers of equal length (e.g., one-two, nine-four) into the uncovered ear. Ask the person to repeat the word(s). Repeat this process for each ear twice, using different words each time. If the client cannot repeat the words, gradually increase your voice intensity until heard. (For more information on client assessment, see Chapter 3.)

---

deafness, especially for low tones. Amplification can assist to a limited degree. Surgical approaches that improve ossicle mobility have resulted in significant improvement.

Sensorineural Loss

Sensorineural hearing loss is caused by a dysfunction of the hair cells or cochlear nerve, a branch of the eighth cranial nerve, in the inner ear that interferes with the transmission of sound from the ear to the brain. There is a decrease in both the air and bone transmission of sound, especially toward higher frequencies.

The onset may be sudden as a result of a vascular event within the inner ear or an adverse effect of medication. This is often accompanied by vestibular (inner ear) symptoms of vertigo (clients may use the term dizziness). Vertigo is the subjective feeling of moving around in space or of objects moving in space around the self when no rotary motion is occurring. It is frequently accompanied by nausea and vomiting. Nystagmus (constant, involuntary, cyclical movements of the eyeball in any direction) and tinnitus may occur. Immediate referral is indicated. The symptoms place the individual at risk for falls and injury.

The onset may also be gradual and is usually accompanied by tinnitus. Causes include presbycusis (old man's hearing), long-term exposure to high intensity noise, and neoplasms of the brainstem or the vestibulocochlear nerve (eighth cranial).

Presbycusis is the most common age-associated hearing loss. There is a degeneration of the inner ear with the exact cause undetermined. It is characterized by progressive, high frequency (higher pitched tones) symmetrical sensorineural hearing loss. As it is progressive, lower pitched sounds are gradually involved. The occurrence, progression, and severity of the hearing loss varies from person to person. Heredity, exposure to excessive noise over time, and hypertension influence the progression of presbycusis. With a decrease in the perception of higher frequency tones, consonants are less audible so words sound like vowels. The person has difficulty understanding speech, especially the higher voices of young children, rapid speech, and foreign accents. Background noise (e.g., at receptions, in restaurants) further impairs the ability to understand speech. A disabling distortion of multiple sound is heard. The most important aspect of management is the person's recognition that a hearing loss has occurred followed by appropriate assessment by a primary care provider or professional nurse. A mix of strategies including referral to appropriate health professionals, amplification, speech/lip reading, and environmental adjustments can enhance hearing.

Exposure to excessive noise places one at risk for hearing loss. The Environmental Protection Agency has proposed that industrial workers be exposed to no more than 85 dB per 8 hours. The exposure time should be cut in half for every 3 dB over this amount. Millions of people use headphones (110 dB or more) to listen to music while jogging, working, or on long plane trips. Listening for 1.8 minutes with headphones is equivalent to working 8 hours at the recommended maximum level.

Metabolic causes of hearing loss include drugs (furosemide, nonsteroidal antiinflammatory drugs [NSAIDS], salicylates, vancomycin) and endocrine diseases (hypothyroidism, diabetes mellitus, renal disease).

Central Loss

Central hearing loss is an auditory processing problem secondary to higher brain level dysfunction, as found in strokes and neoplasms. A major problem seems to be speech discrimination. The older person has difficulty hearing soft voices and sounds at a distance, in groups, and over the telephone. Direct questions can often identify hearing loss undetected by the physical examination.

HEARING SPECIALISTS

Generally, an ear examination by a medical doctor can determine if medical or surgical treatment is indicated. If so, the client is referred to an otolaryngologist or an otologist. Both of these specialists are primary care providers—the former an ear, nose, and throat specialist; the latter an ear specialist.

If indicated, a referral is then made to a certified clinical audiologist who has a graduate degree in the measurement and treatment of hearing deficits. The audiologist tests hearing, evaluates for hearing aids, and can recommend and provide audiologic rehabilitation services. Services can include auditory training, speech/lip reading, counseling for the client and family, and dispensing of assistive devices. Medicare covers all but the purchase of a hearing aid.

A hearing aid specialist is a business person who may perform hearing aid evaluations and whose main purpose is selling hearing aids, accessories, and batteries.

MANAGEMENT OF HEARING LOSS

It is very difficult for people with impaired hearing to compensate for this loss by themselves. They depend on others to speak in ways that they can hear or speech-read. The home health nurse can instruct clients and family members in ways to improve hearing by using the two complementary strategies of enhancing nonverbal communication and using hearing amplification devices. Strategies to improve communication for the client with a hearing loss and for family members and other caregivers are provided in Boxes 9-2 and 9-3.

Hearing aids are the most common amplification devices. Research suggests they improve communication, cognition, and mood. Only

---

BOX 9-2 • STRATEGIES FOR THOSE WITH HEARING LOSS

- Do not ignore mild hearing loss.
- Participate in hearing rehabilitation: Learn speech reading, improve listening skills, and practice identifying speech in different situations. Speech/lip reading expands listening by encompassing the recognition of lip movements, facial expressions, body movements, and gestures. It is best learned in a structured program.
- Ask people to repeat or slow down if you do not understand them.
- Reduce background noise (turn off TV, radio). Use carpets and curtains to absorb background noise.
- Place furniture to facilitate conversation.
- In noisy places, try to sit near sound-absorbent surfaces (curtains, books, upholstery).
- Wear glasses, if necessary, because a speaker's visual cues aid comprehension.
- Wear false teeth or partial plates, if necessary, because teeth enhance bone conduction of sound.
- Let others know what makes conversation better or worse.
- Investigate amplification devices and close-captioned TV

10–15 percent of clients who could benefit from a hearing aid actually use one (USDHHS/PHS, 1994). Hearing aids require manual dexterity for correct use and have limitations. Older adults with arthritis may have difficulty or be unable to adjust volume, change batteries, or insert it in the ear.

Types of hearing aids include: (1) behind-the-ear—this is the most durable and easiest to adjust; (2) in-the-ear—this is the most popular; (3) in-the-canal—worn entirely within the ear canal; (4) eyeglass unit—this is the least popular; (5) on-the-body—aids worn on the body are for those with the most severe hearing loss.

Hearing aids are discreet, are adaptable for phone use and for specific frequencies, are cosmetically appealing, and have a relatively low battery drain. They do require a custom fitting and a great amount of manual dexterity, and they are expensive ($500 or more). Medicare pays for the audiology evaluation but not for the hearing aid itself.

Assistive listening devices, sometimes called pocket talkers, are set up and worn by the person with a hearing loss. They are similar to a SONY Walkman and utilize a microphone. The advantages are that they are directional, are relatively inexpensive, and loud amplification is possible. The disadvantages are that they are bulky, are visible in use, and batteries are rapidly drained.

BOX 9-3 • STRATEGIES FOR THE HEARING IMPAIRED CLIENT'S FAMILY MEMBERS AND CAREGIVERS

- Get the listener's attention first.
- Face the listener directly; have the light on your face.
- Avoid having the sun's glare or bright light behind you so the listener can see your visual cues.
- Do not hide your mouth with your hand or an object.
- Ask the person what you can do to make hearing you easier.
- Use facial expressions and gestures.
- Speak slowly and clearly with more pauses than usual.
- Use short, simple sentences.
- Rephrase rather than repeat a misunderstood sentence.
- Try to lower your voice. Don't shout.
- Maintain the same voice level to the end of the sentence.
- Do not turn and walk away while talking.
- Do not talk with your mouth full; it makes it difficult to see and hear what is being said.
- Converse in an area with sound-absorbing qualities.
- Cut out background noise by turning off the radio, TV, or running water.
- Use touch to gain attention.
- Use the listener's name to alert the person before speaking.
- If in a group, give clues to the hearing impaired person as to the topic of conversation.
- Write important information.
- Be relaxed and attentive.
- Be patient.

Hand-held telephone amplifiers and volume controls are available to attach to phones at home. These devices may be obtained from local telephone companies and many stores. Legislation requires that telephones be compatible with hearing aids.

Visual-alerting systems are available to use for smoke or fire detectors and as indicators that the telephone or doorbell is ringing. Regional telephone companies often have products for rent, lease, or purchase. These products may include loud tone ringing devices, impaired hearing handsets, amplified volume handsets, and light-signaling devices. The latter connects to an ordinary house lamp, which then flashes on and off each time the phone rings.

Closed-captioned television programs are available. Closed captioning provides a print output of the program's speech at the bottom of the TV screen. Decoders to access these programs are available through a variety of outlets.

RESOURCES FOR THOSE WITH HEARING LOSS

The following resources are available for professionals, clients, caregivers, and family members to contact for additional assistance in maximizing hearing ability (V = voice, TDD = telecommunications device for the deaf):

- American Speech-Language-Hearing Association (ASHA), 10801 Rockville Pile, Rockville, MD 20852. (800) 638-8255; (301) 897-5700 (V/TDD). A professional organization of speech and language pathologists and audiologists. Provides information on hearing aids, communication problems, and a *free* list of certified audiologists for each state.
- American Tinnitus Association, P.O. Box 5, Portland, OR 97207-0005. (503) 248-9985; (800) 634-8978 (V). A membership organization that carries out and supports research and education on tinnitus and other ear disorders. Provides resources to both professionals and patients on seeking help and information. Also provides cassette tapes of environmental sound that may provide relief from tinnitus. It has self-help groups for members.
- Hear Now, 9745 East Hampden Avenue, Suite 300, Denver, CO 80231-4923. Reconditions hearing aids, donates hearing aids, and funds hearing aids.
- League for the Hard of Hearing, 71 West 23rd Street, New York, NY 10010. (212) 741-7650 (V/TDD). Provides information and referrals, audiological exams, speech and language therapy, advocacy, and other services for the hearing impaired.
- National Association of the Deaf, 814 Thayer Avenue, Silver Spring, MD 20910. (301) 587-1788 (V/TDD). A membership organization with state chapters. Advocates for members and acts as an information clearinghouse. Request membership information and a *free* catalogue of publications.
- National Captioning Institute. (703) 998-2462. Provides captions for commercial, cable, and public television.

Manufactures and distributes closed-caption decoders for television.

- National Information Center on Deafness, Gallaudet University, 800 Florida Avenue NE, Washington, DC 20002. (202) 651-5051 (V); (202) 651-5052 (TDD). Provides information on a wide variety of topics related to deafness and hearing loss, referrals to local and community services, and a *free* catalogue of publications.

- Bell Atlantic Communication Center for Individuals With Disabilities, 280 Locke Dr., 4th floor, Marlborough, MA 01752. (800) 974-6006 (V/TDD).

- Self Help for Hard of Hearing People (SHHH), 7910 Woodmont Avenue, Suite 1200, Bethesda, MD 20184. (301) 657-2248. National membership organization with local and regional chapters. Provides information, support, and individual referrals. Has special program for elders and uses volunteers to provide support, teach coping skills, and train in the use of amplification.

- Telephone companies. Local telephone companies sell and lease assistive devices.

◆ ◆ ◆

VISION LOSS

Vision changes can begin slowly and go unnoticed for some time, especially among older adults. Vision loss may be related to the normal changes of the aging eye or to eye disease. Glaucoma, cataracts, and macular degeneration are the prevalent eye diseases in the later years of life. Many are unaware of their vision loss. Up to 25 percent of elders have incorrect corrective lens prescriptions, and over 90 percent of elders need corrective lenses (USDHHS/PHS, 1994).

The *Clinician's Handbook of Preventive Services* reports that approximately 13 percent of those 65 years of age and older report vision impairment. This increases to 28 percent of those 85 years of age and older, with over 25 percent reporting blindness or low vision (USDHHS/PHS, 1994). Low vision, or partial sight, is the term used to describe residual vision. Low vision acuity is determined by the best possible correction in the better eye. Moderate low vision is an acuity of

20/70 to 20/100. Severe low vision is an acuity of 20/200 to 20/400, or a visual field of 20 degrees or less. Legal blindness is defined as an acuity of 20/200 or less in the better eye with the best possible correction, or a visual field of 20 degrees or less.

IMPACT ON THE ELDER

Vision loss can impair the elder's physical, social, and emotional life. To meet the demands of daily living, new coping skills are needed at a time when other senses of touch, smell, and hearing may also be diminished. Routine tasks can be more troublesome, fatiguing, and frustrating. Leisure activities such as knitting, woodworking, reading, and watching TV may be compromised. Vision loss can lead to medication mayhem when one is unable to read the medication label. If curbs or stairs are less visible, the fear of falls may increase and force the person to remain in familiar surroundings. The risk for falls, hip fractures, automobile crashes, and other unintentional injuries increase. Grooming problems can affect personal appearance. Frustration with the inability to read newspapers, travel signs, and telephone dials can contribute to social isolation and depression.

NORMAL CHANGES OF THE AGING EYE

The home health nurse can help older adults and their families understand the ocular changes that occur with longevity. With this knowledge, the client and family can work with the nurse to manipulate the environment and improve visual acuity.

Impaired lens accommodation, decreased sensitivity to color and light, decreased tear viscosity, and increased eyelid laxity occur with aging. The pupils become smaller in size, and there is a 65 percent drop in the transmission of light through the lens from 25 to 65 years of age.

Impaired lens accommodation, or presbyopia, results from the loss of elasticity in the lens. The ability to focus sharply on close objects diminishes. The change is progressive, begins in a person's early 40s, and usually stabilizes around age 60. Vision can be corrected by using magnifying lenses (common reading glasses). Persons who wear prescriptive lenses can improve near and central vision with bifocals or trifocals. Decreased lens accommodation can also impair the older person's visual acuity in a darkened room, as well as vision when a bright light is turned on.

As aging occurs, it is more difficult to discriminate the short wave length light of blues and greens. This is also compromised by a yellowed, aging lens. The generous use of warm, contrasting colors (longer wave length light of red, orange, yellow) can help elders navigate their environment and manage their activities of daily living.

Small opacities can develop on the aging lens. Too small to cause vision loss, the opacities can cause the light entering the eye to scatter. Scattered light causes glare. Glare is usually a problem at night, as the pupil of the eye dilates in darkness. More of the lens is exposed. Oncoming headlights appear as blinding flashes of light, which affect the ability to see.

Tear secretions decrease, causing dry eyes. The wearing of contact lenses may be more uncomfortable and require frequent wetting of the contacts. The eyes may be more easily irritated and reddened. Lubricating the eyes with over-the-counter artificial tear drops is helpful.

VISION ASSESSMENT AND SCREENING

Responsibilities of the home health nurse include assessment, screening, and referral to an ophthalmologist for vision loss. A thorough assessment is imperative as the nature and extent of vision loss among older adults varies. The nurse is able to observe the older adult at home for signs of vision loss, which include squinting, holding reading materials close to the face, bumping into objects, and difficulty recognizing faces. Poor grooming reflected in stains on clothing, mismatched clothes, and uncombed hair may be due to visual deficits. The home care nurse should complete a vision health history and conduct a physical assessment of the eyes (see Boxes 9-4 and 9-5).

EYE DISEASES PREVALENT IN THE LATER YEARS

The three prevalent eye diseases of the later years are glaucoma, cataracts, and macular degeneration. Summaries of these diseases' incidence, signs and symptoms, and management are presented here. This generalized information is useful for home health nurse when assisting clients who experience vision loss.

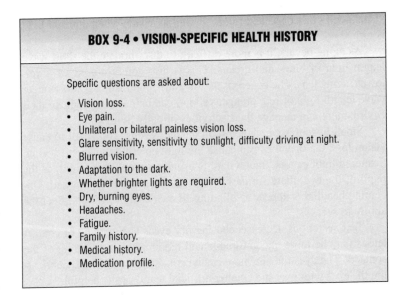

BOX 9-4 • VISION-SPECIFIC HEALTH HISTORY

Specific questions are asked about:

- Vision loss.
- Eye pain.
- Unilateral or bilateral painless vision loss.
- Glare sensitivity, sensitivity to sunlight, difficulty driving at night.
- Blurred vision.
- Adaptation to the dark.
- Whether brighter lights are required.
- Dry, burning eyes.
- Headaches.
- Fatigue.
- Family history.
- Medical history.
- Medication profile.

Glaucoma

Glaucoma is the leading cause of preventable blindness in the United States and the leading cause of blindness among African Americans. Glaucoma has been called the "sneak thief of sight" because it has no symptoms.

Glaucoma is an increase in intraocular pressure (IOP). IOP is determined by the ratio of fluid (aqueous humor) produced by the eye to the amount of fluid that leaves the eye. Normal IOP ranges between 10 and 21 mmHg. This fluid is necessary for the eye to function, that is, to keep the eye inflated and round. When all is well, the fluid made inside the eye equals the amount of fluid leaving the eye. If there is inadequate outflow of fluid from the eye, the fluid builds up and the eye's IOP increases. This damages the optic nerve; over time peripheral (side) vision is impaired. Central vision (the ability to see straight ahead) is not usually altered until much later and is followed by blindness.

Glaucoma is found in 5 to 10 percent of older adults in their 70s and in 2 percent of the population over 40 years of age. It causes 10 percent of all blindness in the United States (Ferri, 1997a). Glaucoma has no symptoms and develops over time.

Early detection and treatment of glaucoma is essential. The home health nurse assesses the client's risk factors for glaucoma. The risk fac-

---

BOX 9-5 • PHYSICAL EXAMINATION OF THE EYE

- Examine eye structures.
- Test pupillary reaction to light and accommodation.
- Assess for extraocular movements.
- Test visual fields for peripheral vision.
- Use a Snellen chart to test distant central vision.
- Use the Rosenbaum hand-held chart to test near central vision.
- Refer for ophthalmoscopic examination of red reflex, lens, and internal eye structures.
- Refer to ophthalmologist for glaucoma screening.

---

tors include: being over age 60, being nearsighted, family history, diabetes, previous eye injury, long exposure to oral cortisone products, and being of African American or Asian American descent. Armed with this knowledge, the nurse can help the client understand the need for periodic vision exams for early detection of an increase in IOP. The home health nurse must instruct all older adults in the importance of having a comprehensive eye exam, including screening for visual acuity and glaucoma, every one to two years by an ophthalmologist. Diabetic clients, at any age, should have exams at least yearly. Screening for glaucoma includes tonometer measures, a visual field test, and an ophthalmoscopy to directly visualize the optic nerve.

There are two types of glaucoma, chronic open angle glaucoma and acute angle closure glaucoma. Chronic open angle glaucoma is the most common. There are no symptoms, not even pain. Although there is no cure, it can usually be controlled with either eye drops or oral medication. Treatment must be continued for the rest of life. The home health nurse monitors the client's medication regimen, which may include instruction in the accurate instilling of eye drops. Some clients find it helpful to store eye drop medications in the refrigerator, since the coldness of the drop will tell them when the medicine makes contact with the eye. If more than one eye drop medication is taken, space the doses by allowing fifteen minutes between doses. The nurse can help the client and family develop a disciplined schedule. Laser surgery may be indicated if medication does not help.

Acute angle closure glaucoma is much less common. The IOP suddenly rises to very high levels as the eye drainage system is suddenly closed off or blocked. Symptoms are the sudden onset of eye pain, eye redness, nausea, vomiting, seeing halos around light, and a blurring of vision. Central vision is damaged rapidly. This is a medical emergency requiring immediate treatment by an ophthalmologist. Prompt management with medication and often laser surgery can resolve the problem.

Cataracts

A cataract, a normal consequence of aging, is an opacity or clouding in the lens of the eye. This usually results from an alteration of the metabolism and distribution of nutrients within the lens. A cataract usually occurs in a combination of the three layers of the lens: the nucleus, cortex, and capsule.

Some stage of cataract develops in over 50 percent of those 65–74 years of age, and in 65–70 percent of those over 75 years. Risk factors include aging, excessive exposure to sunlight, cigarette smoking, diabetes, high cholesterol/triglycerides, longtime use of oral cortisone medication, eye injury, and glaucoma. Knowledge of these risks empowers the home health nurse to inform the client of prevention measures.

Changes in vision can be related to the location and stage of the cataract. A nuclear cataract is the most common type of cataract related to the aging process. As the nucleus gradually becomes opaque, there is difficulty identifying colors and seeing at a distance. A cataract of the cortex is the next most common type, often affecting those with diabetes. Wedge-shaped opacities in the cortex result in problems with glare, loss of contrast vision, and difficulty with near and distance vision. A cataract under the capsule, or elastic covering, of the lens is common in people with diabetes, high myopia, and those taking cortisone. Glare sensitivity and blur occur.

Vision changes reported as a cataract develops include blurry distance vision, especially outdoors; seeing rays of light from headlights and stop lights; faded print lacking in contrast; and colors faded or changed in hue. Blue may appear green, and yellow may look like white. The person may instinctively shade eyes from the sun. Some people who wore glasses report being able to read the newspaper without glasses. This "second sight" occurs as the sclerotic lens causes myopia, which temporarily corrects presbyopia.

Diagnosis is made by the ophthalmoscopic examination. This permits assessment of the red reflex, direct visualization of the lens opacity, and the ability/inability to visualize details of the fundus of the eye.

The application of yellow-tinted filters to corrective lenses improves vision by reducing the blue components of light entering the eye. The wearing of sunglasses and wide-brimmed hats reduces daytime glare.

Surgical correction is indicated when corrected visual acuity in the affected eye is greater than 20/50, glasses no longer increase acuity, and normal activities are compromised. Cataract surgery is the most frequent surgical procedure in older adults. The objective is to remove the opaque lens and restore vision with an intraocular lens implant, removable contact lens, or glasses. The home health nurse guides the client in the management of the vision changes and decision for surgery.

Macular Degeneration

The macula on the retina of the eye provides the highest degree of visual resolution. Deterioration of the macula gradually leads to the loss of central vision and the detailed vision needed to read.

Thirty percent of adults 75 years of age and over are affected, but only 10 percent have significant loss (Heath & Hoepner, 1997; Ferri, 1997b). It is more prevalent in women than men and is the most common cause of legal blindness.

Macular degeneration is a painless, progressive loss of central vision. The first change noticed is reading difficulty. A complete loss of central vision means one cannot read at all, watch TV, play cards, drive a car, recognize faces, or do handwork. Peripheral vision remains intact and total blindness does not occur. The person can get around, do some cooking, cleaning, and gardening, but quality of life and mobility is severely restricted. An important role of the home care nurse is to recognize the extreme modifications that must be made with such an eye disease and to empathize with the client's possible anger, frustration, and depression over attempting to manage with such limitations.

MANAGEMENT OF VISION LOSS

The home health nurse assists elder clients and their families in managing vision losses. The nurse can help them understand vision changes that are occurring and ways to improve vision by manipulating the environment and using assistive devices to enhance vision. The nurse provides information about available community resources and encourages their use. The latter is especially important for elders with limited capabilities who do not have the assistance of family, friends, and neighbors.

BOX 9-6 • STRATEGIES TO ENHANCE VISUAL ACUITY

- Utilize contrasting light and dark colors to see things more easily.
- Use large-print books, clocks, timers, thermometers, and telephone dials. Use talking watches.
- Move nearer to things you wish to see better.
- Place chairs so you can easily see visitors.
- Use magnification devices.
- Use prisms and mirrors to decrease the impact of peripheral vision loss.
- Have corrective lenses evaluated by an ophthalmologist to ensure prescription is correct.
- Use community resources and national organizations whose purpose is to assist those with vision loss.

Coping with vision loss is difficult for those who have had problems dealing with impediments throughout their lives. Elders with other disabilities, such as arthritis or diabetes, may need additional healthcare supports. The home health nurse, in collaboration with other health professionals, can play a key role in helping these people be as independent as possible with the necessary supports to remain in their homes.

Older adults can alter their environments and their behaviors to enhance existing vision. Lighting changes include increasing the wattage of light bulbs, using indirect lighting, having a combination of fluorescent and incandescent lights, adding glowing light switches, and using night lights to illuminate hallways, bedrooms, and stairs to help adjustment to decreased light at night. Encourage elders to keep a small flashlight at the bedside to assist them to venture safely out of bed at night. A flashlight is also helpful when in dark areas outdoors. The use of sheer and lightweight curtains throughout the home to emit more natural light is a helpful suggestion.

Glare reduction is important, as most elders are severely affected by glare. Indoors, clients can use curtains and blinds to diffuse sunlight and decrease glare from windows. Changing or avoiding shiny surfaces that reflect light, such as waxed floors, reflective fixtures, and mirrors, helps if this if feasible in the client's environment. Using dimmer switches and indirect lighting reduces glare. At times, the client's TV is located where glare from windows and lamps block out the screen; rearranging the furniture and location of the TV can eliminate this annoy-

---

BOX 9-7 • GUIDELINES FOR FAMILY MEMBERS AND CAREGIVERS OF CLIENTS WITH IMPAIRED VISION

- Encourage independence.
- Identify yourself when approaching someone with impaired vision.
- State when you are entering or leaving the room.
- Offer help when light is inadequate.
- When in doubt, ask if assistance is needed.
- Use sighted-guide technique as necessary: The person with vision loss holds the arm of the sighted person and follows a few steps behind.
- Use community resources for information and assistance.

---

ance. Instruct clients to let people know if they cannot see their faces because of glare. Arrange seating during home visits so that the client is not facing a window.

There are also modifications that will make the outdoors more pleasant. Wear sunglasses, a wide-brimmed (3-inch) hat, or a hat with a visor when in sunlight. When dining out, select a seat to avoid glare. At nighttime, avoid looking into headlights of oncoming cars, and avoid driving at night if necessary. Many elders make modifications in their social lives by having luncheon rather than dinner dates and going to movie matinees (a better time of day for a large meal, and food and entertainment are less expensive as well) to avoid night driving. See Box 9-6 for ways to enhance visual acuity and Box 9-7 for family member and caregiver guidelines.

RESOURCES FOR THOSE WITH VISION LOSS

Local telephone companies and libraries are good, beginning resources to contact when dealing with vision loss. The following resources are also available for professionals, clients, caregivers, and family members to contact for additional assistance.

- Association for Macular Diseases, 210 East 64th Street, New York, NY 10021. (212) 605-3719. A membership organization that produces a newsletter and provides public education, support, and a hotline.

- The Glaucoma Foundation, 33 Maiden Lane, New York, NY 10038. (800) glaucoma (an eight-digit number, 4528-2662). Offers free information and referrals.
- The Lighthouse, Inc., 111 East 59th Street, New York, NY 10022. (800) 334-5497; (212) 821-9713. Provides special low vision services, rehabilitation services for blindness/vision impairment, and free information.
- LS&S Group, Inc., P.O. Box 673, Northbrook, IL 60065. (800) 468-4789. Offers catalogue specializing in products for visually impaired persons. Products include magnifiers, low vision and talking watches, devices with tactile markings, and household items. Single print copy is free; cassette is $3.00, applied to first purchase.
- National Center on Vision and Aging, 111 East 59th Street, New York, NY 10022. (800) 334-5479. Provides information on vision problems faced by older people and how these problems can be treated. Sells community education material. Conducts conferences and training programs.
- National Eye Institute, 31 Center Drive, MSC 2510, Bethesda, MD 20892-2510. (301) 496-5428. Offers free brochures on many eye diseases and conditions, such as glaucoma, cataracts, diabetic retinopathy, and age-related macular degeneration.
- National Library Services (NLS), 1291 Taylor Street, Washington, DC 20542. (800) 424-8567. Provides services for all print-handicapped people. Special talking books for seniors program. Provides machines to play audiocassettes for free. Each state has at least one NLS regional library.

◆ ◆ ◆

SUMMARY

This chapter covers the two most common changes adults experience as they age. Hearing and vision loss alters the elder's quality of life by limiting communication and mobility patterns. Hearing and vision losses also have a profound impact on an elder's ability to adapt to other medical problems.

Again, because of the intimate nature of the home health nurse's role, which allows entry into the client's environment, the nurse has the responsibility to assess the client's hearing and visual acuity. This is done both incidently as part of a home visit, by picking up on clues, or specifically, by gathering the information on a hearing and vision health history and physical examination.

Hearing and visual acuity can be enhanced through modifications in communication patterns and environmental changes. In addition, there are many community resources available to professionals, clients, families, and caregivers to enhance existing hearing or vision. There are eye diseases of specific concern to older adults, and the home care nurse can initiate definitive medical follow-up as needed, once the risk factors for them are recognized and the signs and symptoms are known.

The causes and progression of many hearing and visual losses cannot be prevented. However, the home care nurse can assess, educate, refer, and reassure the client, listening to the client's perception of the loss and providing the appropriate assistance based on the client's individual needs and the resources available.

REFERENCES

Editors of University of California–Berkeley Wellness Letter. (1991). *The Wellness Encyclopedia* (p. 322). Boston: Houghton Mifflin.

Ferri, F. (1997a). Glaucoma. In F. Ferri, M. Fretwell, & T. Wachtel (Eds.), *Practical Guide to the Care of the Geriatric Patient* (2nd ed., p. 208). St. Louis: Mosby.

Ferri, F. (1997b). Macular degeneration. In F. Ferri, M. Fretwell, & T. Wachtel (Eds.), *Practical Guide to the Care of the Geriatric Patient* (2nd ed., p. 210). St. Louis: Mosby.

Heath, J., & Hoepner, J. (1997). Vision. In R. Ham & P. Sloane (Eds.), *Primary Care Geriatrics* (3rd ed., pp. 378–382). St. Louis: Mosby.

Heath, J. M., & Waters, H. (1997). Hearing. In R. Ham & P. Sloane (Eds.), *Primary Care Geriatrics* (3rd. ed., pp. 383–388). St. Louis: Mosby.

Kenny, R. A. (1989). *Physiology of Aging*. Chicago: Year Book Medical.

La Visso-Mourey, R. J., & Siegler, E. L. (1992). Hearing impairment in the elderly. *Journal of General Internal Medicine*, March/April, 191–198.

USDHHS. (1991). *Aging America: Trends and Projections* (DHHS Publication No. [FcoA] 91-28001). Washington, DC: U.S. Government Printing Office.

USDHHS/PHS. (1994). *Clinician's Handbook of Preventive Services*. Washington, DC: U.S. Government Printing Office.

Wallhagen, M. (1996). 6-year impact of hearing impairment on psychosocial and physiological functioning. *Nurse Practitioner, 21,* 11–12, 14.

DEALING EFFECTIVELY WITH PHYSICALLY AND VERBALLY ABUSIVE ELDERLY CLIENTS AND FAMILIES

Margaret Walsh

◆ ◆ ◆

Defining and Differentiating the Level of Abuse
Investigating and Assessing Individual Incidents of Abuse
Interventions
Summary

One of the most significant challenges in home care is caring for the elderly client who is verbally and physically abusive. At times, a member of the household other than the client may be the abuser.

In order to address abuse, the nurse, other caregivers (volunteer and professional), client, and family members can all be considered participants in a complex set of relationships that either support or limit abuse. This chapter identifies the levels of abusive behaviors and the key steps in assessing abuse in the home. An important part of the chapter discusses interventions to contain or eliminate the abuse. These issues are of concern to both professional and paraprofessional caregivers.

DEFINING AND DIFFERENTIATING THE LEVEL OF ABUSE

It is important to bear in mind the wide range of abusive behavior. Four possible levels of abuse are considered here in defining and differentiating abuse:

1. Annoying, provocative, obnoxious, and compulsive behaviors.
2. Demeaning, humiliating, and emotionally hurtful behaviors.
3. Physically hurtful acts.
4. Physically dangerous, life-threatening situations.

Throughout the situations and discussion presented below, the term *caregiver* is used when the example provided may fit the home care nurse, another professional caregiver, or a paraprofessional, such as the home health aide or homemaker. Likewise, the *client's* behavior can apply instead or as well to the client's family members.

Level 1: Annoying, Provocative, Obnoxious, and Compulsive Behaviors

This is the least intense behavior category, and in many situations it is not abusive. However, these behaviors can be very difficult to deal with and the caregivers may feel abused. The following examples illustrate some typical behavioral patterns in this category. None of the following clients or family members have psychiatric diagnoses.

Situation 1. Clients with compulsive tendencies may have routines and rituals that require the home health aide to perform care in a specific way. These clients have an extraordinary need for control and may require such actions as putting items away in a specific cabinet, in a specific order; and using two squirts of furniture polish, not more. The precision required may make caregivers feel as if they are expected to act like robots. Often the only way for caregivers to successfully serve these clients is to accommodate their ritualistic demands. The caregivers are not actually being abused as much as they have entered into a rigid controlling system that requires them to give up their individuality.

Situation 2. In other situations, the client manipulates the caregivers by threatening not to accept care. The staff inadvertently feels more responsible for the client than the client does for self. One client insisted that the nurse who visited on Sundays bring the newspaper and pay for it herself or she would not be let in the apartment to do the wound dressing. Another client kept caregivers waiting at the door for half an hour before letting them in. Other clients may allow caregivers in the apartment but keep them waiting an hour before they permit their wounds to be dressed. These clients usually respond to firm limits, such as when caregivers state how long they will wait before assuming the client has refused the visit.

Situation 3. There are clients who are more interested in control than in service. Some clients may send caregivers away if they arrive 15 minutes early or will not permit caregivers into the apartment until exactly the right time. If the caregiver arrives 10 minutes after that time, the client may refuse service for the day. When these behaviors occur, it suggests the client may be over-serviced. It is wise for the case manager to have all caregivers keep a log to evaluate the exact tasks performed. Usually the evaluation reveals that service can be reduced or terminated with these clients.

Situation 4. Other clients demonstrate a reckless disregard for the caregivers. A client may insist that an aide push the client's wheelchair on very long walks (e.g., 30 city blocks) or go out in inclement weather or in the middle of the night. Limits can be set that reduce the number of blocks that the aide is permitted to push the client. Limits can also be set on outings with regard to weather and time of night.

Level 2: Demeaning, Humiliating, and Emotionally Hurtful Behaviors

Very often, a client masters the ability to zero in on the frailty of each caregiver. The client may verbally attack caregivers in ways that penetrate their defense systems and reduce them to tears or frustration. A client may talk to caregivers with such contempt that it induces humiliation, anger, and shame. Sometimes the abuse is not in the specific words used, but in the tone of voice, body language, and delivery. It is commonly believed that only 7 percent of communication is in the words spoken, 38 percent is in the voice tone, and 55 percent is in the body language. This means that 93 percent of the message is not in the words. Whenever a caregiver appears to overreact to what is said, the nonverbal behavior of the client may be carrying the aggressive aspect of the message. These types of abuse happen more frequently with paraprofessional caregivers. The home health aide spends more time in the home than the nurse and provides personal and housekeeping tasks. Some clients may interpret the aide's caregiving as maid or butler service, expecting a different level of care. Other clients may treat all people in service professions in hurtful ways.

Specific examples of demeaning, humiliating, and emotionally hurtful behaviors are:

- Cursing at caregivers, making demeaning racial remarks, or calling them names such as "stupid" or "dumb."
- Yelling and screaming at caregivers in the street or at the store, thereby publicly humiliating them.
- Threatening caregivers with lawsuits and with getting them in trouble so they will never work again.
- Creating "no win" situations for caregivers: If caregivers ask how the client wants something done, the client responds that the caregivers do not know what they are doing; if the caregivers do not ask, the client criticizes them, saying they are trying to take over the house. No matter what the caregivers do, they are wrong.
- Accusing a caregiver of stealing as a way to punish the caregiver for not doing exactly what the client wanted.
- Threatening to replace the caregiver who is carefully following the plan of care with a different caregiver (one who will do what the client wants despite the plan of care).
- Making verbal sexual overtures, comments that have sexual innuendos, or inappropriate requests. For example, the caregiver is asked to massage genitals or perform extensive perineal care when the client can do the care.

Most of these behaviors can be dealt with if the caregiver is firm and consistent with limits specifically defining the abusive behavior that will not be tolerated. If these behaviors occur with an aide, the nurse must be informed quickly and kept informed as the situation unfolds. Since the majority of abusive clients and families will disregard limits on abusive behavior, it is imperative that the caregiver back the limit up with a consequence, such as "time-out." With time-out, the caregiver stops performing tasks until the abuse stops or limits visits to when a nonoffending family member is present. These techniques are described in detail later.

Level 3: Physically Hurtful Acts

In homes where physical violence toward family members is permitted, a firm, speedy response from the nurse is crucial in preventing a pattern of abuse from becoming the norm in the relationship between client and caregivers. The response must communicate to the client and family that *under no circumstances* will workers be subjected to harm. Examples of hurtful behaviors include:

- Throwing something at the caregiver, such as water or food. A more serious variation is throwing urine or feces at the caregiver.
- Trying to hit caregivers with an object, such as a cane, walker, or wheelchair, or striking caregivers with their hands.
- Driving an electric wheelchair in a menacing way or trying to run over the caregiver.
- Biting or spitting at the caregiver.
- Sexually harassing caregivers by physically touching, propositioning, or threatening them. One client licked an aide from her ear to her throat during a stand-and-pivot transfer.

There are two hidden risks to the abusive client. One danger to the client who strikes out at a caregiver (even if the client is frail and cannot physically injure the person) is the ever-present possibility that the client may catch the caregiver off guard and the caregiver may actually strike back in an automatic, unconscious gesture of self-defense that could be hurtful to the client. Another possibility is that a caregiver may lose balance and drop the client if attacked during a transfer or wound treatment or when practicing ambulation.

Case conferences between staff and the client and family are useful in decreasing abusive behavior. It is imperative that agency staff "make a big deal" about the abuse. The message must be loud and clear that care cannot be rendered if caregivers are abused or threatened. In cases of sexual harassment and hitting, it is sometimes effective to replace female caregivers with male caregivers, if possible. If case conferences, time-out strategies, and changing the genders of the caregivers does not stop the abuse, then the client may need psychiatric evaluation and treatment. The client may not be appropriate for home care.

Level 4: Physically Dangerous, Life-Threatening Situations

A physically dangerous situation involves the use of force and is a police matter. In these situations, the caregiver may be threatened with a weapon or an actual physical trauma may be inflicted. Physical force may also be used to subdue the caregiver. Many of these situations have the potential to be life threatening. In other situations, the caregiver may witness physical violence toward members of the household and get hurt by being caught in the middle. Usually these cases will have Level 2 and 3 symptoms before a Level 4 event occurs. If caregivers are attentive, they may prevent a possible escalation to Level 4. Sometimes, however, events unknown to the caregiver will occur, such as when a family member returns from jail looking for revenge, or when a family member who is high on crack attacks the caregiver who will not give money. In homes where drug deals occur, there is always a possibility that violence can erupt due to deals gone bad.

In physically dangerous situations, agencies tend to take quicker action if the professional nurse, social worker, or physical therapist is in danger, as opposed to an aide. There seems to be hesitancy on the part of agencies to truly act on an aide's report. This common tendency should be acknowledged and compensated for by the home care nurse carefully investigating any and all complaints of potential danger.

The process of identifying the actual abuse taking place in the home is very complex, as is the planning of a strategy that will work with a particular client and family. This role usually belongs to the case manager, home care nurse, or supervising nurse. The goals are always to provide safe care to the client, continue service, and ensure the safety of staff.

INVESTIGATING AND ASSESSING INDIVIDUAL INCIDENTS OF ABUSE

There are basic steps that should be a part of each investigation of alleged abuse. The following information outlines how to investigate and assess incidents of abuse.

Define and Identify the Abuse

Define and identify the abuse as objectively as possible. It is very important for representatives of an agency to avoid righteous indignation and dramatic, emotional interventions. The assessment must be carefully done with meticulous attention to all the details. It is difficult to know whom to believe when there are conflicting stories. Thoroughness and avoidance of premature conclusions are the most useful skills in uncovering the truth. It is equally important that the investigation and intervention be done quickly, usually within 24 to 72 hours. All data should be documented explicitly, even curses and insults quoted exactly as heard.

When identifying behavior as abusive, the specific behavior should be described in detail. If the abuse is physical, a role play (portrayed as realistically as possible) is necessary to discern what happened. Many of the words used to describe a physical incident evoke powerful images in the listener. With role play, the report of abuse is sometimes found to be overly dramatized.

Identify Precipitating Events

What transpired up to the point at which the abuse occurred? Try to identify patterns causing stress for the client. Explore whether the client experienced the caregiver's behavior as objectionable. during a period of agitation, severely cognitively impaired clients may become violent if caregivers approach them in a particular way. Sometimes staff may unnecessarily provoke a client. If a precipitating event can be identified, a plan can be created that avoids such situations. For example, if the behavior only occurs in public, perhaps the aide should stop taking the client to the grocery store. If the behavior takes place when friends are present, the client should be requested to have friends visit after the service is given. If a certain family member is the cause, caregivers can be instructed to leave when that family member arrives. If the abuse only happens during a stand-and-pivot transfer, a mechanical lift can be used or the client can be transferred by a family member rather than an aide. If the abuse was precipitated by a caregiver provoking the client, the caregiver may need counseling or education (depending on whether the act was mean and deliberate or due to a lack of training).

Discern If the Perpetrator Intended to Hurt the Caregiver

Some acts are truly accidental. Others are a client's defense against perceived harm. It must be discerned if the client wanted to injure the caregiver. It is useful for caregivers to distinguish whether the abuse is directed at them personally or if it has nothing to do with them as human beings. Sometimes the abuse would be done to anyone performing a particular task. Caregivers are often able to recover from the emotionally hurtful effects of abuse when they realize it was not directed at them personally. This allows caregivers to detach in a way that is useful for psychological recovery.

Predicting the Potential for Violence

In assessing a family's potential for abuse, it is important to consider prior behavior. If an individual has a history of striking out, having altercations with neighbors, punching the mailman, or having been jailed for violent behavior, the likelihood is greater that the individual will resort to violence. If a client has been a victim of family violence, there may be a need for measures to protect the client. The presence of unsecured weapons should be carefully assessed. When families have a violent history and continue to brag about whom they are going to hurt in the neighborhood, caregivers should be concerned for their own safety. This alertness is sometimes missing in caregivers and should be cause for alarm.

Seeing What Is Really There

There is an old story that if one tries to cook a live frog by putting it in boiling water, the frog will immediately jump out. However, if the frog is put in tepid water and the heat is slowly turned up, the frog will relax and go to sleep and allow itself to be boiled. There is a comparable phenomenon that is known in home care. When the home health aide becomes a part of a home environment for a period of time, the aide loses the ability to discern what is dysfunctional because certain behaviors are found normal and acceptable in that particular home. For example, one nurse visited a family whose young adult son was disabled as the result of a shootout involving drugs. The father, a heavy drinker, had several guns on display above the son's bed. The nurse and aides took no notice of the guns. Later at a case conference, an aide reported that she found a five-year-old playing with a rifle one morning. Neither the aides nor the nurse had recognized the pattern of danger that was emerging given the family volatility and the presence of unsecured weapons.

The presence of all weapons should be documented and discussed with a nursing supervisor. Immediate action may be required if the caregiver is afraid or, as in this case, a young child is unsupervised. Depending on the nature of the danger a quick, firm response is necessary.

Assess the Meaning of the Abuse to the Caregiver

The degree of hurt inflicted by verbal abuse depends a great deal on the meaning the caregiver attaches to the abuse. If the caregiver is able to remain detached and not personalize the verbal abuse, then the abuse does not hit its mark and is not effective. Some caregivers can laugh at the absurdity of some of their client's behaviors. However, when a caregiver is in a situation for long periods of time (10–24 hours), the ability of the abuse to penetrate the caregiver's emotional boundaries increases. Even if the caregiver does not take it seriously, the constant haranguing can negatively affect self-esteem and mood.

Assess the Client's Self-Control Capacity

In designing an intervention, it is crucial to assess the client's ability to control the behavior. This is accomplished by diagnosis, history, and observation. There are mental illnesses and dementing conditions that severely impair or destroy the client's ability to control behavior.

It is important to observe clients to see if they can control their behavior under any circumstances. If one finds that the client can act appropriately in front of primary care providers, psychiatrists, or when at the store, it is possible that the client can exercise control in the home. However, when assessing ability, it is important to remember that part of the nature of dementia is the day-to-day fluctuation in capacity. When in doubt, it is often useful to assume that the person has control and institute behavior modification techniques that may engage the internal control mechanisms. If the client has been judged as not having control or if the behavior modification techniques do not work, the only answers to relentless or serious abuse may be medication, nursing home placement, or reduction of service and reliance on family.

Assess the Client's Capacity for Relationship

Assess the client's relationships with friends, family, and caregivers. The client who has friends and family who care and keep in touch has learned how to be in a relationship. The client who is isolated and without friends may be unable to sustain any relationship. In these situations, the client has often driven people away. If the client is attached to the caregiver and displays behavior that suggests it is important for the client to preserve the relationship, there is a much better prognosis that the client can learn to control the abuse than if the client is detached from the caregiver and unable to permit anyone to get close. The latter frequently dismiss caregivers, especially if the caregiver does a good job. For them, closeness must be avoided because it makes them too vulnerable and anxious.

INTERVENTIONS

There are a few clinically sound interventions that work to contain or eliminate abuse. The following suggestions are the most useful.

Caregiver Logs

One of the best ways to closely monitor a difficult situation is to have the caregivers keep detailed logs. This gives accurate data about the situation. Paying attention to the incidents in this way is itself a very powerful and subtle intervention. Caregivers feel more connected to solving the situation because they are working together to track the abuse. The client may self-correct the problematic behavior if the client is aware that notes are being kept.

The logs can also be used to assess whether the hours of care match the tasks performed and, more importantly, to assess the client's needs. Tensions can increase between the client and caregiver when the caregiver does not have enough work to do.

To maximize the usefulness of the logs, case managers need to be very clear about what they want reported. They may be interested in food intake, verbal abuse, a client's sleep/wake patterns, or the level of client's independence in personal care. Some caregivers need special training in writing logs. If there is verbal or physical abuse, the case manager must ask the caregiver to describe incidents explicitly.

Debriefing Caregivers Outside of the Home

Caregivers may be reluctant to fully report incidents to a case manager (nurse) while in the home of the client. It has been found that nearly every interview conducted in the office elicits new information that was never shared with the nurse. Why is this? One explanation is that the client and family members punish the caregiver if they "tell their business." The punishment inflicted on caregivers may take the form of complaining to them and making their day miserable, or they may ask for their removal. Most people can appreciate how it must feel to report required information to a supervisor and have one's integrity questioned because of telling the truth and doing the job correctly.

Additionally, there seems to be a common phenomenon that caregivers shut down and do not speak up near the home of a client, even if the case manager walks with caregivers to the car or out to the elevator, or takes them into a private room in the home. This "shut down" is observed frequently. It is hypothesized that caregivers adopt a coping style that is in part characterized by a passive mental state that limits assertive language. Psychodynamically, this is akin to a counter-transference response. Clearly, it is found that the best information is obtained when the caregiver and case manager have time to sit together and talk in a neutral, safe atmosphere. Caregivers become more verbal and assertive when they feel safe and treated as colleagues. New information is shared that the caregiver may not even realize is significant. Caregivers should always be compensated for debriefing time in the office.

A Contract for Care

When discussing limits, it is useful to establish a contract. The contract must be specific, and it should be very clear what consequences will ensue if the contract is violated. The process of establishing a contract begins with the nurse clarifying the home care expectations of the client and family. A plan of care is devised that matches the realistic expectations of the client, with caregiver duties outlined. The nurse must be able to supervise each part of the contract. Therefore, it is useful for the home health team to identify how they will track each item in the contract. Contracts are usually established at a case conference. It is imperative that the understandings, the contract, and the consequences be summarized in a letter to the client and family. A copy should go to the primary care provider and a copy should be kept in the agency.

Consequences for Abusive Behavior

The key to eliminating abusive behavior is to develop therapeutically appropriate consequences. Telling clients and their families that they cannot do something is meaningless unless there is an immediately felt consequence. The use of consequences, however, assumes that clients can exercise control over their behavior; if they cannot, the following techniques may not be appropriate for them.

A powerful and simple consequence for clients who have the capacity to enter into a relationship is to reduce contact with the nurse and other caregivers. When the client is abusive, the caregiver withdraws to a safe distance and refuses to assist the client until the abuse stops. Time-out is a form of this. Basically, the caregiver asks the client to stop the offensive behavior. The client is then told if it does not stop, the caregiver is going to go into the next room (or out in the hallway or apartment lobby) for a period of time (anywhere from 5 to 15 minutes, depending on the client's mentation, ability to wait, and degree of abuse).

The nurse must give very clear guidelines for time-out. The caregiver must act accordingly and remain in contact with the home health agency office. It is important not to use time-out for clients who are unsafe alone or for clients who are so vindictive and masochistic that they will deliberately hurt themselves to express rage. Administration and legal counsel should be consulted if a situation seems risky. The primary care provider should be consulted and agree on the use of time-out.

After the time-out, the caregiver returns and asks the client if it is all right to continue with the service. If the client again resumes the abusive behavior, the caregiver repeats the steps, but increases the amount of time-out. If the client is abusive a third time, the caregiver should call the office. Depending on the case, the office will decide how to handle the situation, which may include calling a family member to stay with the client until alternative arrangements can be made. Alternatively, The office may send the nurse out for a supervision visit to determine options available.

Time-out is also useful for caregivers because it takes them away from the full force of the client's rage and can help the caregivers stay in control. In 95 percent of cases, time-out works when it is applied consistently. However, for clients with very powerful personalities, it may be necessary to use time-out on each caregiving visit for two weeks before the client stops testing the limits and comes to the realization that no means no.

With clients who are demented, psychiatrically ill, or so committed to abuse that they would rather jeopardize themselves, time-out may not be appropriate. In these situations a psychiatric evaluation, intense counseling (3–5 times the first week), and medication may be the best option. Sometimes these interventions can be combined with time-out.

If a client refuses psychiatric intervention and if the abuse is significant, then it is imperative that an assessment of the client's competency be made. If the client is competent, then the agency might consider administrative discharge with a referral to the local governmental agency that is responsible for "Protective Services for Adults." It is also possible to offer to refer the client to a skilled nursing facility or to discharge the client to the care of the family. Discharge proceedings should be carefully done after all other options have failed. The administrator and legal counsel should give final authorization to the administrative discharge. Home health agencies are private organizations, and to discontinue service is always an option and should not be overlooked. To risk the health and safety of good employees for the sake of one client or family is not sound judgement. The primary care provider must be informed and consulted throughout all stages.

Another effective consequence is a conference that includes the client, family, case manager, administrator, and all caregivers to discuss the abuse. This is very labor intensive for the agency, but the sheer unpleasantness of being "called on the carpet" for abusive behavior may serve as a deterrent. At the case conference, it is important that the staff make a "big deal" and be outraged by the abusive behavior, but do so in an appropriate and therapeutically sound manner. Remember, often less is more. A few powerfully delivered sentences by the nurse or administrator may be enough. This process serves to define the "rules of the game," the norms of working together. When not done overtly, then, by default, the norm becomes the abuse.

The home health team should always prepare before meeting with the client and family. Team members should prepare for the client conference with the exact details about the abuse, clarity regarding outcomes to be accomplished during the conference, and specific consequences that will ensue if the abusive behavior continues. When there are several family members involved, it is useful to include all of them in the case conference. It is important to ask the family to select one person who will be the spokesperson for the family. It may also be necessary to limit who the client or spokesperson may contact at the agency, usually the case manager or nursing supervisor.

Another form of consequence is to allow the client some degree of inconvenience. For example, a family member may be called at work to come to the client's home to cover for an aide who leaves before an eight-hour shift is over, or to have family members take the client for physical therapy because the agency's therapist refuses to visit the client at home. This disrupts family members' lives and may motivate them to put pressure on the client to stop the abuse. Family pressure is very effective with clients, even those with compromised mentation.

Another possibility is to suspend service if it is safe for the client to be alone or to get services outside of the home. This creates inconvenience and a loss of comfort and may motivate a change in behavior. Usually the service is put on hold until a case conference can be held to renegotiate the situation.

Publicizing the misbehavior within the confines of confidentiality may also serve as a deterrent. As many authority figures as possible should be involved, such as the primary care provider, social worker, psychologist, psychiatrist, and any family members who may be able to convince the client to eliminate the behavior.

Refusing to allow caregivers to participate in specific tasks or having caregivers do so at inconvenient times is another possible deterrent. For example, if a client runs the wheelchair too fast and the home health aide cannot keep up, the client may lose the privilege of having the aide's company. If a client fondles a female PT, a male PT who can only visit at inconvenient times may be substituted.

When there is difficulty with a family member, a common consequence is to negotiate that service only be provided so long as the family member is not in the house. This is especially necessary if the family member has threatened or sexually harassed the caregiver.

Whenever a client apologizes for being mean or abusive, it is important for the caregiver not to relieve the client's guilt. The caregiver acknowledges the apology and accepts it, but at the same time is clear that the behavior hurt and should not happen again. Note the following example of an interchange between caregiver and client: The client says, "I'm sorry I gave you such a hard time yesterday." The caregiver responds, "I appreciate your apology, and you did give me a hard time. When you spit in my face, I felt humiliated and very angry. Please don't ever do that to me again." Or, "When you threw your food on the floor, I felt frustrated. Please don't do that again."

When a client apologizes, the aide is often moved to say, "It's all right. I know you were having a bad day." The client may interpret this response as permission to continue to act abusively. Many clients have no guilt when they abuse. If a client does demonstrate guilt, the caregiver should reinforce the guilt and not relieve the client of it. The presence of an apology or guilt is a good prognostic sign for change in the abusive behavior. It is a sign of someone who has the capacity to be aware of "the other"—a necessary ingredient in relationships. Do not undermine this healthy guilt.

Understanding and Depersonalizing Abuse

Attempting to discern the psychodynamic purpose of the abusive behavior is an internal intervention by which the caregiver seeks to achieve or maintain a therapeutic openness. It is especially important when a caregiver is working with a client for a long period of time or for extended hours in a day.

Example 1. A home health aide was working with a very abusive client. When the time came for the aide to go on vacation, she decided not to tell the client because she believed the client would harass her. The aide just did not show up one day, and the agency sent a replacement. Only then was the client told that the aide was on vacation. The client was distressed that the aide had left him and was appropriately angry that he had not been told. When the aide returned, the client punished her by giving her an exceptionally difficult day. The aide was devastated. She had been working for him for about two months. She cared deeply about this client and could not believe how he was treating her. When she understood the following underlying psychodynamic causes, the aide found it much easier to accept the client's behavior.

The reason the client treated her with such bitterness and hostility was because he was attached to her and found her leaving painful. With this understanding, the aide could then interpret the client's behavior objectively. Consequently, she was able to reach a state of equanimity regarding the punishment. The aide was able to weather the bad day, knowing it would pass and recognizing it was payback for not preparing the client for her vacation.

Example 2. Another aide had a client who yelled and screamed at her the day before she went on vacation. This aide recognized how painful her vacation was to the client. She turned to the client and told him she was going to miss him, too. The client started to laugh. He recognized that the aide's message was, "I understand that you are yelling at me because you are going to miss me and my leaving makes you angry."

Understanding the causes frees caregivers from the tendency to personalize the client's struggle. Caregivers may need help interpreting some difficult behaviors. They should be taught to understand the complex process of a client's attachment to them.

Self-Evaluation of Care

Examples of sadistic behavior on the part of the client have been described above. It is equally important to realize that caregivers (professional and paraprofessional) can also be sadistic, sometimes in very subtle ways, toward clients. This is a dance of the shadow side of the personality that gets very little attention in professional literature or nursing investigation. Everyone has a shadow or dark side—despite how caring, loving, and selfless one is, the opposite is also true within one's personality. All people carry the potential to be sadistic, dominating, and hurtful. Caregivers sometimes behave in ways that unnecessarily provoke anger in clients and families. Typical behaviors that may have a sadistic theme include keeping clients waiting, creating inappropriate expectations by not being clear, making promises that are not kept, exaggerating a client's behaviors, taking incidents out of context, posturing as a victim (blaming the client for things that are not the client's fault, such as the staff's inability to say no or a lack of communication among team members).

When a client is abusive or difficult to manage, it may in part be due to staff performance issues. This is not to say that when caregivers perform inappropriately they deserve to be verbally or physically abused. There are many times, however, when passively aggressive maneuvers are used toward clients against which the clients have no recourse. People with undiagnosed psychiatric disorders or who are experiencing intense helplessness may resort to verbal and physical abuse when they see no other option.

Sometimes the client's verbal or physical abuse precedes the staff's passively aggressive maneuvers. The staff justifies this behavior as a necessary response to the client's difficult behavior. Oftentimes, it is difficult to decide who initiated the dysfunctional dynamic, but this is not necessarily important. What is important is that the caregivers, both professional and paraprofessional, assume responsibility to behave therapeutically and professionally. The caregiver, by virtue of the role, is responsible for taking the lead in ending the dysfunctional pattern.

SUMMARY

It is clinically useful to think of abuse on a continuum. This gives the nurse perspective and reduces the tendency to overreact to the provocative nature of abuse. It also helps keep the nurse alert and to avoid becoming lulled by the chronicity or subtleness of the abuse.

It is important for the nurse to avoid premature conclusions by carefully assessing reports of abuse. This chapter provides a variety of interventions that give the nurse accurate and substantive information, that create a document trail, and that limit abusive behavior so care can be safely rendered to clients. These steps also serve as a base for prudent administrative discharge if it is found that a client cannot be serviced and is a danger to self or staff.

By doing a thorough investigation of reports of abuse, the nurse can identify: the possible purpose served by the abuse, the precipitating events, the client's ability for self-control, the degree of client attachment to the caregiver, the client's capacity to be in a relationship, the intent of the perpetrator to hurt the caregiver, and the potential for violence in the home.

In-office debriefing is a key technique for obtaining thorough information and for solidifying the relationship among team members. This form of communication enhances the likelihood that caregivers will report incidents to the case manager quickly and in entirety. In addition, daily logs of selected issues keep the nurse up to date with the events of the case as they unfold.

Strategies for eliminating abuse include time-out, contracts, case conferences, and therapeutic consequences. Managing a case that involves abuse of the staff is very complex and necessitates as deep an understanding of the psychodynamics of the client and family as possible.

After completing the investigation and detailing reports from the caregivers, the nurse must discern which strategies to apply. The goal is to intervene in such a way that the client or family is motivated to stop the abuse. Compliance with the service contract must be monitored so there is no doubt in the client's and family's minds that the agency means what it says. The primary care provider should be kept informed of all developments and initiatives. The primary care provider's direction and permission may be needed for interventions.

While assessing the abuse and possible interventions that might be useful in a case, the case manager should continually evaluate the possibility that the dysfunctional interactions may be in part due to unsuitable behaviors of caregivers. Effective remediation by counseling and training should enable the staff to support a plan of care that maximizes the possibility the client can continue to be served by caregivers who work free from abuse.

11

CARING FOR THE ELDERLY CLIENT WITH URINARY AND BOWEL PROBLEMS

Janice H. Hentgen
Marilyn Oppong-Addae
Victoria D. Tanico

◆ ◆ ◆

NORMAL URINARY CHANGES ASSOCIATED WITH AGING
Strategies for Maintaining Normal Urinary Patterns
Urinary Pattern Problems and Nursing Care

NORMAL BOWEL CHANGES ASSOCIATED WITH AGING
Strategies for Maintaining Normal Bowel Patterns
Bowel Pattern Problems and Nursing Care

SUMMARY

This chapter assists the home care nurse in promoting the continuation of bladder and bowel patterns that are normal for the client. At times, as people age, changes occur in the lower GI system and urinary tract system that cause more disconcerting distress than many healthcare professionals realize.

Ideally, if the home care nurse can promote regular elimination patterns, it will enhance the client's self-esteem and promote independence in other health areas. First, the nurse needs to know the normal age-associated changes in these systems and ways to promote control and regularity. With some clients, changes in patterns are caused by disease or surgery, and teaching, monitoring, and completing adaptive treatments are part of the home care nursing role. Becoming familiar with ways to help clients restore control of elimination patterns or cope effectively with temporary or permanent elimination adaptations is the goal of good home care nursing.

◆ ◆ ◆

NORMAL URINARY CHANGES ASSOCIATED WITH AGING

As with all other bodily systems, the urinary tract system undergoes age-related changes. However, age alone does not cause incontinence. There are changes that may contribute to making it more difficult to maintain bladder control. Older adults have a mild increase of residual urine, a slight decrease in bladder capacity (often first noted in late middle age with trips to the bathroom at night that were not needed when younger), increased involuntary bladder contractions, and a decreased ability to postpone voiding. It is not understood why, but elders produce and excrete more urine at night.

In women, there is a decrease in estrogen levels after menopause that affect pelvic floor musculature and sphincter support. The decrease in estrogen levels can cause atrophic vaginitis and urethritis, both of which affect continence. The pelvic supporting tissues may also be affected secondary to perinatal trauma occurring in childbirth. Women are generally more susceptible to urinary tract infections (UTIs) than men due to the shortness of their urethras.

Among men, the incidence of benign prostate enlargement causes pressure on the urethra, which results in decreased urinary flow and obstruction. If clients have a history of UTI and chronic urinary retention, the detrusor muscle may become fibrotic, resulting in a compromised bladder with less control (Staab & Hodges, 1996).

STRATEGIES FOR MAINTAINING NORMAL URINARY PATTERNS

When conducting the physical assessment, the home care nurse can determine if the client is experiencing any voiding pattern problems or bladder control occurrences that are new, problematic, or indicative of other health complications. By listening to the client's concerns, the nurse can begin to discover the underlying cause and plan strategies that are appropriate.

Strategies for regaining healthy voiding patterns are many and varied and more will be covered later in this chapter (Box 11-1). There are strategies that the home care nurse can recommend to maintain urinary tract health if retraining the body to respond to a pattern is the strategy of choice. The strategies listed can be used with all adults, regardless of age, and can be used in conjunction with items mentioned for clients with incontinence issues addressed in the next section.

1. Maintain hydration: This takes six to eight eight-ounce glasses of fluid a day—preferably water, but other liquids can be counted, such as tea, juice, decaffeinated coffee (caffeine is both a bladder irritant and a diuretic), soda, and nondairy-based soups. If there are no dietary restrictions, any favorite fluids can be figured into the requirements. Milk is considered a food and does not meet fluid requirements.

2. Establish a voiding pattern: This is important to assist the client with comfort and to avoid infections and incontinence episodes. Voiding no more frequently than every two hours in conjunction to eating or drinking is a helpful guideline to follow. Voiding more frequently involves additional trips to the bathroom (which take energy and effort on the part of the client and caretaker) and doesn't allow the bladder a chance to feel full enough to stimulate an urge response. A pattern also eliminates the chance that the client will forget when the last was, which can eliminate accidents at worst and uncomfortable episodes of urgency at best.

3. Establish proper perineal hygiene habits: Cleaning the perineal area after voiding should always be done from front to back. This should be routinely taught to female clients. Teach clients to wash hands *after* voiding to protect others, and it should be recommended to wash hands *before* voiding as well. Clients who have unclean hands may infect themselves by accidentally touching the perineal area when cleaning after voiding.

4. Treat signs and symptoms of UTI immediately: For many elders, the early signs and symptoms of UTIs may go unrecognized. Younger adults experience the local symptom of burning upon urination, but this is not a symptom among most elders.

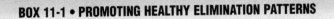

BOX 11-1 • PROMOTING HEALTHY ELIMINATION PATTERNS

- Drink at least 6 to 8 glasses of water per day
- Implement a toileting routine that incorporates the daily routine (voiding approximately every 2 to 4 hr)
- Increase dietary fiber and bulk in the diet
- Respond as soon as possible to the urge to move bowels or empty bladder
- Daily bowel movements are not essential for good health; bowel movements every 2 to 3 days are more common
- Avoid prolonged use of laxatives or enemas
- Avoid using mineral oil; it can interfere with vitamin absorption
- Engage in physical activity within personal limitations
- Report any changes in bladder or bowel habits, blood in urine or feces, abdominal pain, or weight loss

---

Symptoms may only be recognized when the infection spreads to the bladder or kidneys and the client experiences back or flank pain, fever, confusion, or disorientation. Maintaining adequate fluid intake and proper perineal hygiene are the best preventive measures.

URINARY PATTERN PROBLEMS AND NURSING CARE

Incontinence

The most common urinary tract problem is incontinence. All urinary tract issues that home care nurses deal with revolve around bladder training techniques; assistive or modification devices, such as bladder catheterization (intermittent or continuous); and surgical modifications, such as managing elimination through a urostomy. The nursing interventions in client urinary management include client and family teaching; supervising, monitoring, and implementing interventions; and evaluating outcomes.

Steps to Incontinence Management

The choice of urinary management strategy depends on the problem's cause and the client's potential and prognosis. If it is possible to retrain the bladder, the following steps are useful for the home care nurse to follow:

Step 1—Assessment. Identify the problem by completing a detailed history, performing a complete physical examination, and evaluating the functional status of the client. The assessment includes the diagnoses (both primary and secondary), the symptoms (urgency, dysuria, frequency and episodes of leakage), and the type, onset, and pattern of urinary incontinence. Also, note mobility (whether the client uses a commode or urinal) and mental status (is the client alert to recognize bladder fullness and know where the toilet is located). Determine if the client is motivated to self-toilet. Assess diet and fluid intake, and note if the client is dehydrated, constipated, or consuming drinks with caffeine.

Evaluate the relationship of incontinence to the client's diagnosis. If the client has diabetes, glycosuria can cause incontinence. Review the client's medications, including side effects. Follow up with the primary care provider regarding any significant rectal, abdominal, or pelvic examination findings. Review the client's urinalysis and any other test results that may have implications for urinary status.

Step 2—Establish a nursing diagnosis. Some examples of nursing diagnoses that address alterations in urinary function by type of disorder are stress incontinence, related to decreased outlet resistance; urge incontinence, related to detrusor instability or irritation; urinary retention, related to enlarged prostate and medications; and functional incontinence, related to decreased physical or cognitive capability.

Step 3—Gather baseline voiding information. Have the client, family, or other caregiver record voiding time, amount, and continence status. The fluid intake (time, amount, type of fluid, especially caffeinated beverages) is also noted. Remember, the home care nurse is the key to successful data collection and, subsequently, the appropriate program selection and successful treatment outcome. It is critical that the same caregivers remain with the client's program for at least two weeks. This data collection process may take a week or more to gather enough data to observe a pattern and determine the plan of action.

Step 4—Plan an individual program for the client. Information gathered from the nursing assessment and the voiding record will help determine which, if any, program a client is most appropriate for. The program options include habit training (scheduled toileting), relaxation training,

Kegel exercises, bladder retraining, and dietary management (primarily increasing fluid intake).

Step 5—Implementing the program. After determining the appropriate management program, establish goals and expected outcomes with realistic time frames for implementation. The client, family, and caregiver should be involved in the interventions and goal setting. Continue monitoring voiding patterns and adjust toileting times as necessary. Time may need to be increased or decreased between toileting activities. Fluid intake should be regulated to six to eight eight-ounce glasses (1,400–1,900 cc) per day at designated times, unless contraindicated by a medical condition. All fluids should be caffeine free, as caffeine is both a bladder irritant and a diuretic.

Step 6—Evaluation. Continue to monitor the client's progress based on meeting specified objectives. Redefine goals and timing if necessary. Periodic reassessment of urinary function is needed to ensure that the intervention and program choice continues to be the appropriate one for the client. Schedules, diet, fluids, medication, and the environment may need to be adjusted.

Treatment Programs

Behavioral management is very effective for clients who are diagnosed as having stress, urge, or functional incontinence. Habit training, relaxation training, instruction in pelvic floor muscle exercises (Kegel exercises), and bladder retraining increase the client's awareness of the lower urinary tract and can enhance control of the detrusor and pelvic muscular function. These techniques are participatory, relatively noninvasive, and generally free of side effects. Highly motivated individuals without cognitive deficits appear to benefit most and are the best candidates for inclusion in behavioral programs. According to the National Institute of Health's consensus statement on *Urinary Incontinence in Adults,* "As a general rule, the least invasive procedures should be tried first."

Habit training. This training is defined as determining an interval during which the client can be continent and gradually increasing this interval to approximate a normal voiding pattern of every three to four hours. This is also called scheduled toileting.

The objective is to keep the client dry and avoid incontinence, not to modify bladder function. To perform this procedure, keep accurate voiding records for 72 hours. Based on the pattern observed in the voiding record, establish a toileting interval, usually every two to four hours. In general, a typical toileting schedule for 24 hours includes toilet upon awakening, after breakfast, lunch, and dinner, and before bedtime, and once or twice during the night, depending upon when the client went to sleep and the toileting interval established. Void on schedule in the toilet, commode, or bedpan/urinal, whichever is most suitable (even when incontinence episodes occur), to assure bladder emptying. Increase fluid volume to at least six to eight eight-ounce glasses of fluid per day, unless restricted for medical reasons. This helps to increase bladder capacity and dilute urine, which helps in preventing UTIs.

When establishing the interval between voiding, negotiate the interval with the client and family to reflect lifestyle patterns and to increase compliance. Provide consistent encouragement and positive feedback. When there are no episodes of incontinence for 24 hours, increase the toileting interval by one-half to one hour.

Relaxation training. This training involves practicing relaxation techniques in response to the urge to void. Urgency with urine leakage is a significant cause of incontinence in the elderly. The objective is to help the client control the urge to void, thereby creating time to reach a toilet and reducing the incidence of urinary incontinence. Instruct the client in how to relax in response to the urge to void. Success in controlling the urge should be noted on the voiding record. Some suggestions for effective relaxation techniques include taking several deep breaths or thinking of a pleasant situation. When reduction or elimination of the urge to void occurs, the client should walk unhurriedly to the bathroom, bedside commode, or receive assistance with the bedpan/urinal to void. Accidents are more likely to occur when rushing to the bathroom. The home care nurse and care providers should give consistent encouragement and positive feedback.

Kegel exercises. Kegels involve improving urethral resistance and urinary control through the use of active exercise of the pubococcygeus (PCG) muscle. The objective is to strengthen the voluntary periurethral and pelvic floor muscles to reduce the incidence of incontinence in women and men. The PCG muscle is also used to hold back the passing of flatus.

To identify the correct muscle, voluntarily stop and start the stream of urine. This is a helpful exercise in itself. To determine if the muscle is contracted, place a gloved finger inside the vagina or rectum and squeeze the PCG muscle around the finger. The abdominal, thigh, and buttock muscles should be relaxed if the PCG is appropriately contracting during Kegel exercise. The client can place a hand on the abdominal muscles to ensure that there is no movement. Most clients prefer to sit or lie down when doing these exercises, but they can be performed anytime, anywhere, since the muscle is internal and there is no visible sign of exercising.

These exercises will be effective when they are taught properly and reinforced often. They require the client's understanding, cooperation, compliance, and participation. Instruct the client to squeeze the PCG muscle and hold for a count of ten seconds. Then relax for ten seconds. It is just as important to relax as it is to contract this muscle. Repeat the exercise 15 times in the morning, 15 times in the afternoon, and 20 times at night, or exercise for ten minutes, three times a day. A kitchen timer can be used to let the client know when ten minutes have elapsed. The client should work up to 25 exercises at a time. Initially, clients may not be able to contract the PCG muscle for ten seconds, but, slowly, over several weeks, they should be able to work up to ten-second holds. After two weeks of consistent daily exercise, fewer incontinence episodes should be noticed. In a month, a bigger improvement will be seen. Once clients have identified and are developing strength in this muscle, they must be instructed to use this muscle during any behavior or activity that causes incontinence, such as coughing, lifting, and laughing. Continue to track accidents on the voiding record to help the client and caregiver note progress and provide encouragement to continue the exercises.

Bladder retraining. This helps to promote continence by gradually increasing the intervals between voiding in an attempt to correct the habit of frequent voiding, to suppress bladder instability, and eventually diminish urgency. The objective is to restore normal bladder function by adjusting voiding patterns. Unlike habit training, in which the voiding schedule is adjusted to the needs of the client, bladder training encourages the client to adopt an expanded voiding interval.

Bladder retraining is individualized and is a time-consuming process. Voiding records should be accurately kept for 72 hours. When usual voiding times have been established, arrange for the client to be toileted one-half hour prior to the next expected time. If there is no observable voiding pattern, toilet the client at one-hour intervals, beginning upon wakening in the morning and continuing hourly until bedtime. The client should be awakened to void at less frequent intervals during the night.

Timing is crucial to success, and the client, family, and caregiver need to be aware of the intense time commitment this program requires. When the client has remained dry most of the time for one week, the toileting interval should be increased to two hours, and finally to three hours. Some clients will never be able to retain urine longer than two or three hours, but others will regain more control. The program is based as much as possible on the client's pattern before voluntary control was lost, is designed to reestablish or begin a pattern, and is flexible enough to be modified to the client's needs. Toilet on schedule in the toilet, commode, or bedpan/urinal, whichever is most suitable, even when incontinence episodes occur, to assure bladder emptying. Increase fluid volume to at least six to eight eight-ounce glasses per day, unless restricted for medical reasons. This helps to increase bladder capacity, and the urge to void can be felt more easily with a full bladder. Restrict fluids after dinner to minimize nighttime incontinence. Continue to record intake and output on the voiding record. Monitor progress and make adjustments to the voiding schedule and fluid intake as necessary.

Some triggering techniques to help the client void when toileting include running water at the sink, placing hands in a basin of warm water, drinking warm fluids, pouring warm water over the perineal area, or applying light pressure over the bladder area with the hands (Crede). Provide the client privacy during toileting and place toilet tissue within easy reach. Help the client relax by offering a magazine to read, since relaxation is important to elimination. Do not rush the client. Allow the client to sit on the toilet, commode, or bedpan for about 15 minutes. A shorter time is too rushed and more time defeats the purpose. Give consistent encouragement and positive feedback. If an accident or relapse occurs, focus the attention on every success that is achieved each day.

Types of Persistent Urinary Incontinence

There are different types of persistent urinary incontinence: urge, stress, overflow, and functional. In the elderly, these types may be seen in combination and referred to as "mixed." It is important to determine the types of incontinence in order to select the best method of management.

Urge incontinence. Most commonly seen in the elderly, urge incontinence is the involuntary urine loss associated with a sudden, strong desire to void. It is caused by an unstable bladder or detrusor instability, isolated or associated with central nervous system disorders such as stroke, parkinsonism, Alzheimer's disease, brain tumor or aneurysm, and spinal cord injury. It can also result from detrusor hyperexcitability due to cystitis, urethritis, atrophic vaginitis, tumors, stones, prostatic hypertrophy, and diverticulitis.

The sudden urge to void, called urgency, does not allow enough time for a client to reach a toilet or obtain a bedpan or urinal. The volume of urine loss is usually several hundred milliliters with complete bladder emptying. The timing of incontinence is usually predictable and can occur in any position and at any time, day or night. Urge incontinence is frequently associated with other voiding complaints, most often frequency, nocturia, and suprapubic discomfort. Dysuria (painful urination) indicates the presence of infection or inflammation of the bladder or urethra. Urge incontinence is usually managed by placing the client on bladder retraining, using pads, and using a bedside commode or bedpan/urinals. Adjusting the intake of fluid, planning a schedule of voiding, and prompted voiding may also alleviate this. The major objective is to reduce the chance of triggering an uninhibited detrusor contraction by regulating the frequency of voiding and preventing the bladder from being overdistended.

Stress incontinence. Stress incontinence is the involuntary loss of urine associated with sneezing, coughing, laughing, lifting, walking, and other forms of exertion that increase intra-abdominal pressure. In women, it results from sphincter dysfunction due to relaxation and weakness of the pelvic floor musculature and to reduction in urethral resistance. Accounting for about 50 percent of all incontinence, stress incontinence is most common in women, especially those with multiple childbirths, estrogen deficiency, or trauma to the external urinary sphincter. It also occurs in men due to pelvic trauma or sphincter injury after prostatectomy. It is characterized by small to moderate amounts of urine leaking simultaneously with exertion when intra-abdominal pressure exceeds urethral resistance. The voiding record will usually show frequent wetting in small amounts during the day while the client is active and reduced or absent incontinence at night while the client is in bed.

Stress incontinence is best managed with urethral sphincter exercises, along with Kegel exercises, to strengthen the pelvic musculature. These exercises consist of contracting and relaxing the external sphincter to increase its tone and urethral resistance. The success of these exercises is predicated on locating the pelvic muscles and practicing 100–200 contractions per day, which may not be practical for the frail, confused elderly client. An absorbent pad may be required until control is achieved. Dietary restriction of caffeine may also be helpful. Surgical intervention to suspend the bladder, remove a tumor, or implant an artificial urinary sphincter can be beneficial for some. However, surgery may be contraindicated in the elderly.

Overflow incontinence. Overflow incontinence is involuntary urine loss associated with an overdistended bladder. This implies that the bladder cannot empty completely, retains urine, becomes overdistended, and then overflows. A hypotonic detrusor from neurologic dysfunction or a bladder that does not contract due to diabetes or spinal cord injury can lead to chronic urinary retention and overflow incontinence. Bladder outlet or urethral obstruction due to enlarged prostate, urethral stricture, or bowel impaction can lead to urinary retention and produce overflow incontinence. The chronic use of tranquilizers can also create a hypotonic bladder. Overflow incontinence is characterized by leakage of small amounts of urine, either periodically or continuously. This will be evident in the incontinence record. Signs may include a palpable or percussable bladder, suprapubic tenderness, and a hesitant, interrupted urine flow.

Pharmacologic management may include decreasing or eliminating tranquilizers, as they can cause urinary retention. Muscle relaxants may be helpful in decreasing bladder outlet resistance. Cholinergics will increase the pressure within the bladder, but are not always effective and can result in permanent kidney damage in the elderly.

Functional incontinence. Functional incontinence occurs when a normally continent individual is either unable or unwilling to get to the toilet in time. Bladder and urethral function is essentially normal. Immobility, due to impairment of cognitive or physical functioning, psychological unwillingness, or environmental barriers to toilets are associated with the problem. With functional incontinence, large volumes are voided with total emptying of the bladder in inappropriate situations. It is typically seen with impairment of mobility or dexterity (e.g., with arthritic or stroke patients), making toileting difficult. The unavailability of assistance with toileting, unfamiliar settings, lack of accessible toileting facilities, and cognitive impairment or confusion around toileting procedures may also lead to functional incontinence. Other causes include medications that impair mobility, dexterity, or awareness; physical or chemical restraints; environmental barriers to the toilet (clutter, inadequate lighting in and around the bathroom); and sensory impairment, including poor vision, hearing, and speech (to communicate the need to toilet).

Treatment should focus on removing the physical or psychological barriers to continence. If the client requires assistance with toileting, prompt attention should be provided to calls for help. Bedside commodes, bedpans, and urinals should be made available if toilets are inaccessible or if the client is unable to reach one. Lowered dosages or changes in medications that contribute to confusion, drowsiness, or incontinence may solve the problem. Physically painful disabilities should be treated with analgesics and physical therapy, if appropriate, to regain or maintain mobility and dexterity. Clients who have dementia or who are incontinent due to psychologic disorders often respond to habit training or scheduled toileting. Absorbent pads and pants or external collection devices (mainly for men) may be the appropriate management device if the client fails to respond to other treatment modalities.

Reversible Causes of Incontinence

There are four major categories of medications that can cause incontinence: sedative hypnotics, diuretics, drugs with anticholinergic properties, and adrenergic agents. Sedative hypnotics are metabolized poorly by the elderly. They can cloud the sensorium and may leave traces that are measurable in the client's urine for two weeks after one pill has been given. Diuretics may deposit, suddenly, two liters in the bladder and overload the urinary tract system, causing incontinence. Anticholinergic drugs—which include antipsychotic medications, antidepressants, antihistamines, and drugs used for diarrhea—can produce urinary retention and allow the urine to build up until it overflows. Adrenergic agents either stimulate the sympathetic nervous system or block it; the sympathetic nervous system controls the bladder outlet. Nose drops, such as oxymetazoline hydrochloride (Afrin) and phenylephrine hydrochloride (Neo-Synephrine), will tighten the bladder neck and can result in urinary retention. Drugs used for hypertension block the sympathetic nervous system and thereby open up the bladder neck, producing stress incontinence.

Irreversible Incontinence

Detrusor instability is a common type of incontinence among the elderly. Due to underlying illness or physiological changes, the client loses control over the detrusor muscle in the bladder. With this disorder, the bladder contracts when it shouldn't or fails to contract when it should. Brain damage caused by diseases such as Alzheimer's, CVA, or Parkinson's disease can result in this type of incontinence.

Other causes unrelated to brain damage may fall in this category. Irritation of the bladder from radiation, a bladder stone, or cancer of the bladder may cause incontinence. Neurologic damage could be the cause, such as a slipped disc, a surgical procedure that damaged the nerves, or a peripheral neuropathy due to diabetes or syphilis.

In overflow incontinence, the bladder doesn't empty properly when full and the urine begins to leak from a full bladder. This can be caused by an anatomic obstruction, such as prostate, stricture, or cystocele. A contractile bladder due to diabetes or spinal cord injury may also cause overflow. Surgery, medication, or catheterization may help.

Bladder outlet obstruction is common in elderly males and is usually due to prostate enlargement or urethral stricture. Women who have had multiple deliveries may have outlet incontinence. This type of obstruction is frequently corrected surgically.

Urinary Retention

Urinary retention is the accumulation of urine in the bladder with inability of the bladder to empty fully. Urine collects in the bladder, stretching its walls, causing feelings of pressure, discomfort, tenderness over the symphysis pubis, restlessness, and diaphoresis. Urine production slowly fills the bladder and prevents activation of stretch receptors. After distending beyond a certain point, the bladder becomes unable to contract.

A key sign of urinary retention is the absence of urine output over several hours and the formation of bladder distention. The client under the influence of anesthetics or analgesics may feel only pressure, but the alert client has severe pain as the bladder distends beyond its normal capacity. In severe urinary retention, the bladder may hold as much as 2,000 to 3,000 mL of urine. As retention progresses, overflow may develop. Pressure in the bladder builds to a point that the external urethral sphincter is unable to hold back urine. The sphincter temporarily opens to allow a small volume of urine (25 to 60 mL) to escape. As urine exits, the bladder pressure falls enough to allow the sphincter to regain control and close. With retention overflow, the client voids small amounts of urine two or three times an hour with no real relief of distention or discomfort. Bladder spasms may occur with the voiding. Retention occurs as a result of urethral obstruction, surgical trauma, alternations in motor and sensory innervation of the bladder, medication side effects, and anxiety.

Bladder muscles weaken with age, which may promote the retention of large volumes of urine. The most common cause of retention in women is fecal impaction. Hypertrophy, present to some degree in most older men, is the primary cause in men. Symptoms of retention include urinary frequency, straining, dribbling, palpable bladder, and a feeling that the bladder has not been emptied.

Retention can predispose older individuals to the development of urinary tract infections. Good fluid intake and efforts to enhance voiding should be emphasized, including voiding in an upright position, massaging the bladder area, running water while attempting to void, and soaking hands in warm water.

Catheterization

The purposes for using catheters to empty bladders include relieving discomfort of bladder distention and providing decompression, obtaining a sterile urine sample when the bladder empties incompletely, and long-term management of clients with spinal cord injuries, neuromuscular degeneration, or incompetent bladders.

Intermittent catheterization is considered when the client has an obstruction to urine outflow (for example, prostate enlargement) or undergoes surgical repair of the urethra and surrounding structures. Intermittent catheterization is also indicated for the client with urethral obstruction from blood clots, for the client who is critically ill or comatose (as a means to measure output), and for the client who needs continuous or intermittent bladder irrigations.

Long-term use is indicated for clients with skin rashes, ulcers, or wounds that are irritated by contact with urine; clients who are terminally ill; clients with a neurogenic bladder; and clients for whom bed liner changes are painful.

The catheterization technique used for older adults is no different from the technique used for younger clients. The only difference is that the client may not be able to assume a sustained position for insertion of the catheter. Assistance is often needed, and a family member or caregiver can help to hold the client's legs apart or maintain a certain position while the home care nurse inserts the catheter. Home care nurses must remember that adaptations for all nursing care are frequently necessary, and catheterization may require the ultimate in improvision in a client's home.

Urostomy Care

Urostomy, a surgical alteration of the normal urinary tract to attach a ureter to the abdominal surface (very much like a colostomy), is a permanent alteration in the urinary system. It is used as a last resort for clients with severely compromised urinary systems due to a diseased state. As with intermittent and continuous catheterization, urostomy care in elders is no different than in younger clients. However, their skin is much more fragile and all the usual skin protection routines must be implemented.

◆   ◆   ◆

NORMAL BOWEL CHANGES ASSOCIATED WITH AGING

To maintain bowel function in the elderly, it is necessary to keep in mind that bowel patterns are established at 30–36 months of age and are affected by many variables throughout the life span. Some of the variables are the type and amount of food and fluid intake, activity, amount of rest, medications, emotional state, stress, and disease. It is essential for the home care nurse to know what elimination pattern existed for the major part of the client's adult life (see Box 11-1).

In the elderly, changes may occur in the gastrointestinal system that impair digestion and elimination. Loss of teeth and problems with dentures can cause discomfort and affect the ability to chew food. Partially chewed food is not properly digested. With aging, peristalsis declines and slow emptying of the esophagus occurs. The older person may lose muscle tone in the anal sphincter and perineal floor.

Problems with bowel elimination are displayed as constipation, diarrhea, or impaction. Bowel incontinence is the inability to control passage of feces and gas from the anus. Both bowel elimination problems and incontinence require a thorough assessment of the client.

STRATEGIES FOR MAINTAINING NORMAL BOWEL PATTERNS

The home care nurse completes a GI assessment as part of the physical assessment (see Box 11-2). If it is determined that the client has bowel pattern problems, then a program to regain the client's normal pattern needs to be instituted.

As a part of the client teaching, the home care nurse reinforces healthy habits that encourage normal defecation patterns. These include such measures as establishing a time of day for bowel evacuation. Most people find that they have a natural urge to evacuate their bowels at a particular time

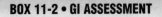

BOX 11-2 • GI ASSESSMENT

Conduct GI assessment including medical history and physical examination as follows:

- Food and fluid intake
- Symptoms—constipation, diarrhea, frequent bowel movements
- History of the use of enemas, laxatives, or suppositories
- Medications and their effects upon the GI tract
- Past history of bowel activity*
- Current history of bowel activity (7–10 days)*
- Rectal exam—to check for fecal impaction and also to test anal sphincter (normally, a tightening of the sphincter as the finger is inserted is noticed; ask the client to squeeze the finger tightly and note response)
- Stethoscope check of abdomen to assess bowel motility
- Observe for presence of hemorrhoids, since hemorrhoids can interfere with defecation primarily due to pain. Treatment is indicated for hemorrhoids

Once the GI assessment is completed and the current bowel pattern known, identify the specific bowel problem as follows:

- Incontinence with normal stool consistency
- Incontinence with constipated stool
- Incontinence with diarrhea
- Chronic constipation

Specifically include consistency, frequency, usual time of day, and if every day.

---

of day. It may be in the morning after breakfast or before bedtime. What is important is to establish a pattern and allow time to evacuate the bowel at the established time. Toileting time needs to be private and unrushed. Suggest the client have a comfortable environment (warm, well-lighted, etc.) and be relaxed (some clients may like to read or look at a magazine).

The client's diet needs to be rich in high fiber foods (see Chapter 6) and plenty of fluids. The older client should be encouraged to be as mobile as physically possible. Increased activity promotes peristalsis, and this helps the stool move naturally through the GI tract.

BOWEL PATTERN PROBLEMS AND NURSING CARE

It is important to regulate bowel patterns by developing a pattern specific to the client's needs. As shown in Box 11-2, there are several patterns of bowel consistency and each demands a different program of management. For all bowel programs, have the client, family, or caregiver keep accurate records of results. The home care nurse must review records regularly and adjust the program based on bowel activity.

Diarrhea

For clients who experience diarrhea on a regular basis, the cause needs to be determined. The GI assessment as outlined should reveal information important in determining the cause. A stool specimen for occult blood and for ova and parasites may be indicated. Frequently, an elder's GI system is more susceptible to the effects of foreign organisms. Also, the older adult may have other chronic diseases that compound the effects of an aging bowel.

If no impaction is found upon physical examination and laboratory reports are negative, develop a program that includes toileting after each meal. Consider the use of bulk laxative fiber products and adjust the dosage as indicated on the package for the client's age and weight.

Chronic diarrhea can be as critical in the older adult as in infants. Their systems cannot tolerate prolonged loss of electrolytes, and definitive medical management may be needed until the cause can be determined or until the diarrhea ceases. Diarrhea is not a problem that can be overlooked.

Constipation

More frequent than diarrhea, the older adult will complain of signs and symptoms of constipation. What is important is to regulate the bowel patterns with a program that is specific to the particular complaints. For clients with normal stool consistency but who have difficulty evacuating the bowel, the pattern includes establishing a program based on the client's usual bowel activity. Toileting once or twice a day at times the client is used to may be successful. Also, drinking some liquid while on the toilet, commode, or bedpan may be helpful. A glycerine suppository may stimulate bowel activity and should be administered 20–30 minutes before the client sits on the bedpan, toilet, or commode. If there are still no results, consider using a bisacodyl (Dulcolax) suppository, which stimulates peristalsis of the bowel track and lubricates as well. Always encourage a "squatting " position for defecation (the body itself will act to push out the stool). These approaches are also effective if the client is incontinent of stool of normal consistency.

For clients with constipation of hard or dry stool, increase fluid intake to achieve six to eight eight-ounce glasses per day. Educate the client about appropriate food intake and discuss and encourage activity, such as leg and arm exercises (if in a wheelchair) and walking (if ambulatory). Arrange to check the client at least once a week for impaction. A caregiver can be instructed in this procedure. Decide on the best time of day for bowel movement and the method to use for "squatting" position. Provide privacy. Instruct the client to lean forward if possible and apply manual pressure to the abdomen, gently massaging side to side. Consider using a suppository (glycerine or bisacodyl).

Colostomy Care

The home care client with a colostomy may have received limited teaching and support while in the hospital and may not have been provided with appropriate supplies or equipment. Since a colostomy can have a strong emotional impact because of the dramatic change in lifestyle, the home care nurse must be sure the client understands that the colostomy takes on the function of waste elimination; the client will not be having bowel movements rectally because a part of the colon and the rectum were bypassed.

The colostomy may be temporary or permanent. This information needs to be obtained from the referring primary care provider, as it will either mean another surgery to reattach the colon or the need to adapt to the colostomy for the rest of the client's life. These may be difficult concepts for the older adult to comprehend. Recognition of the client's personal feelings and emotions is necessary. A colostomy can cause serious body image changes, especially if the colostomy is permanent. The client may fear there will be foul odors and leakage, affecting self-esteem. If the client is dependent upon others to assist with caregiving, this can cause ongoing embarrassment.

Physically caring for a colostomy is no different when the client is elderly, except for greater attention to skin care needs. Evaluation of the equipment and fit will assure prevention of accidents and untoward skin irritation. Washing around the stoma and applying a skin barrier (e.g., stomahesive, hollihesive, and Karaja paste or powder) to prevent skin breakdown is a necessary step with every appliance change. Most elders do not have firm abdominal tissue, which is needed for most products to adhere well. An elder client's abdomen may have folds of loose skin that encumber an adequate appliance fit.

In many instances, it may be family members or caregivers that are responsible for the care of the colostomy. They become the home care nurse's primary "students" when teaching colostomy care. Caregiving instruction includes colostomy irrigations, changing appliances, and caring for the skin. Caregivers may need teaching and encouragement about cleaning around the stoma. They may fear causing pain or damaging the colostomy. Reassurance and reinforcement of previous teaching needs to be ongoing, especially if the caregiver is elderly.

◆　◆　◆

SUMMARY

Bladder and bowel pattern management problems are common concerns among clients receiving home health care. They are frequent enough that the home care nurse will find the topic presents itself on a daily basis. This chapter has provided an overview of ways to assess for and promote normal bladder and bowel functioning. Common variations from normal that are seen in the elderly home care population were discussed. The psychosocial aspects of elimination, especially when caregivers are involved with this very personal experience, should not be overlooked.

The chapter also examined more permanent bladder and bowel adaptations the elderly client may be experiencing. Caregiving for elders with urostomies or colostomies is not much different than among younger clients. Most issues remain the same. The biggest difference in providing appropriate care to clients with bladder and bowel pattern alterations in the home setting is that the nurse is required to use creativity and improvision in very different environments to ensure that care is safe and client-centered.

REFERENCE

Staab, A. S., & Hodges, L. C. (1996). *Essentials of gerontological nursing: Adaptation to the aging process*. Philadelphia: Lippincott–Raven.

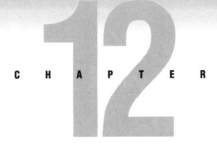

C H A P T E R

PROMOTING SKIN INTEGRITY AND PRESSURE ULCER HEALING IN THE ELDERLY CLIENT

Maureen Dailey

◆ ◆ ◆

Anatomy and Physiology of Skin
Promoting Skin Integrity in Older Adults
Pressure Ulcer Risk Assessment
Description of Pressure Ulcers
Risk Factors and Appropriate Interventions
Pressure Ulcer Healing and the Older Adult
Documenting Pressure Ulcers
Managing Peripheral Circulatory Problems
Managing Ulcer Care With Wound Care Products
Summary

T
he physical, emotional, and economic costs of an elderly client developing a pressure or vascular ulcer or the advancement of an existing ulcer is devastating to the client and caregivers. There are many elderly clients with chronic diseases or other risk factors who are at an increased risk for developing ulcers or who have already experienced ulcers. Successful home care agencies will be skillful at identifying clients at risk for ulcers and efficient in healing existing ulcers in their elderly clients.

The number of home care visits reimbursed for all types of care is less in a managed care market, which also influences the number of visits reimbursed for ulcer care. The potential to demonstrate nursing value in a multidisciplinary approach to prevent and care for ulcers is significant, as managed care continues to influence the practice of nursing in home health agencies.

With the physical, emotional, and financial costs in mind, the purpose of this chapter is twofold. First, it emphasizes the importance of maintaining the integrity of an elder's skin. This can best be accomplished by reviewing the anatomy, physiology, and function of the layers of skin and underlying tissue. The goal of the home health nurse is to prevent pressure ulcers among all clients, but especially among the most vulnerable and at highest risk, elderly clients. Second, the chapter identifies the major categories of ulcers in elderly clients encountered by the home care nurse. Pressure ulcer clinical guidelines are becoming the standard of practice in home care. Information from these guidelines included in this chapter reflects current research on prevention and optimal practices in the care of pressure ulcers. This information will assist the clinically based home care nurse to translate current pressure ulcer prevention and care research into practice.

ANATOMY AND PHYSIOLOGY OF SKIN

There are two principle layers of skin—the five outer layers, called the epidermis, and the two inner layers, called the dermis. The major appendages of skin—hair, nails, and sweat and sebaceous glands—are present primarily in the dermis, as are capillaries, lymph vessels, and nerve endings. Some extend into the epidermis or originate in the epidermis and extend down into the dermis. The major functions of the largest organ, the skin, include:

1. Protection from the sun (UV light).
2. Protection from pathogens (bacteria and fungal infections).
3. Protection from toxins (chemicals).
4. Thermal and fluid regulation (temperature and fluid-electrolyte balance, or homeostasis).
5. Synthesis of vitamin D via photoconversion (involved in metabolism and absorption of calcium, important for bones).

6. Providing sensation or communication (transmission of the sensation of touch, heat, or pressure) and facilitating appropriate response (e.g., to prevent injury).
7. Providing social and body image (i.e., a visual clue to ethnicity and chronological age).
8. Nutrition (the skin keeps nutrients within the body).

In the aging skin, the tissue wrinkles, loses turgor, acquires an increased translucency, becomes thinner and more fragile, and has a greater propensity for tear-type injuries. There is a decrease in number, production, and activity of sebaceous and sweat glands. Atrophy of subcutaneous fat in the dermis and a change in fat distribution result in less body insulation and lack of protective cushion. Fatty distribution is increased over the hips and abdomen and around the viscera and muscles. Poor nutrition and vitamin deficiencies contribute to changes in the elder's skin. Protein and calorie deficiencies cause the skin to become dryer, to become more pallid and grayish in color, and to lose elasticity (Staab & Lyles, 1990).

The underlying tissue is the subcutaneous tissue and components of the muscular and skeletal systems. The loose subcutaneous tissue consists of fat and both connective and elastic tissue. Skeletal muscle is below the fascia—the white fibrous plane of tissue separating the subcutaneous tissue with muscle. The skeletal system, consisting of bones, joints, and supportive connective tissue, such as ligaments and cartilage, is beneath muscle. The nervous, muscular, and skeletal systems work in concert to produce voluntary movement.

The major functions of subcutaneous tissue are:

1. Shock-absorption and cushioning.
2. Thermal regulation.
3. Energy storage.

The major functions of the voluntary muscular and skeletal systems are:

1. Movement.
2. Posture or muscle tone.
3. Heat production.
4. Supportive framework.
5. Protection of delicate structures under bone.
6. Storage of important minerals for homeostasis (calcium and phosphorus in bone).
7. Hematopoiesis (blood cell formation in red bone marrow).

PROMOTING SKIN INTEGRITY IN OLDER ADULTS

Home care nurses need to be comfortable identifying the layers of skin and the underlying subcutaneous tissue, muscle, and bone. The changes in an elder's skin increase the risk for insult and breakdown. Familiarity with the layers of skin, as well as the subcutaneous tissue and underlying muscles, tendons, and bones, empowers the nurse to collaborate effectively with primary care providers and other home care team members to effectively advocate for the best ulcer prevention and care for their elderly clients.

In addition to understanding the anatomy, physiology, and function of the skin, is the important task of promoting the elder's skin integrity. As a home care nurse, the roles of clinician and teacher are equally important. Implications for nursing care of elders who are at high risk for a compromised integumentary system include:

1. Teaching about clothing and dressing to decrease constriction. Waist elastic should be loose enough not to constrict. Eliminate the use of knee-high hose and socks with tight elastic.
2. Teaching about safe traveling. When traveling by automobile, they should stop frequently and get out of the car and walk. When flying, they should walk in the aisle every one to two hours.
3. Teaching about avoiding skin and deeper tissue injuries— scrapes, burns, cuts, and blisters (break in new shoes slowly).
4. Being alert for chemical toxicity from dermal patches and pastes that may pass through the thin outer layer of the skin more rapidly.
5. Being aware that heat intolerance problems, such as heatstroke and sunstroke, occur more frequently in older adults due to a reduced ability to perspire and reduced insulation quality.
6. Encouraging elder clients to wear hats, light clothing, and sunscreen products, and to drink large amounts of fluids in hot weather.
7. Pinching the skin of the client's forehead or sternum (instead of the back of the hand) to test for dehydration.
8. Protecting bony prominences from pressure so as to avoid skin breakdown.

9. Getting skin rashes diagnosed and treated and teaching clients to avoid scratching, which can cause breaks in the skin.
10. Understanding that the elderly have a propensity for skin cancers, owing to the increasing cytoarchitectural disarray present in their epidermal cells and their more significant exposure to carcinogenic agents, such as ultraviolet light.
11. Instructing older adults not to use topical bleaching creams, as they may cause local reactions.
12. Using lanolin-based preparations to replace natural oils.
13. Decreasing the number of full baths per week, especially in cold weather.
14. Using small amounts of nonalkaline soaps—they are less drying to the skin.
15. Observing the skin should be a daily task. Concentrate on sagging skin folds, behind the ears, between the digits, in the anal and genital regions, at bony prominences, around the sacrum, and around the feet, especially the heels and between the toes. Keep toenails trimmed neatly straight across and filed to eliminate scratching while sleeping. (Adapted from Staab & Lyles, 1990.)

PRESSURE ULCER RISK ASSESSMENT

The key to pressure ulcer risk identification and prevention of pressure ulcers is the appropriate use of a risk assessment tool and knowledge about risk factors and effective interventions. Many home care agencies are utilizing the Braden Risk Assessment Scale (AHCPR, 1992; see Table 12-1).

A risk assessment tool assists the home care nurse to identify specific risk factors and, by scoring the tool, to identify the degree of the risk. Some home care agencies have made it their policy to do a risk assessment for pressure ulcers on all adult clients upon admission. However, a home care nurse can utilize an assessment tool even if it is not standard practice in the home care agency. A pressure ulcer risk assessment tool takes about five minutes to complete. It is invaluable in focusing the nursing care plan of elderly clients at risk. Research has shown risk assessment tools improve the quality of elderly client care and assist in preventing the formation of new ulcers.

(Text continues on p. 234)

TABLE 12-1 • BRADEN RISK ASSESSMENT SCALE

NOTE: Bed- and chair-bound individuals or those with impaired ability to reposition should be assessed upon admission for their risk of developing pressure ulcers. Patients with established pressure ulcers should be reassessed periodically.

Patient name _____

Date _____

(Indicate appropriate numbers below) _____

SENSORY PERCEPTION Ability to respond meaningfully to pressure-related discomfort	**1. Completely Limited:** Unresponsive (does not moan, flinch, or grasp) to painful stimuli, due to diminished level of consciousness or sedation, *or* limited ability to feel pain over most of body surface.	**2. Very Limited:** Responds only to painful stimuli. Cannot communicate discomfort except by moaning or restlessness, *or* has a sensory impairment that limits the ability to feel pain or discomfort over half of body.	**3. Slightly Limited:** Responds to verbal commands but cannot always communicate discomfort or need to be turned, *or* has some sensory impairment that limits ability to feel pain or discomfort in one or two extremities.	**4. No Impairment:** Responds to verbal commands. Has no sensory deficit that would limit ability to feel or voice pain or discomfort.
MOISTURE Degree to which skin is exposed to moisture	**1. Constantly Moist:** Skin is kept moist almost constantly by perspiration, urine, etc. Dampness is detected every time patient is moved or turned.	**2. Very Moist:** Skin is often, but not always, moist. Linen must be changed at least once in 8 hr.	**3. Occasionally Moist:** Skin is occasionally moist, requiring an extra linen change approximately once a day.	**4. Rarely Moist:** Skin is usually dry. Linen only requires changing at routine intervals.
ACTIVITY Degree of physical activity	**1. Bedfast:** Confined to bed.	**2. Chairfast:** Ability to walk is severely limited or nonexistent. Cannot bear own weight or must be assisted into chair or wheelchair.	**3. Walks Occasionally:** Walks occasionally during the day, but for very short distances, with or without assistance. Spends majority of day/night in bed or chair.	**4. Walks Frequently:** Walks outside the room at least twice a day and inside the room at least once every two hours during waking hours.

(continued)

231

TABLE 12-1 • Continued

				(Indicate appropriate numbers below)
MOBILITY Ability to change and control body position	**1. Completely Immobile:** Does not make even slight changes in body or extremity position without assistance.	**2. Very Limited:** Makes occasional slight changes in body or extremity position but unable to make frequent or significant changes independently.	**3. Slightly Limited:** Makes frequent though slight changes in body or extremity position independently.	**4. No Limitations:** Makes major and frequent changes in position without assistance.	
NUTRITION *Usual* food intake pattern	**1. Very Poor:** Never eats a complete meal. Rarely eats more than a third of any food offered. Eats two servings or less of protein (meat or dairy products) per day. Takes fluids poorly. Does not take a liquid dietary supplement, *or* is NPO or maintained on clear liquids or IVs for more than five days.	**2. Probably Inadequate:** Rarely eats a complete meal and generally eats only about half of any food offered. Protein intake includes only three servings of meat or dairy products per day. Occasionally will take a dietary supplement, *or* receives less than optimum amount of liquid diet or tube feeding.	**3. Adequate:** Eats over half of most meals. Eats a total of four servings of protein (meat, dairy products) each day. Occasionally will refuse a meal, but will usually take a supplement if offered, *or* is on a tube feeding or TPN regimen that probably meets most of nutritional needs.	**4. Excellent:** Eats most of every meal. Never refuses a meal. Usually eats a total of four or more servings of meat and dairy products. Occasionally eats between meals. Does not require supplementation.	

(continued)

TABLE 12-1 • Continued

	1. Problem:	2. Potential Problem:	3. No Apparent Problem:	(Indicate appropriate numbers below)
FRICTION AND SHEAR	Requires moderate to maximum assistance in moving. Complete lifting without sliding against sheets is impossible. Frequently slides down in bed or chair, requiring frequent repositioning with maximum assistance. Spasticity, contractures, or agitation lead to almost constant friction.	Moves feebly or requires minimum assistance. During a move, skin probably slides to some extent against sheets, chair, restraints, or other devices. Maintains relatively good position in chair or bed most of the time but occasionally slides down.	Moves in bed and in chair independently and has sufficient muscle strength to lift up completely during move. Maintains good position in bed or chair at all times.	
			TOTAL SCORE:	

NOTE: Patients with a total score of 16 or less are considered to be at risk of developing pressure ulcers: 15 or 16 = low risk; 13 or 14 = moderate risk; 12 or less = high risk.

Copyright © 1988 Barbara Braden and Nancy Bergstrom. Reprinted with permission. Source: B. J. Braden & N. Bergstrom. (1989, August). Clinical utility of the Braden Scale for Predicting Pressure Sore Risk. Decubitus, 2, 44–51.

The major risk factors for pressure ulcers, using the Braden Scale, include:

1. Decreased sensory perception or the inability to respond meaningfully to pressure-related discomfort. Thus, the critical force of pressure becomes key to tissue damage.
2. Increased moisture or degree to which skin is exposed to moisture is increased.
3. Decreased activity, especially for elderly clients who are chair- or bed-bound.
4. Decreased mobility or the inability to change and control body position.
5. Decreased nutrition or inadequate nutrition due to poor food intake pattern.
6. Friction and shear.

DESCRIPTION OF PRESSURE ULCERS

Pressure ulcers are wounds or injuries to the skin or underlying tissue primarily caused by unrelieved pressure. They usually occur over a bony prominence. If a pressure ulcer is confined to the epidermis or the epidermis and dermis, it is called a partial thickness ulcer. Stage I and II pressure ulcers are both partial thickness ulcers. A stage I pressure ulcer is not an open ulcer. It may appear as nonblanchable erythema of intact skin when pressure is applied. In clients who have darker skin pigmentation, a stage I ulcer may appear as persistently red or blue, or it may have purple hues.

Stage II pressure ulcers extend into but not through the dermis; they do not extend into subcutaneous tissue. Wounds that are not pressure ulcers should not be staged according to the pressure ulcer staging system. Wounds other than pressure ulcers should be called partial or full thickness wounds. A wound that extends through the dermis, the inner layer of skin, into the subcutaneous tissue is called a full thickness wound.

Stage III and IV pressure ulcers are both full thickness ulcers, as both extend deeper than the dermis. Stage III pressure ulcers extend below the dermis into the subcutaneous tissue, but not through the fascial plane. Stage IV pressure ulcers extend through the fascial plane and into the muscle, and they can extend into tendon, bone, and joints as well. If an ulcer is covered by black necrotic tissue or fibrin slough, also necrotic tissue, that is softening or liquefying by debridement and appears as yellow, gray, tan, or green tissue, the ulcer cannot be staged.

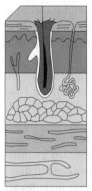 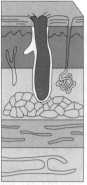 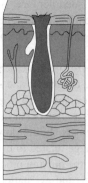 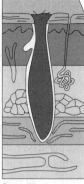

Stage I
The primary sign is redness. The skin does not return to a normal color when the pressure is relieved, but there is no induration—the skin and underlying tissues remain soft.

Stage II
Redness persists, usually accompanied by edema and induration. The epidermis may blister or erode.

Stage III
There is an open lesion and a crater exposing subcutaneous tissue. You may be able to see fascia at the base of the ulcer.

Stage IV
Necrosis may extend through the fascia and may even involve the bone. Eschar is a common finding. Bone destruction can lead to periosteitis, osteitis, and osteomyelitis.

FIGURE 12-1 • Classification of Pressure Ulcers

The ulcer can only be accurately staged when the base of the wound can be visualized (AHCPR, 1992; Staab & Hodges, 1996). The AHCPR *Quick Reference Guideline for Clinicians: Numbers 3 and 15* are available by calling (800) 358-9295. Figure 12-1 depicts the four stages of pressure ulcers.

RISK FACTORS AND APPROPRIATE INTERVENTIONS

The home health nurse's goal is to eliminate or reduce risk factors associated with pressure ulcers. Interventions must be based on the risk factors identified.

Pressure

Pressure is the primary "loading force" causing pressure ulcers. Pressure puts added load or demands on tissue, especially tissue over bony prominences. Pressure is a destructive force when applied over time. Pressure ulcers occur in certain characteristic areas when pressure is applied beyond tissue tolerance. A home care nurse should inspect the at-risk elderly client's skin from head to toe on each visit, paying close attention to bony prominences, for signs of skin or underlying tissue damage.

When an elderly client is essentially bed-bound, the pressure ulcers often occur on the trochanter and may occur on the sacrum if the head of the bed is raised above 30 degrees. When a client is chair-bound, pressure ulcers most often occur in the ischial area and can occur on the sacrum if the client is sliding down in the chair. Preventing skin and deeper tissue damage related to pressure is best accomplished by instituting the steps of the nursing process, which include assessment, diagnosis, intervention, and evaluation. An effective program includes all four steps.

The home care nurse should assess the elderly client for periods of prolonged sitting and lying. Instruct the family or caregiver to turn the bed-bound client every two hours. If repositioning at night is not possible, institute pillow bridging: Use pillows or wedges to bridge bony prominences, such as elbows, knees, and ankles. Bony prominences should be kept off the bed and the areas should not touch each other. Place the client in the side-lying 30 degree angle position, with pressure off the sacrum, trochanter, and hip.

Medicare will cover a pressure-reducing mattress overlay for the elderly client who has at least one additional risk factor for pressure ulcers, such as poor nutritional status. Support surfaces for beds are separated into three categories for reimbursement under Medicare and Medicaid (Medicaid coverage varies from state to state but usually follows Medicare's guidelines). The categories are listed in Table 12-2. Group I items are for prevention and for stage I pressure ulcers. Items in groups II and III provide surfaces for clients with existing pressure ulcers, post–flap surgery, or surgery to repair deeper pressure ulcers.

The chair-bound elderly client and caregiver should be taught to have the client change position every hour. Clients who are able to move are taught to shift their own body weight by raising up with their arms. Chair cushions come in different materials and provide some pressure reduction for clients in wheelchairs. The more expensive cushions are resistant to "bottoming out," or losing their effectiveness in redistributing pressure. The Roho and Jay seat cushions are used at several major rehabilitation centers in the New York area for elderly clients at high risk. It is important to note that once an inexpensive cushion or mattress is purchased, it may be difficult to successfully get reimbursement for another support surface of higher quality within a certain time frame.

TABLE 12-2 • SUPPORT SURFACE: MEDICARE B ELIGIBILITY CRITERIA

Group I	Group II	Group III
Foam, gel, air, water, or APP (alternating pressure pad)	Low air loss (LAL), alternating pressure mattress, powered mattress overlay, or nonpowered adjustable zone	Air fluidized therapy
Criteria: Completely immobile	*Criteria:* Multiple stage II pressure ulcers on the trunk or pelvis	*Criteria:* Has a stage III or IV pressure ulcer on the trunk or pelvis at least 8 sq cm in area
or	*and*	*and*
Has limited mobility and *one* of the following risk factors: 1. Impaired nutrition 2. Incontinence 3. Altered sensory perception 4. Compromised circulation	Has a comprehensive ulcer treatment program (including the use of an appropriate Group I product that has been tried for at least one month)	Bedridden or chair-bound Does not require wet soaks or moist wound dressings that are not protected by an occlusive cover Cannot have a coexisting pulmonary disease
or	*or*	All other equipment has been considered and ruled out
Has any stage pressure ulcer and *one* of the following risk factors: 1. Impaired nutrition 2. Incontinence 3. Altered sensory perception 4. Compromised circulation	Has a stage III or IV pressure ulcer *or* Postsurgical flap/graft within the past 60 days and prior to discharge was on a Group II or III support surface	Absence of air fluidized therapy would require institutionalization Trained adult caregiver is available Conservative treatment was tried for at least one month prior to use of the fluidized bed with worsening or no improvement of the ulcer

The home care nurse should check for bottoming-out by doing a "hand check" of all support surfaces for the at-risk elderly client on each visit. It is a momentary check but very important. The "hand check" involves placing a hand between the bed or the chair and the support surface (the mattress or overlay on a bed or chair cushion). If a bony prominence can be felt through the support surface, pressure reduction is not effective and the support surface needs to be serviced or replaced. Monitoring the correct functioning of support surfaces is an important role of the home care nurse but is often overlooked on visits. The "hand check" should be performed and documented in the visit record and should also be taught to the client's family and caregivers. The home care nurse should observe and document a return demonstration to ensure the caregiver's ability to implement this important check.

The heels of a chair- or bed-bound client should be elevated by using pillows or a heel-lift device. Heel booties should *not* be used; they still leave pressure on the heels and are ineffective in preventing pressure ulcers. A heel ulcer can develop under a bootie, and it may not be noticed until it is a serious ulcer. Because there is so little supportive tissue between the epidermis and bone of the heels, heels break down more rapidly when pressure is exerted.

The client should not sit in a recliner. The "V" position, with the head and legs elevated, puts tremendous pressure on the sacrum and so is contraindicated. Donut devices actually cause more pressure on the sacrum and should not be used. To assess proper seating cushions for chair-bound clients, the home care nurse should consider postural alignment, distribution of weight, balance and stability, and pressure reduction. The nurse can consult physical and occupational therapists, as they have advanced training in assessing clients for the best seating device.

A written plan for the family and caregivers detailing the types of devices and the timing of turning and positioning is helpful in achieving compliance with the plan. For the bed-bound client, it is imperative for the home care nurse to:

1. Teach caregivers to perform turning and positioning every two hours.
2. Teach caregivers to place the client in the side-lying, 30 degree, oblique position.
3. Place the at-risk client on a pressure-reducing mattress, such as a foam, static air, alternating air, gel overlay, or water mattress.
4. Do "hand checks" on all home visits to assess the effectiveness of support surfaces for the bed. Document the check. Teach the family and caregivers to perform this check.
5. Teach the pillow and wedge bridging technique to keep bony prominences off the bed and from resting on another bony area.
6. Teach caregivers to keep the client's heels off the bed by using pillows or a heel-lift device to suspend the heels.

For the chair-bound elderly client, the home care nurse should:

1. Teach caregivers to change the client's position every hour for clients who cannot reposition themselves.
2. Teach clients who can move themselves to do small shifts every 15 minutes.
3. Place clients on an effective pressure-reducing cushion.
4. Do a "hand check" on each visit and teach family and caregivers how to check for cushion effectiveness. Document the check.

Moisture

Increased moisture is most often related to urinary and fecal incontinence, with fecal incontinence being more caustic to skin. Maceration related to moisture increases an elderly client's potential for developing a pressure ulcer and complicates recovery in a client that already has skin breakdown. The chair-bound incontinent client should wear a diaper that is absorbent and keeps excess moisture away from the skin surface. The bed-bound incontinent client should be placed on an open, lightweight diaper that does not interfere with the support surface reducing pressure to bony prominences.

For both urinary and fecal incontinence, the skin must be cleansed and dried gently. Avoid overdrying the skin. Soap and water should only be used once a day; water temperature should be tepid or warm. Condition the skin with a moisturizer and barrier ointment to prevent dryness. For additional episodes of incontinence, use a no-rinse incontinence cleanser. Consider a fecal incontinence collector for bed-bound clients to prevent skin breakdown.

Activity

The elderly client with decreased mobility is at increased risk for skin breakdown and contractures. The home care nurse should assess the elderly client for mobility and whether physical or occupational therapy is appropriate. If it is, then the primary care provider should be consulted for rehabilitation orders. A maintenance program of range of motion (ROM) should be instituted for bed-bound clients to prevent contractures. The home care nurse should check the state's home health aide scope of practice when passive ROM is required to make sure a home health aide or home attendant can perform passive ROM. This is especially important when a contracture already exists. Pain management is another consideration with ROM and rehabilitation programs. The easy-lift day chair electrically lifts the sitting person, such as an elderly Parkinson's client, into a standing position. This can help some chair-bound clients become ambulatory. Although reimbursement is problematic for this chair, rental agreements involving private pay may be a solution the home care nurse can suggest.

Mobility

The elderly client that is not able to change and control body position is at increased risk for pressure ulcers. There are gradations of mobility noted in the Braden Risk Assessment tool, from "no limitations" (the client makes major and frequent changes in position without assistance) to "completely immobile" (the client does not make even slight changes in body or extremity position without assistance). An over-the-bed trapeze can be helpful in assisting an elderly client who has good upper body strength to change positions in bed. The trapeze is available on a frame that is positioned behind the client's regular bed, therefore a hospital bed is not mandatory. Side rails can also be obtained for regular beds to assist elderly clients in repositioning and turning.

Nutrition

Nutrition is key in preventing pressure ulcers. Without adequate nutrition, especially protein and calorie intake, the body begins to break down and the immune system is impaired. Both the breakdown of the body (a catabolic state) and an impaired immune response put the elderly client at increased risk for pressure ulcers and potentiate other risk factors. Protein and calorie intake must be adequate to prevent skin breakdown. The key lab values to evaluate are albumin, transferrin, and lymphocyte count, as well as hemoglobin and hematocrit for elderly clients suspected of having nutritional deficiencies. A client is at risk for skin breakdown when albumin values fall below 3.5 g/dL.

Friction and Shear

Friction occurs when the top layer of skin, the epidermis, is damaged from moving or dragging across a coarse surface. Shear affects deeper tissues and occurs when the surface layer of skin remains in contact with bed linens and the like while the tissues attached to the bone are pulled in one direction because of body weight. Friction and the possibility of shearing must be prevented. Effective measures to prevent friction and shearing should be taught to family members and caregivers.

Measures to prevent friction:

1. Smooth corn starch on susceptible body parts to decrease friction. Avoid sprinkling corn starch in the air. Instead, place it on the hands and thinly smooth over the body parts subject to friction.
2. Obtain assistance to move a client up in bed so the client's heels are not dragging on the bed.
3. Use a film dressing to protect an irritated area to prevent increased damage.
4. Keep skin lubricated to prevent drying and cracking of skin.
5. Avoid laundering the client's sheets with harsh detergents.

Measures to prevent shearing:

1. Avoid massaging over bony prominences that angulates or bends capillaries.
2. Keep the head of the bed below 45 degrees or at the lowest elevation that is safe. This helps prevent the client from sliding down in the bed.
3. Use a pull sheet to move the client from one side of the bed to the other.
4. Whenever possible, have the client assist with positioning by lifting with an over-the-bed trapeze, especially if only one caregiver is available.
5. When clients are sitting, their feet should be on a footrest to reduce pressure at the back of the thighs and knees.

Documentation of pressure ulcer risk assessment and appropriate interventions are important to facilitate continuity of care and meet the quality, regulatory, and accrediting standards that home care agencies must meet. Caregiver or client noncompliance with the prevention program should be documented. Appropriate interventions or contracting with the client and caregivers to enhance participation of the client and caregivers in the skin care program may be helpful.

The Outcomes Assessment Information Set (OASIS) addresses pressure ulcer prevention and healing as quality indicators in home care. Some home health agencies have already participated in a demonstration project with this tool, and Medicare has mandated that all participating Medicare home health agencies implement it by 1999. Thus, effective and efficient pressure ulcer prevention and care of existing ulcers will be used as benchmarks for quality in the home care industry throughout the country.

PRESSURE ULCER HEALING AND THE OLDER ADULT

The phases of pressure ulcer healing are the inflammatory, proliferative, and maturative phases. Healing is a dynamic process and not static. It has been described as a cascade of events that occur in predictable fashion or sequence. One phase may overlap another phase of wound healing. However, with elderly clients, healing can be a slow and tedious process. Often there are health status situations that prolong the resolution of one phase and the beginning of another phase.

It is important that the home care nurse understand the factors that hinder the progression through the phases of pressure ulcer healing in order to initiate actions that are designed to successfully promote the healing process. The risk factors outlined in the previous section, if present, impact the progress.

Documenting the age of the wound and its characteristics are factors the nurse uses to identify the wound healing stage. Pressure ulcers can become "stuck" in a phase of healing and not progress to closure or complete healing if local or systemic factors are not supportive of wound healing. Among elders, there are many factors that can slow the process down.

The home care nurse can best assist clients by working with family members and other caregivers to *prevent* pressure ulcers from forming. Primary prevention is the best way to manage pressure ulcers in the elderly. The home care nurse needs to emphasize all the "savings" that prevention offers. When families recognize the incentives for preventing pressure ulcers, teaching prevention measures can be the primary focus of caregiving that the home care nurse provides. The home care nurse should share the following information to assist families in recognizing the value of instituting primary prevention measures. The benefits include:

1. Quality of life: Pressure ulcers cause limitations to mobility, activity, and clothing choices.
2. Pain prevention: Stage I, II, and III pressure ulcers are painful. Analgesics for pain can be expensive and may have side effects

that can cause additional health risks and stress to the elderly client.
3. Additional caregiving: Pressure ulcers increase the amount of care that the client needs, as well as housekeeping (e.g., washing soiled clothing and bed linens due to drainage from the ulcerated area).
4. Financial cost: Pressure ulcer care requires cleansing products, medicines applied to the ulcer, and dressings. These items are expensive and often need to be used several times a day.

The inflammatory phase of wound healing occurs three to five days after the initial insult and is characterized by erythema (redness), warmth, edema, and pain. At a cellular level, vessels have constricted and platelets have aggregated to form a fibrin clot to seal the wound. Then vasodilation releases plasma into the wound area, causing edema and warmth. White blood cells migrate to the wounded area and engulf bacteria and necrotic tissue. Finally, macrophages begin debriding and revascularizing the wound.

The proliferative phase generally occurs from days 4 or 5 through day 20. The main event during this phase is tissue development. In partial thickness ulcers, epithelial cells migrate across the wound surface in a process known as epithelialization. The wound is covered with a thin layer of silvery cells, which, while fragile, protects from bacterial invasion. Full thickness ulcers, those that extend into subcutaneous tissue or deeper, are characterized by the appearance of collagen, a product of fibroblasts. Also, capillaries develop from nearby vessels to nourish the newly generating tissue, thus giving the wound a granular appearance. The wound edges approximate (come closer together). Finally, the wound is closed by epithelialization.

The final maturative phase occurs 21 days after the insult and may take as long as two years to complete. This is when the ulcer matures and the collagen in the scar remodels. At this point, equilibrium between collagen synthesis and breakdown is in balance, and the fibroblasts and capillary buds retract. The scar becomes less bulky and decreases in redness as the wound gains tensile strength and is better able to withstand stress. With good nutrition and optimal local and systemic factors that affect wound healing, a wounded area can regain up to 80 percent of its prior tensile strength.

The client's risk to develop pressure ulcers and ability to successfully heal an ulcer is profoundly affected by the client's nutritional status. The inflammatory and proliferative phases are prolonged and delayed in elderly clients with poor or inadequate nutritional status. If an ulcer is infected, healing is delayed. An ulcer with extensive depth and circumference will have an extended proliferative phase of healing. It is important for the elderly client to maintain optimal caloric and protein intake, even when the ulcer is closed, because healing continues to take place under the closed skin or scar.

Understanding the timing and events in the phases of ulcer healing is critical for home care nurses. This information enables the nurse to determine if the wound is acute (one that is following a predictable path of healing) or if it is chronic (one that is stuck in wound healing, or delayed wound healing). The home care nurse can make this determination from the client's history, or from the admission data, noting the length of time the wound has existed. An acute wound can heal quickly with efficient and effective wound care. A chronic wound can be "jumpstarted" and heal by implementing appropriate wound healing techniques and addressing local and systemic factors that affect healing.

DOCUMENTING PRESSURE ULCERS

The assessment process for documenting a client's skin integrity begins upon admission to home care. A total head to toe assessment should be performed and documented on the appropriate agency form. Figure 12-2 provides a form that is helpful to use for a client who begins home care services with a pressure ulcer.

An initial assessment of an elderly client should include a total body assessment, paying particular attention to bony prominences. Return visits focus on assessing the existing pressure ulcers and identifying risks for new ones. The skin should be inspected on each home visit for any changes in skin integrity. An episode of skin breakdown can be missed if adequate skin inspection does not occur on the initial assessment and subsequent home visits. Caregivers should be taught to inspect the client's skin daily and to report any alterations to the nurse for early intervention.

The site of the wound should be documented using standard medical terminology. Measuring the ulcer is critical to determine the pace of healing or to signal a delay in the healing progress. Most home care agencies have a policy for nurses to measure wounds once or twice a week. Usually, the policy or protocol notes the measurement system; most often the metric system is used (thus sizes are in centimeters). Length, width, and depth should be noted.

Any undermining, tunneling, or sinus tracts need to be carefully measured and documented. Undermining occurs when the edges of the

PRESSURE ULCER ASSESSMENT GUIDE

Patient Name: _____   Date: _____ Time: _____

ULCER 1	**ULCER 2**
Site _____	Site _____
Stage* _____	Stage* _____
Size (cm)	Size (cm)
Length _____	Length _____
Width _____	Width _____
Depth _____	Depth _____

	No	Yes			No	Yes
Sinus Tract	☐	☐	Sinus Tract		☐	☐
Tunneling	☐	☐	Tunneling		☐	☐
Undermining	☐	☐	Undermining		☐	☐
Necrotic Tissue	☐	☐	Necrotic Tissue		☐	☐
Slough	☐	☐	Slough		☐	☐
Eschar	☐	☐	Eschar		☐	☐
Exudate	☐	☐	Exudate		☐	☐
Serous	☐	☐	Serous		☐	☐
Serosanguineous	☐	☐	Serosanguineous		☐	☐
Purulent	☐	☐	Purulent		☐	☐
Granulation	☐	☐	Granulation		☐	☐
Epithelialization	☐	☐	Epithelialization		☐	☐
Pain	☐	☐	Pain		☐	☐
Surrounding Skin			**Surrounding Skin**			
Erythema	☐	☐	Erythema		☐	☐
Maceration	☐	☐	Maceration		☐	☐
Induration	☐	☐	Induration		☐	☐

Description of Ulcer(s)

_____

_____

Indicate Ulcer Sites

Anterior   Posterior

(Attach a color photo of the pressure ulcer[s] [Optional])

*Classification of pressure ulcers

Stage I: Nonblanchable erythema of intact skin, the heralding lesion of skin ulceration. In individuals with darker skin, discoloration of the skin, warmth, edema, induration, or hardness may also be indicators.

Stage II: Partial thickness skin loss involving epidermis, dermis, or both.

Stage III: Full thickness skin loss involving damage to or necrosis of subcutaneous tissue that may extend down to, but not through, underlying fascia. The ulcer presents clinically as a deep crater with or without undermining adjacent tissue.

Stage IV: Full thickness skin loss with extensive destruction, tissue necrosis, or damage to muscle, bone, or supporting structures (e.g., tendon or joint capsule).

FIGURE 12-2 • Pressure Ulcer Assessment Guide

wound are not fixed and the wound actually extends underneath the edges. The extent of undermining is measured using sterile gloves and a cotton applicator. It is described by position on the clock (e.g., "wound undermined 5 cm at 12 through 3 o'clock, 2 cm from 3 to 9 o'clock"). Tunneling involves wound openings that communicate to another wound opening under the skin. Sinus tracts are openings that communicate to a blind area. They are measured and described similarly to undermining.

The type, color, and amount of drainage is also recorded, as well as the presence of any odor. Odor under an occlusive dressing may be normal and related to the dressing product. However, if an odor persists after the wound is cleansed, it signifies possible infection and the primary care provider should be notified. Note the type and amount of tissue in the wound bed, as well as the condition of the surrounding skin. Maceration indicates that excess moisture is in contact with the surrounding skin and a more absorbent dressing may be needed.

It is very important to place the client in the same position for wound measurement and assessment, as the size and shape of a wound can vary in different positions due to sagging skin. Thus, the home care nurse should note what anatomical position the client is in when weekly or biweekly measurements are taken.

Documenting all aspects of ulcer status is important to provide the next caregiver with a clear picture of the wound's status, as well as to ensure appropriate follow-up and reimbursement. Consistency in wound assessment and documentation in a home care agency contributes to improved wound care outcomes for elderly clients.

Pressure ulcer care is constantly changing and nurses should refer to textbooks, agency protocol manuals, skin care clinical specialists, evidence-based guidelines (such as AHCPR's *Guidelines* noted in the reference list), and wound care product salespersons for the most current management recommendations. Enterostomal therapy (ET) nurses are clinical specialists to consult with in home care for difficult or complex wounds. Their national organization—the Wound, Ostomy, Continence Nurses Society (WOCN)—can identify a local ET nurse according to geographic region. Their toll-free number is (888) 224-WOCN, and their e-mail address is www.wocn.org. The ET nurse collaborates with primary care providers and all home care team members. The ET nurse facilitates communication with sales representatives who have samples of new products for home care nurses to use with clients. Thus, access to ET nurses allows home care nurses to practice on the cutting edge of wound care. The ET nurse can also set up a skin care team within a home care agency to implement a successful ulcer prevention and wound care program.

MANAGING PERIPHERAL CIRCULATORY PROBLEMS

Elderly clients with clotting disorders or peripheral circulatory problems, such as venous or arterial insufficiency, need to have the underlying disease treated to optimize functioning of the circulatory system. It is important for the home care nurse to accurately assess the vascular status of the elderly client and document changes that may indicate significant vascular disease. The home care nurse must be astute at recognizing the signs and symptoms of arterial, venous, and arterial-venous mix diseases and suggest appropriate diagnostic testing and treatment with the primary care provider via nurse collaboration.

The major intervention essential to wound healing for venous systemic circulatory problems is compression. Venous stasis ulcers will usually not progress to healing, or stay healed, unless the venous insufficiency is addressed. The valves that normally prevent the backflow of blood in leg veins become incompetent with venous insufficiency, and prescription support stockings with 30–40 cm pressure mercury are necessary to prevent healed ulcers from recurring. Compression bandages over the primary dressing or other forms of compression are essential during wound healing to achieve therapeutic compression so nutrients and oxygen get to the area of the venous stasis ulcer.

Often a compression boot, known as an "Unna" boot, is utilized. This consists of gauze impregnated with zinc oxide and other compounds, which harden by drying. Usually, a primary dressing is placed over the ulcerated area under the compression boot to absorb drainage and protect the wound. The boot is changed by the primary care provider or home care nurse one to two times a week depending on the amount of drainage. It is important apply the boot properly. If the gauze is not smooth, a new ulcer or circulatory compromise can occur.

To improve venous insufficiency, several interventions can be used:

1. Compression therapy is the most important. The nurse should consult with the primary care provider about the use of some form of compression before a dressing is discussed.
2. Dry and taught skin related to edema must be cared for to prevent cracking and bacterial invasion. Hydrate the skin with a moisturizing lotion and apply a barrier ointment to the peri-wound skin to prevent maceration.
3. The compression boot should be changed in the morning before the client develops lower extremity edema. The client should not remove the boot too far in advance of the nurse's visit.

4. The client's legs should always be elevated when the client is sitting, and prolonged standing should be avoided.
5. Instruct the client to ambulate with a heel-to-toe sequence, activating and strengthening the calf pump mechanism to aid in venous return.

Arterial ulcers are related to poor circulation of the client's lower extremities and tend to be on the lower legs or feet. The home care nurse should instruct the client, family, and caregivers not to apply heat (e.g., with heating pads or soaking in warm water) due to decreased sensation and potential for skin damage and burns. The client should be instructed not to smoke and to avoid caffeine, as these products exacerbate the symptoms.

Leg pain at night can be distressing. The head of the client's bed can be elevated on blocks so the client does not have to get up at night and dangle legs to relieve pain; this also avoids complicating edema.

If the client is advanced in years and has multiple comorbidities, revascularization and bypass surgery may not be appropriate. In this case, conservative wound care management, even allowing a necrotic cap or scab to remain, may be the most appropriate wound care choice. The skin of clients with arterial insufficiency is usually thin, fragile, and dry. Caregivers should hydrate the client's skin with a moisturizer. Scrupulous foot care, including podiatric appointments, thorough cleansing, avoiding moisture between the toes, and always wearing well-fitting shoes, is essential in preventing further injury, infection, or exacerbation of an existing wound. Other classes of wounds also occur in the elderly population. Neuropathic ulcers are foot ulcers related to neuropathy that commonly occur in diabetic patients (Table 12-3). Pressure ulcers and vascular ulcers comprise the majority of wounds encountered by the home care nurse with elderly clients.

MANAGING ULCER CARE WITH WOUND CARE PRODUCTS

Pressure ulcers and ulcers caused by insufficient vasculation heal only when the environment is ideal. Home care nurses follow the same principles for wound healing as nurses in the acute care setting:

1. Provide moisture to the wound.
2. Debride the wound (remove necrotic tissue by irrigating the wound bed).

TABLE 12-3 • QUICK ASSESSMENT OF LEG ULCERS

Venous Insufficiency (Stasis)	Arterial Insufficiency	Peripheral Neuropathy
HISTORY		
Previous DVT and varicosities	Diabetes	Diabetes
Reduced mobility	Anemia	Spinal cord injury
Obesity	Arthritis	Hansen's disease
Vascular ulcers	Increased pain with activity or elevation	Relief of pain with ambulation
Phlebitis	CVA	Paresthesia of extremities
Traumatic injury	Smoking	
CHF	Intermittent claudication	
Orthopedic procedures	Traumatic injury to extremity	
Pain reduced by elevation	Vascular procedures/ surgeries	
	Hypertension	
	Hyperlipidemia	
	Arterial disease	
LOCATION		
Medial aspect of lower leg and ankle	Toetips or web spaces	Plantar aspect of foot
Superior to medial malleolus	Phalangeal heads around lateral malleolus	Metatarsal heads
	Areas exposed to pressure or repetitive trauma	Heels
		Altered pressure points/ sites of painless trauma/ repetitive stress
APPEARANCE		
Color: base ruddy	Color: base of wound, pale/pallor on elevation; dependent rubor	Color: Normal skin tones; trophic skin changes, fissuring or callus formation
Surrounding skin: erythema (venous dermatitis) or brown staining (hyperpigmentation)	Skin: shiny, taut, thin, dry, hair loss on lower extremities, atrophy of subcutaneous tissue	Depth: variable
Depth: usually shallow		Wound margins: well defined
Wound margins: irregular	Depth: deep	Exudate: variable
Exudate: moderate to heavy	Wound margins: even	Edema: cellulitis, erythema, and induration common
Edema: pitting or nonpitting; possible induration and cellulitis	Exudate: minimal	Skin temp: warm
	Edema: variable	Granulation tissue: frequently present
Skin temp: normal; warm to touch	Skin temp: decreased/cold	Infection: frequent
Granulation: frequently present	Granulation tissue: rarely present	Necrotic tissue variable, gangrene uncommon
Infection: less common	Infection: frequent (signs may be subtle)	Reflexes usually diminished
	Necrosis, eschar, gangrene may be present	Altered gait; orthopedic deformities common

(continued)

TABLE 12-3 • Continued		
Venous Insufficiency (Stasis)	**Arterial Insufficiency**	**Peripheral Neuropathy**
PERFUSION		
Pain	**Pain**	**Pain**
Minimal unless infected or desiccated	Intermittent claudication	Diminished sensitivity to touch
Peripheral pulses	Resting	Reduced response to pin prick, usually painless
Present/palpable	Positional	**Peripheral pulses**
Capillary refill	Nocturnal	Palpable/present
Normal—less than 3 seconds	**Peripheral pulses**	**Capillary refill**
	Absent or diminished	Normal
	Capillary refill	
	Delayed—more than 3 seconds	
	ABI < 0.8	
INTERVENTIONS		
Measures to improve venous return	**Measures to improve tissue perfusion**	**Measures to eliminate trauma**
Surgical obliteration of damaged veins	Revascularization if possible	Pressure relief for healed ulcers
Elevation of legs	Medications to improve RBC transit through narrowed vessels	"Offloading" for plantar ulcers (bedrest *or* contact casting *or* orthopedic shoes)
Compression therapy to provide at least 30 mmHg compression at ankle	Lifestyle changes (no tobacco, no caffeine, no constrictive garments, avoidance of cold)	Appropriate footwear
Options:		**Tight glucose control**
Short stretch bandages (e.g., Setopress, Surepress, Comprilan)	Hydration	**Aggressive infection control**
	Measures to prevent trauma to tissues (appropriate footwear at *all times*)	Debridement of any necrotic tissue
Therapeutic support stockings	**Topical therapy**	Orthopedic consult for exposed bone
Unna Boots	Dry uninfected necrotic wound: keep dry	Antibiotic coverage
Profore 4-layer wrap	Dry infected wound: immediate referral for surgical debridement, aggressive antibiotic therapy	**Topical therapy**
Compression pumps		Cautious use of occlusive dressings
Topical therapy	Open wound:	Dressing to absorb exudate, keep surface moist
Goals:	Moist wound healing	
Absorb exudate	Nonocclusive dressings (e.g., solid hydrogels) or *cautious* use of occlusive dressings	
Maintain moist wound surface (e.g., alginate, foam, hydrocolloid dressings)	Aggressive treatment of any infection	

Reprinted by permission of the Wound, Ostomy, and Continence Nurse Society, Costa Mesa, California.

3. Implement wound packing and dressing changes.
4. Prevent infection, and manage infection if it occurs.

Moisture is needed to promote granulation and epithelialization. Foreign bodies (such as necrotic debris: black eschar or fibrin slough) must be removed to promote efficient wound healing and prevent infection. Mechanical, chemical, or autolysis debridement is implemented to maintain a clean wound bed. Irrigation is the most common form of mechanical debridement and is often used by nurses in the home. Dressing changes vary with the phase of wound healing, wound size and depth, and amount of drainage. Throughout treatment, infection is prevented. The home care nurse implements these procedures and teaches them to the client, family members, and caregivers. Even when the most careful procedures are performed, infection may occur. Identification of an infected ulcer and managing the infection are also part of the home care nurse's caregiving responsibilities.

Wound care products are numerous. The decision to use a product is dependent on several factors. First, determine whether the goal of wound care is to heal or to provide palliative treatment. Second, choose the dressing based on the wound's size, depth, and location, the amount and type of drainage, comfort, and cost. Table 12-4 lists dressing categories, actions and indications for each dressing category, and special considerations when making a dressing choice. This information is presented to demonstrate the variety of products available to treat and manage pressure and vascular insufficiency ulceration in the elderly home care population.

Medicare Part A covers 100 percent of wound care supplies while the client is receiving home care. Legislation has been enacted to change Medicare Part B coverage, and this may affect wound care supply coverage. Some home care agencies already have vendors billing wound care supplies directly to Part B. Unlike Medicare, Medicaid coverage varies by state. Commercial and managed care coverage varies for wound care supplies—both between companies and over time with one company. In addition, product brands can vary greatly within a wound product category.

Because healthcare insurance coverage for wound care supplies is in flux, it is imperative the home care nurse verify what the client's costs will be for any product chosen. Most older adults are on fixed incomes, and wound care can extend over a protracted length of time. As a client advocate, the home care nurse must find wound care products that meet the needs of healing the wound but that don't unnecessarily burden the client financially.

(Text continues on p. 254)

TABLE 12-4 • MAJOR WOUND PRODUCT CATEGORIES

Dressing Category	Actions and Indications	Considerations
Cotton mesh	Used for wet-to-dry debridement or packing (should be opened to single layer and molded into wound loosely) Used as a secondary dressing Moderately absorptive	Bulky Inexpensive May be used on partial or full thickness wounds May be combined with normal saline (or gel) to create a moist dressing or antibiotic for infected wounds
Gauze packing	Used in tunneling or sinus tracts to fill dead space	Should be packed loosely to prevent pressure necrosis
Gauze wrapping	Used on extremity wounds as a secondary dressing	Eliminates the need for tape on the skin Do not use for packing
High absorbency	Specialized to wick away excess exudate and prevent maceration and infection	Can be more costly but presents strikethrough drainage
Impregnated gauze	Can be impregnated with white petroleum or immersed in oil	Nonadherent and can prevent bleeding or trauma to wound bed (especially helpful in wounds with tumor growth) Protects wound from unnecessary loss of body fluids Petroleum-impregnated gauze often used at donor sites
Nonadherent	More occlusive than gauze Less traumatic to wound bed and less painful to client Minimally absorptive	Usually requires a secondary dressing
Films	Minimally absorptive Moisture retentive Reduces pain at wound site Promotes epithelialization Transparent for easy inspection Water resistant	Appropriate to protect lacerations, abrasions, blisters, and stage II pressure ulcers that are blistered Can be used for autolytic debridement Does not require use of secondary dressing Can wrinkle and be difficult to apply to certain body areas

(continued)

TABLE 12-4 • Continued

Dressing Category	Actions and Indications	Considerations
Hydrocolloids	Most moisture retentive Occlusive or semipermeable Less pain at wound site Water resistant Minimally to moderately absorptive Melt-out of dressing occurs Excellent barrier to pathogens	Can be used under compression bandages for venous stasis ulcers Some forms are more absorptive than others Some adhere better with innovations (e.g., tapered edges) Usually cannot visualize wound Daily removal is not recommended Can be used for autolytic debridement Can be used over primary dressing, such as a wound filler May be used on full thickness wounds, such as stage III and IV pressure ulcers
Hydrogels	Moisture retentive Moderately absorptive Less pain at wound site Cooling sensation for burn wounds Can be impregnated into gauze or used as the primary dressing Can be water resistant when used with a secondary film dressing	Comes in liquid or solid sheet form Can visualize wound through some solid forms Now available in economic, multiple-dose, liquid forms Can be used when infection is present As with any wound exposed to air, liquid gel must be covered well with secondary dressing to prevent wound contamination and parasitic infestation (e.g., maggots)
Exudate absorbers	Can be beads, powder, paste or alginates Moisture retentive Highly absorptive	Requires a secondary dressing Important to consider compatibility with secondary dressing Helps to prevent maceration of surrounding skin and frequent dressing changes with heavy exudate Promotes autolytic debridement
Foams	Moderately to highly absorptive Moisture retentive	Can be used under compression bandage for venous stasis ulcer Cushions the wound from trauma

(continued)

TABLE 12-4 • MAJOR WOUND PRODUCT CATEGORIES (continued)

Dressing Category	Actions and Indications	Considerations
Foams (continued)	Less pain at wound site Nonadherent	Facilitates autolytic debridement May require a secondary adhesive to secure dressing Can contain charcoal filler for odor control
Composite or combination	Multilayer dressing combining multiple types, such as gel, foam, and film Moderately to highly absorptive	Can be costly in price Decreases frequency of wound care Can be used under compression bandaging for venous stasis ulcers

Special considerations: There are thousands of wound care products that perform multiple functions, and some can be used concurrently. Listings of products are available on the Internet and via local and national vendors. Before using a product, the nurse should read the manufacturer's instructions on product interactions and on the category, action, precautions, and stage of the wound that the product is indicated for.

Wound care experts in home care agencies can assist in wound product decision making. If resources are limited, manufacturers have representatives to answer questions on appropriate uses and precautions for their products.

SUMMARY

The integumentary system is the largest system in the body. Over a lifetime, insults to the system take its toll. In addition, changes in aging skin impact the system's ability to protect the underlying tissue. Wounds or ulcerations may occur, especially if a client has a poor nutritional state or is inactive or immobile. Ideally, the home care nurse works to prevent skin damage in clients by teaching healthy skin care habits. However, if an ulceration occurs, the caregiving focus expands.

In the acute care setting, wounds can be managed only briefly because the hospital stay is short. Therefore, pressure ulcer management becomes a major role of home care nurses. Management of ulcerations depends on the goal of care and the cause, location, and size of the ulcer bed. Many wound care products are available for the nurse to use for palliative care and for healing. Home care nurses have many resources to assist them in providing the best product for the ulcerations being treated. Considering the changes in the Medicare home care reimbursement system, the proliferation of managed care across the nation, and how frequently wounds are encountered in home care, wound care expertise for all home care nurses is essential to the success of wound healing and the reputation of home care agencies. Any reduction in the inconvenience, discomfort, pain, and length of time that accompanies an ulcer should be included in the caregiving goal.

REFERENCES

Bolton, L., & Rijswick, L. (1991). Wound dressings: Meeting clinical and biological needs. *Dermatology Nursing, 3*(3), 146–160.

Brown-Etris, M., & Hardy, G. (1993). The wound care puzzle. *Ostomy Wound Management, 39*(2), 45–60.

Bryant, R. (Ed.). (1992). *Acute and chronic wounds*. St. Louis: Mosby.

Bryant, R. A guide to selection of a support surface. Costa Mesa, CA: WOCN (Wound, Ostomy and Continence Nurses Society).

Clinical fact sheets. (1996). Quick assessment of leg ulcers, arterial ulcers, venous ulcers and neuropathic ulcers. Costa Mesa, CA: WOCN.

Doughty, D. (1992). Topical therapy: From concepts to results. *Ostomy Wound Management, 39*(8), 16–24.

Feinglass, J., & Tang, L. (1996). The intermittent claudication research study: Vascular outcomes research using home health nurses. *Journal of Vascular Nursing, XIV*(1), 8–11.

Grant, J., & Russell, M. (1996). Malabsorption associated with surgical procedures and its treatment. *Nutrition in Clinical Practice, 11*(2), 1996.

Hanson, D. (1996). Decreasing the prevalence of pressure ulcers using agency standards. *Home Healthcare Nurse, 14*(7), 525–531.

Krasner, D. (1991). Resolving the dressing dilemma: Selecting wound dressing by category. *Ostomy Wound Management, 35,* 62–70.

Krasner, D. (Ed.). (1990). *Chronic wound care: A clinical source book for healthcare professionals*. King of Prussia, PA: Health Management Publications, Inc.

Loescher, L. (1995). The dynamics of skin aging. *Progressions, 7*(2), 1–13.

Nutrition interventions manual for professionals caring for older Americans: Nutrition Screening Initiative. Washington, DC: Greer, Margolis, Mitchell, Grunwald & Assoc., 1991. 24 pp. Available from: The Nutrition Screening Initiative, 2626 Pennsylvania Ave., NW, Suite 301, Washington, DC 20037.

Pressure ulcers in adults: Prediction and prevention. Quick Reference Guide for Clinicians & Patient Guide. (Clinical Practice Guideline, No. 3.) U.S. Department of Health & Human Services, Public Health Services, Agency for Health Care Policy and Research; 1992, May. AHCPR Pub. No.: 92-0047 & 0048. Available by calling AHCPR, 800-358-9295.

Pressure ulcer treatment. Quick Reference Guide for Clinicians & Patient Guide. (Clinical Practice Guideline, No. 15.) U.S. Department of Health & Human Services, Public Health Services, Agency for Health Care Policy and Research; 1994, December. AHCPR Pub. No.: 95-0653 & 0654. Available by calling AHCPR, 800-358-9295.

Staab, A. S., & Hodges, L. C. (1996). *Essentials of gerontological nursing: Adaptation to the aging process*. Philadelphia: Lippincott–Raven.

Staab, A. S., & Lyles, M. (1990). *Manual of geriatric nursing*. Glenview, IL: Scott, Foresman/Little Brown Higher Education.

Thomas Hess, C. (1993). Wound care products. *Ostomy and Wound Management, 39*(3), 79–86.

Treatment of pressure ulcers: Quick Reference Guide & Consumer Guide: AHCPR Guidelines, U.S. Department of Health & Human Services, Dec. 1992.

Wysocki, A. B. (1995). A review of skin and its appendages. *Advances in Wound Care, 8*(2), 53–70.

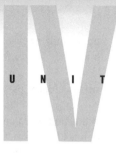

HOME CARE MANAGEMENT OF ELDERLY CLIENTS WITH SPECIFIC MEDICAL AND SURGICAL DIAGNOSES

This unit focuses on caring for elders who have been diagnosed with specific medical and surgical diagnoses. The information found in these ten chapters is helpful to the home care nurse who needs information about case management for a client with a specific diagnosis.

For nurses who are new to home healthcare, each chapter will provide important information to successfully manage elderly clients with some of the most common health problems related to aging. At times, the case load of a home health agency may be fairly stable with clients who have diabetes or cardiac or respiratory problems. When the agency provides care for clients with Alzheimer's or rheumatoid disease, even the experienced nurse may need an update on current information. All home care nurses will find information in this unit that will make caregiving easier.

The unit begins with postoperative caregiving and rheumatoid disease management. Older adults experience surgery different from younger clients. They have a longer healing time, mobility issues that may complicate recovery, and different ways of expressing pain. The client with chronic rheumatoid disease has needs that focus on pain management, mobility, and safety issues.

As the unit continues, four major disease categories are discussed; diabetes, cardiac insufficiency, respiratory maladies, and neurological incidents. These four diagnoses and the systems involved affect the greatest number of elders and make up the bulk of cases in most home care agencies. Nurses need current, up-to-date, and useful information when managing these clients.

The home care needs of the elderly psychiatric population is addressed in the next chapter.

The last three chapters in this unit focus on three different client care diagnoses, however, they are ones that have had recent changes affecting home caregiving and the role of home health agencies. Cancer, as a diagnosis, may be treated surgically, and the information on postoperative care in Chapter 13 may be helpful. In addition, the home care nurse is provided with current information on chemotherapeutic and radiologic treatment, along with pain management. The chapter on Alzheimer's disease shares the latest caregiving techniques. As people experience increasing longevity, Alzheimer's disease will affect more and more elders. The last chapter in this unit discusses palliative caregiving, regardless of the original medical or surgical diagnosis. Many home health agencies are certified to provide hospice care and to deliver palliative care to elderly clients. The needs of the family as the unit of service are shared in this final chapter.

13

CARING FOR THE ELDERLY POSTOPERATIVE CLIENT

Sheryl Mara Zang

◆ ◆ ◆

P:	Principal Diagnosis
O:	Orders for Frequency and Duration
S:	Services Ordered
T:	Treatment Ordered
O:	Ordered Medication and Other Medications in the Home
P:	Prognosis
E:	Emergency or Elective Surgery
R:	Rehabilitation Needed
A:	Assessment—Physical and Mental
T:	The Medical History
I:	Instructions/Teaching
V:	Verbal Coordination and Case Management
E:	Evaluation of Plan of Care
	Summary

Clients who at one time were thought to be surgical risks because of their age are now having all types of surgical procedures performed. Nurses need to be aware of the very acute needs of the surgical client, as well as the special needs of the elderly client. This chapter focuses on the elderly client who has had a surgical procedure. It also guides the home care nurse in using the Health Care Financing

Administration (HCFA) Form 485 (see Figure 13-1). This form helps the nurse focus the visit and understand what to look for when planning the care. Form 485 directs the individualized plan of treatment, also known as the "plan of care" (POC), and is developed in consultation with the primary care provider. This important form is required for all clients receiving home healthcare. This chapter outlines the essential fields to be familiar with (boxes on the form to be completed) when planning the care for an elderly client and uses a postoperative client as an example. It also guides the nurse when the findings of the home visit do not match Form 485. The reader will notice that this chapter is formatted in a manner that uses "postoperative" as a mnemonic device to organize the information.

P: PRINCIPAL DIAGNOSIS

The principal diagnosis is located in field 11 on Form 485. The principal diagnosis should be the primary reason why the nurse is visiting the client at home. The principal diagnosis may be related to the surgical procedure or the result of the surgical procedure. An example would be wound dehiscence following abdominal surgery. Wound dehiscence would be the principal diagnosis as this is the diagnosis that justifies skilled nursing services.

After completing a full physical exam, the nurse needs to evaluate all significant findings. As an example, a client is referred for home care with a postsurgical diagnosis of appendectomy. The client has a healed incision and no abdominal pain. The client's blood pressure is elevated at the initial visit. The nurse continues to monitor the incision site and surrounding area and to monitor the client for any complications from the surgery. The client's blood pressure and vital signs are also monitored closely. If the blood pressure continues to remain elevated, the principal diagnosis may need to be changed to hypertension. The elevated blood pressure would then continue to be monitored and the home care nurse would focus teaching on diet, medication use, and lifestyle changes, along with postoperative teaching.

The nurse should always ask: Which diagnosis justifies the need for skilled nursing service? An elderly client may have a significant history in addition to the recent surgery. The surgery may be new in onset, but at times it will be the medical history that justifies close monitoring. A client may have had a cholecystectomy, but if unstable diabetes is the acute problem at the time, the unstable diabetes should be the principal diagnosis. The nurse must understand that the plan of care

Department of Health and Human Services
Health Care Financing Administration

Form Approved
OMB No. 0938-0357

HOME HEALTH CERTIFICATION AND PLAN OF CARE

1. Patient's HI Claim No.	2. Start of Care Date	3. Certification Period From: To:	4. Medical Record No.	5. Provider No.

6. Patient's Name and Address	7. Provider's Name, Address and Telephone Number

8. Date of Birth:	9. Sex ☐ M ☐ F	10. Medications: Dose/Frequency/Route (N)ew (C)hanged

11. ICD-9-CM	Principal Diagnosis	Date	
12. ICD-9-CM	Surgical Procedure	Date	
13. ICD-9-CM	Other Pertinent Diagnoses	Date	

14. DME and Supplies	15. Safety Measures:

16. Nutritional Req.	17. Allergies:

18.A. Functional Limitations

1 ☐ Amputation	5 ☐ Paralysis	9 ☐ Legally Blind
2 ☐ Bowel/Bladder (Incontinence)	6 ☐ Endurance	A ☐ Dyspnea With Minimal Exertion
3 ☐ Contracture	7 ☐ Ambulation	B ☐ Other (Specify)
4 ☐ Hearing	8 ☐ Speech	

18.B. Activities Permitted

1 ☐ Complete Bedrest	6 ☐ Partial Weight Bearing	A ☐ Wheelchair
2 ☐ Bedrest BRP	7 ☐ Independent At Home	B ☐ Walker
3 ☐ Up As Tolerated		C ☐ No Restrictions
4 ☐ Transfer Bed/Chair	8 ☐ Crutches	D ☐ Other (Specify)
5 ☐ Exercises Prescribed	9 ☐ Cane	

19. Mental Status:

1 ☐ Oriented	3 ☐ Forgetful	5 ☐ Disoriented	7 ☐ Agitated
2 ☐ Comatose	4 ☐ Depressed	6 ☐ Lethargic	8 ☐ Other

20. Prognosis: 1 ☐ Poor   2 ☐ Guarded   3 ☐ Fair   4 ☐ Good   5 ☐ Excellent

21. Orders for Discipline and Treatments (Specify Amount/Frequency/Duration)

22. Goals/Rehabilitation Potential/Discharge Plans

23. Nurse's Signature and Date of Verbal SOC Where Applicable:	25. Date HHA Received Signed POT

24. Physician's Name and Address	26. I certify/recertify that this patient is confined to his/her home and needs intermittent skilled nursing care, physical therapy and/or speech therapy or continues to need occupational therapy. The patient is under my care, and I have authorized the services on this plan of care and will periodically review the plan.
27. Attending Physician's Signature and Date Signed	28. Anyone who misrepresents, falsifies, or conceals essential information required for payment of Federal funds may be subject to fine, imprisonment or civil penalty under applicable Federal laws.

Form HCFA-485 (C-4) (02-94) (Print Aligned)

Privacy Act Statement

Sections 1812, 1814, 1815, 1816, 1861, and 1862 of the Social Security Act authorize collection of this information. The primary use of this information is to process and pay Medicare benefits to or on behalf of eligible individuals. Disclosure of this information may be made to: Peer Review Organizations and Quality Review Organizations in connection with their review of claims, or in connection with studies or other review activities, conducted pursuant to Part B of Title XI of the Social Security Act; State Licensing Boards for review of unethical practices or nonprofessional conduct; A congressional office from the record of an individual in response to an inquiry from the congressional office at the request of that individual.

Where the individual's identification number is his/her Social Security Number (SSN), collection of this information is authorized by Executive Order 9397. Furnishing the information on this form, including the SSN, is voluntary, but failure to do so may result in disapproval of the request for payment of Medicare benefits.

Paper Work Burden Statement

Public reporting burden for this collection of information is estimated to average 15 minutes per response and recordkeeping burden is estimated to average 15 minutes per response. This includes time for reviewing instructions, searching existing data sources, gathering and maintaining data needed, and completing and reviewing the collection of information. Send comments regarding this burden estimate or any other aspect of this collection of information, including suggestions for reducing the burden, to Health Care Financing Administration, P.O. Box 26684, Baltimore, Maryland 21207, and to the Office of Information and Regulatory Affairs, Office of Management and Budget, Washington, D.C. 20503. Paperwork Reduction Project 0938-0357.

FIGURE 13-1 • HCFA Form 485

for frequency, duration, and services ordered has to be relevant to the principal diagnosis.

All diagnoses pertinent to the plan of care are listed with date of onset or date of exacerbation. Insurance companies and case managers understand that elderly postoperative clients require close monitoring, but if a client had an uneventful outpatient procedure or a routine postoperative hospital experience, it is the nurse's responsibility to justify why home care visits continue to be needed. The nurse must always document and support the services provided in the home. By understanding which diagnosis should be the principal diagnosis, the insurance surveyors can easily determine the need for skilled services and how they are being met.

O: ORDERS FOR FREQUENCY AND DURATION

The orders for frequency and duration are located in field 21 on Form 485. The home care nurse uses this information to be aware of the primary care provider's orders for frequency and duration of visits. Depending on the client's insurance coverage, or if the client is in a managed care company, the nurse plans for the assessment and teaching to fit into a specified amount of visits. The client's physical and mental status are assessed and realistic goals are planned.

The nurse may find that the elderly client is very confused or very anxious, especially after a surgical procedure. This may slow down the teaching process and necessitate that the nurse visit more often, especially when the case is newly opened. If extra visits are indicated, this must be documented and at times verbally reported. All changes have to be made in consultation with the primary care provider.

The situation that the nurse finds in the home may be completely different than what is listed on Form 485. A home care nurse may visit a client and find the client to be incontinent, unable to ambulate independently, and very forgetful and agitated. However, the functional limitations in field 18A describe the client as continent, the activities permitted in field 18B describe the client as up as tolerated, and the mental status in field 19 lists the client as oriented but forgetful. The plan of care in this case, especially the frequency of visits, has to be addressed with the primary care provider. The nurse has to evaluate the functional needs of the elderly client, as well as the acute postoperative needs. The frequency of visits should be designed to ensure client safety between visits and client safety at home.

The nurse addressing the postoperative care of an elder realizes that the client may also be at great risk for new problems. The incontinent client who is confused and unable to ambulate independently can experience skin breakdown and contractures. A plan of care should be put into place that addresses these concerns in addition to the presenting needs. Visits may need to occur more frequently due to the client's functional limitations and level of orientation. The duration of service may need to be increased as well. Addressing each functional limitation with a plan that reflects skilled nursing is the home care nurse's goal. The postoperative period may progress without any significant findings, but documenting the other care the elderly client needs is important so that visits can be justified.

If an elderly client develops a postoperative infection or complication, the nurse needs to notify the primary care provider immediately and closely monitor the client. An increase in frequency of visits may be indicated. The nurse consults with the primary care provider to ensure that the frequency of visits and duration of care match the needs of the client.

S: SERVICES ORDERED

The elderly postoperative client, as well as clients with other diagnoses, must need at least one skilled service to receive home care services that are reimbursed by Medicare. The services ordered are located in field 21 under *disciplines*. At the initial visit, the nurse evaluates the client for services. On every following visit, the nurse reevaluates to see if there are any changes necessitating additional skilled services or if any change in home health aide status is indicated.

Additional or reduced services may be in order if there is a significant change in the client's condition. For example, a client who had a surgical procedure with complications is very weak from prolonged bedrest and hospitalization. The only service ordered at the time of discharge was skilled nursing. On the initial visit, the nurse and client felt that restorative therapy was indicated. The nurse consulted with the primary care provider, and physical therapy was ordered. Another client was very confused during her hospital stay. She had had a surgical procedure and kept pulling at all the tubes and removing the IVs. The client was sent home with an order for 24-hour home health aide service. When the nurse met the client during the initial visit, the client was oriented and very comfortable in her surroundings. She was able to perform all her own ADL. The nurse reduced the home health aide service to four hours times five days a week for assistance with shopping, laundry, and personal care. In the third week of home care service, the home health aide visits were reduced to three times a week for two hours of assistance with personal care. These examples demonstrate how the nurse ensures that the functional needs of the client match the services ordered.

Services for the elderly postoperative client are regularly reassessed for either an increase or decrease in the frequency and duration of services. Elderly postoperative clients should be monitored for changes in alertness and cognition, responses to the care given, changes in condition, new problems, or changes in the diagnosis. The environment and support system are also monitored, as well as any other change in personal care needs.

T: TREATMENT ORDERED

The treatment orders for the home care client are located in field 21 of Form 485. The home care nurse evaluates the client's response to the treatment ordered for appropriateness at the initial visit and on every revisit. As an example, a client may have had a postoperative incision that required follow-up at-home treatment at the time of discharge from the hospital. On the initial home visit, the home care nurse evaluates for a change in treatment needs and for complicating environmental factors. The nurse assesses the client for the ability to complete treatment independently or with help from others. If the client cannot be independent in a certain treatment, this is documented, along with the reasons why, what alternative plan (including family and caregiver teaching) was implemented, and arrangements for future visits. Each notation includes the client's response to the treatment.

A client who undergoes an outpatient surgical procedure or an emergency procedure may have a very involved medical history that complicates what might otherwise have been a simple procedure. For example, on an initial home visit, a nurse finds the client using oxygen and nebulizer treatments in the home. If the surgeon is unaware of these treatments, the nurse coordinates care with the primary care provider who prescribed the treatments and includes it in the surgeon's plan of care. Ideally, treatments found in the home correlate to a diagnosis. If oxygen or nebulizer treatments are needed, there should a respiratory diagnosis justifying these treatments.

Some clients use home remedies or folk treatments that are part of their cultural, religious, or regional practice. The primary care provider should be made aware of this and the practice incorporated into the plan of care, once it is determined that the practice either has a neutral or beneficial effect on the client's treatment and recovery. In some instances, the home remedy potentiates the effect of the original medication or prescribed treatment, which may need to be reduced or changed. If the practice is determined to be harmless and the client has faith in it, following its use may support the client emotionally and assist in recovery.

O: ORDERED MEDICATION AND OTHER MEDICATIONS IN THE HOME

The home care nurse needs to compare the primary care provider's orders very carefully with the medication that the client is taking at home. The client's surgeon may be unaware of the complete medication profile. The nurse needs to follow up with the primary care provider who ordered the medication and inform the surgeon about what medication the client is taking. Some medication may be contraindicated in the postoperative state.

Postsurgically, pain medication and medication for sleep may have been ordered in the hospital and automatically written on prescriptions for the client to take at home. The nurse reviews each medication with the client. If the client does not need or want it, the nurse needs to coordinate this with the surgeon and discontinue the medication.

Another concern is whether the elderly client can independently manage the medication routine. The nurse completes a medication assessment, emphasizing medications that are new or changed since the surgery. The nurse will gain more accurate information about a client's medication understanding if the client is given an opportunity to explain what the medication is used for, when it is taken, and the effects expected. If the client is able to read the label and tell the nurse what the prescription is and how to take it, the nurse can provide a written medication tool to help the client remember dosage schedules. If the client needs to open the bottle to look at the medication, the teaching should be focused on what the medication looks like for identification purposes. The nurse can develop a schedule tool that incorporates pictures of the medication for this type of learner. If the client needs to smell or touch the medication to identify it, the nurse can include one of the pills taped to the teaching tool so the client can clearly identify what medication to take at what time. The nurse should reinforce medication instruction at each visit.

If the elderly client is unable to self-manage the medication, the nurse must involve the family and other caregivers as much as possible. If the medication regimen is very complex, the nurse should discuss this with the primary care provider. A medication that was ordered for four times a day may be changed in dose so that it can be given two times a day. Family members may need to call the client at the time the medication is to be taken to remind the client. If there is no significant other, the nurse helps the client identify if there are any neighbors that can assist. If there is no reasonable assistance available, the nurse needs to coordinate with the primary care provider; depending on the client's insurance, the nurse may need to visit weekly to prefill a medication dispensing device that the client can safely manage throughout the week.

A medication list is a necessary tool for nurses to refer to in the client's home, and it will also assist the surgeon and the various primary care providers that the client needs to see. The client should be instructed to take the medication list on each visit to a primary care provider. The list should be updated as needed.

When reviewing the medications with the client, the nurse asks if there are any medications taken due to religious or cultural beliefs. Just as with treatments, the primary care provider needs to be aware of any nonprescription medications the client is taking. These medications should be incorporated into the plan of care if possible. If a folk medicine or over-the-counter remedy is contraindicated by the primary care provider, the nurse should incorporate this instruction into revisits and stress the reasons why it is not recommended with their present medication schedule. If clients understand the "why" for things, it helps them make informed decisions.

P: PROGNOSIS

Many elderly clients who undergo surgical procedures are unprepared for the extent and involvement of the diagnosis and outcome of the surgery. A typical case situation involves a client who has had abdominal pain and difficulty moving her bowels. Results of various tests revealed that there was an obstruction. The surgeon told the client of the possibility of different outcomes, depending upon the findings during the surgery. During the surgery, it was determined that the client needed to have a colostomy. The client may have heard the surgeon say this preoperatively, but postoperatively it was very hard for her to cope with the actual outcome. The client had a typically short hospital stay and came home completely unfamiliar with all the care needed to manage the colostomy and the emotional effects of the body image changes. The surgeon also found that the tumor causing the obstruction was malignant, and the client was informed that she would need outpatient chemotherapy. These changes were sudden, permanent, and would have been difficult for the client to cope with without instruction and much needed support, both of which the home care nurse provided.

Once a client is aware of the diagnosis and prognosis, many concerns are expressed and need to be addressed. The skilled nursing needs of the elderly postoperative client have to be addressed immediately so that the client can effectively manage self-care between nursing visits. The nurse has to ensure that each visit reflects a skilled nursing need.

The home care nurse needs a complex set of skills to assist the client who is very overwhelmed with the prognosis or outcome of the surgical procedure. Caregiving needs should be coordinated with the primary care provider and social work intervention may be indicated. The nurse also needs to be familiar with the different community resources and support services available to the client. The client may do very well in a support group with people that are going through a similar process. The nurse always considers contingency planning. If other resources or services are more appropriate for the client, the client is discharged from the home care program and referred to the appropriate services. Such options include moving to an assisted living center or a residential care facility, or enrollment in a hospice program if the client's prognosis is poor and life expectancy is less than six months (see Chapter 22).

It is imperative that the nurse understand how involved the client wants the nurse to be in the decision-making process regarding healthcare choices. Depending upon cultural or religious practices, the client may not want to involve the nurse or other healthcare providers. The nurse also needs to ask clients if there are other people that they would like involved in the plan of care. Some clients may pick a relative or neighbor, and some may prefer a religious leader be involved.

On the initial home visit, the nurse includes in the assessment the client's understanding of the type and outcome of the surgery. Many family members do not want the elderly client to know the diagnosis and prognosis. The nurse should provide the necessary skilled care and consider the family's wishes. However, it is the responsibility of the nurse to discuss this decision with the family, as the client has a right to be informed. Frequently, the client is aware of the diagnosis and prognosis and is protecting the family by not mentioning it. An elderly client may ask the nurse, "What is really wrong with me?" The best response is to ask what the client thinks is wrong. Based on the response, either confirm the seriousness of the surgery or, if the explanation shared is nowhere near the direction the illness will be taking the client, suggest the client ask the primary care provider for the particulars about the surgery and long-term expected outcome.

Frequently, the family tries to "protect" the client, not realizing the client may be much more ready for the information than the family gives the client credit for. Clients may want to make decisions regarding distribution of valuables, people they want to see, and places they want to visit, or to complete their funeral plans. When family members keep the truth to themselves, they take these choices away from the client.

Family members may be very anxious and find that their coping patterns may be ineffective at times. The nurse may need to assist with referrals to meet their needs, as well as the clients. There are many support services and groups designed to include family members. The nurse should always ask the client if family members can be involved in the visit. If the client agrees, family members should be prepared for the changes the client will be going through and given concrete ways in which they can assist the client, considering each one's physical and emotional ability.

E: EMERGENCY OR ELECTIVE SURGERY

Many elderly clients have emergency surgery because an immediate intervention is indicated. These clients do not have time to prepare for the surgery, either physically or mentally, and may take a longer time to adjust to any changes. Some clients may not even understand afterward why the surgery was conducted. The nurse will be better prepared to assist the client if the client understands the events leading up to the surgery. Then, a plan of care can be formulated based on the client's readiness to learn.

Some elders choose to have planned, elective surgery. These clients had choices to make and felt that surgery was the best choice. They may be more prepared to take an active role in any new self-care practices needed as a result of the surgery.

When the nurse visits a postoperative elderly client, a detailed history is obtained (see Chapter 3). The history and physical findings that led to the decision to have surgery gives the nurse a more complete picture of the client. Many clients have chosen surgery for the relief of symptoms and an improvement in their physical status. The clients who choose to have a surgical procedure tend to cope better when the surgery involves body image changes or causes some new acute problem. Clients who have emergency surgery may be overwhelmed by any change in body image or any a new treatment or procedure needed as a result of the surgery.

The nurse visits more frequently in the beginning postoperative phase to monitor the client's health status and any signs of inability to cope. An inability to cope will affect the self-care practices of the client. The nurse has to plan for the client's care until the client can care for self.

When a client with a detailed medical history has planned the surgery, the client has time to ensure that all other health problems are monitored and under control. A client who has diabetes or hypertension may have needed medical intervention and stabilization before the surgery took place. The client may also have needed to adjust medications or change lifestyle behaviors. This preoperative monitoring of the client's medical status and lifestyle changes will have a positive effect on the outcome of the surgery.

For clients who have emergency surgery, the medical conditions may not be under control. The postoperative considerations may include conditions that need close monitoring, readjustment of medication, and lifestyle changes. The nurse not only monitors the postoperative state but the underlying medical condition as well. If a client has had no time to prepare for surgery or feels overwhelmed with the diagnosis, change in body image, or new self-care practices, the client may benefit from a variety of community support services.

R: REHABILITATION NEEDED

Surgery may alter functional status and place the older client in a temporary state of weakness. Whether the surgery was emergency or elective, the nurse needs to find out the functional status prior to surgery and incorporate a plan of care that will help the client regain that status.

Depending upon the client's condition after surgery and the type of surgery that the client underwent, physical therapy may be indicated. The nurse needs to be involved in the functional status assessment of the client and evaluate whether nursing rehabilitation is sufficient or if physical therapy is indicated.

Home care nurses recognize that the elderly client becomes more independent in ADL as a result of being home and back in a familiar setting. However, the client is usually in a weakened state, both from the surgery and the hospitalization, and realistic rehabilitation goals need to be incorporated into the plan of care. In some situations, the client's condition is indicative of needing restorative therapy. Rehabilitation nursing must be a part of every nursing visit.

The home health aide is an essential part of the nursing rehabilitation plan. Initially, when the client comes home from the hospital, the home health aide's plan of care reflects all the assistance needed with ambulation, transfer, and range of motion exercises. As the client's condition changes, the home health aide's plan of care incorporates the improvement or decline in the client's functional status.

An elderly client may only have had ambulatory surgery and been in the hospital for just a few hours, but if anesthesia was involved, the client will be weakened and need time to recover from the combined effects of anesthesia, surgery, and stronger or more frequent doses of medication for pain, especially in the first hours after the surgery. The surgeries that are now performed on an outpatient basis were once performed as inpatient procedures and clients had time to recover in the hospital. Clients are now discharged sooner, and as a result they must address postoperative concerns in addition to meeting ADL and IADL needs.

Home care nurses must cooperate with the surgeon and ensure that the ambulation and activity orders are clear and that the client has a very good understanding of restrictions and limitations. Depending upon the surgeon and the specific needs of the client, postoperative activity orders and restrictions may vary greatly from client to client.

On the initial visit, the home care nurse asks to see any discharge papers from the hospital and any guidelines for exercises or restrictions. A client who has had a mastectomy will need special arm exercises, which usually are started within 24 hours after surgery. An elderly client who has had an above the knee amputation needs to know not to stay in a semi-Fowler's position in order to prevent a contracture of the hip. If specific orders are not written on the primary care provider's plan of care, the nurse follows up with the surgeon and instructs the client appropriately. Written instructions that the client and family can refer to between home health nursing visits and after services are terminated can be very helpful.

A: ASSESSMENT—PHYSICAL AND MENTAL

The elderly postoperative client needs to be followed very closely at home, especially if the client had a short hospital stay. The home care nurse uses the same basic principles of postoperative care that nurses assesses for in the hospital.

The nurse conducts a full systems review as part of the history and physical. The referral for home care indicates the purpose of the visit, and the surgeon may have written on discharge papers to be notified of certain parameters (e.g., a temperature above 101 degrees or a blood pressure below or above a certain range). The nurse needs to speak with the surgeon after the initial visit to discuss the findings. If there are untoward findings, the surgeon may change the parameters. One client situation involved an elder with a transurethral resection of the prostate. The nurse discussed the findings of the initial visit with the surgeon and verified the client's medications. The nurse asked the surgeon if she wanted to be notified if any findings occurred. The surgeon said she wanted to be notified if the client had excessive clots or any active bleeding five days after the surgery. The nurse then visited the client on the fifth postoperative day and found that the client had excessive bleeding and clots. The nurse called the surgeon and an appointment was made for the client to see the surgeon later that day.

In addition to the initial assessment, the nurse's role includes close monitoring and a full systems review at each visit (see chapter 3). Even if the client had no significant findings on the previous visit, there are many possible changes during the postoperative period that need monitoring. Checking vital signs and comparing them to previous visits and the hospital discharge record guides the nurse in decision making. For the client's well-being, a stable cardiovascular system must be maintained. The nurse also assesses for complications, such as a pulmonary embolism or hypovolemic shock. The respiratory system is assessed to make sure that the client does not have symptoms of pneumonia or atelectasis. Urinary output (quantity and quality) and bowel status is assessed. The nurse assesses the surgical wound site for any signs of infection such as redness, purulent drainage, or fever.

If the surgical incision is open and a treatment is ordered, the nurse visits for the treatment until the client, family, or caregiver can learn the wound care. Nursing visits are then tapered off. The nurse continues to visit to monitor the status of the wound, the client's overall health status, and the caregiver's ability to manage care. The nurse should discharge the client when the incision is healed.

The primary care provider must be notified if there is any dehiscence-separation or splitting open of layers of the surgical wound. The surgeon may want to order a different type of treatment, see the client, or have the client readmitted to the hospital. The nurse has to make sure that the client and family members understand the signs and symptoms of infection and postoperative complications and know to call the nursing agency or primary care provider if changes are observed.

The home care nurse evaluates the ambulation and functional status of the elderly postoperative client and assesses the client's ability to function safely throughout the day and night. Becoming familiar with the client's routine helps the nurse determine if the client will need in-home assistance, professional or otherwise.

One example of assessing functional ability involves an 81-year-old female client who came home from the hospital after having a surgical repair of the right hip. The client was discharged from the hospital with a walker and orders for full weight bearing. The nurse assessed the client and documented that she was able to ambulate with a slow and steady gait using the walker. The nurse was told the next day that the client fell during the night and broke her other hip. The client fell while ambulating to the bathroom. Perhaps this could have been prevented if the nurse had assessed the 24-hour routine of the client. If the nurse had asked the client about nighttime habits, the client may have revealed that she gets up at night to use the bathroom. The nurse could have evaluated the environment and the client's ability to get to the bathroom safely at night to determined if a commode was indicated. Home care nurses evaluate for any services or devices that would make the client's road to recovery an easier one.

A client may have a very uneventful immediate postoperative recovery. Typically, the nurse visits more frequently in the beginning and tapers visits as the postoperative period progresses. The nurse is always aware, however, that surgical complications can occur many days after the surgery. The nurse ensures that the client has a follow-up appointment with the surgeon and is able to keep it.

T: THE MEDICAL HISTORY

The home care nurse enters the client's home with the primary care provider's orders and, at times, a hospital discharge report. However thorough, these may not give the nurse a complete medical history of the client. When obtaining the medical history, it is important to get the present history and then progress backwards. If an elderly client has had diabetes for twenty years, the nurse will certainly incorporate it into the plan of care, but the instruction needed and the affect on the surgical outcome may not be as great as that of a client with new, unstable, insulin dependent diabetes. The dates of onset are very important, as the medical history may have been the reason the client needed surgical intervention. If a client has a long history of cardiac complications that resulted in cardiac surgery, the client has had time to prepare for this. If the client has a new colostomy with no past history of bowel complications, this may require a greater adjustment.

As mentioned earlier, the nurse needs to review each medication the client is taking, both prescribed and over-the-counter. The nurse matches each medication to a condition or diagnosis. By asking the client when each medication was ordered and why, the nurse can help piece together the client's medical history. If a client cannot remember and there is no family member to assist, the nurse can coordinate information with the primary care provider who is listed on the medication bottle. If the client is unaware of the primary care provider's address or phone number, the home care nurse should call the pharmacy as that information is kept on file there.

After coordinating care with the primary care provider, the nurse has an understanding of the status of the client's medical conditions. The extent and severity of the illness are important to be aware of so that goals can be realistically planned. If the client has a history of angina and is aware of the medications and possible complications, the number of nursing visits that focus on monitoring and teaching cardiac management are quite limited. If the client has just been diagnosed with diabetes, the nurse needs to realistically plan how long it will take to teach every step of diabetes management, regardless of the surgical diagnosis.

Many nurses find it helpful to use the agency's initial form and complete as much of the form as possible while taking the history. The medical history certainly has an impact on the surgical outcome. If the client has a known medical history of diabetes, understanding the effect of diabetes on the client's overall health is imperative. If a client has a history of peripheral vascular disease and had a toe amputated, the healing process may be slower and close monitoring of the vascular status is indicated.

At the initial visit, the nurse asks what the client's major medical concerns are at this time. Concerns may not be related to the surgery or the client's medical history. The client could be concerned with dizziness or frequency with urination. Sometimes the symptoms of other health problems, and the need to eliminate them, are more important to the client than the surgical problem. The nurse has to follow up with the primary care provider as these concerns may not have been addressed in the pre- or postoperative period. The client's chief complaint is one of the most important parts of the assessment, and the complaint can certainly change from visit to visit. The nurse follows up with the primary care provider to help the client meet these immediate needs.

I: INSTRUCTIONS/TEACHING

Many home care agencies are using clinical pathways that outline how many nursing visits a client can receive, depending upon the diagnosis and what is to be assessed, taught, and monitored. Clinical pathways work very nicely when the client is "routine" and the pre- and postoperative periods are uneventful. The home care nurse soon realizes that most clients do not fall into the routine category. After the nurse does a complete physical, mental, and environmental assessment, the goal is to accurately outline the client's problems with specific teaching interventions. Teaching can only take place when the client is ready to learn. As mentioned earlier, the elderly client may have had emergency surgery, still be in a weakened state, and possibly in denial of the outcome. If a client had a mastectomy or a colostomy or part of a toe removed, the client may be focused on the loss and not what the home care nurse is teaching. Because of shorter hospital stays, clients may come home in pain, weak, and angry, feeling that they should still be in the hospital.

Clients may not be aware of what Medicare or other insurance companies cover and feel that they need more than four hours of home health aide service daily. The nurse must prioritize goals and assess the client's ability to understand and carry out a treatment plan.

The most important concern is to find out how the client functioned prior to surgery and hospitalization. The home care nurse may determine that the client is forgetful or confused, but revise the intervention when the client says he remembers to take his medications because he puts them by his coffee cup. The client's routine may not have to change if teaching focuses on incorporating modifications. For instance, to fit deep breathing into the client's routine, the nurse can ask what television show the client watches at 10:00 o'clock. If the client can remember and tells the nurse what show is on what channel, perhaps the nurse can instruct the client to do deep breathing exercises every time a commercial comes on. This strategy works well for many rehabilitation exercises (e.g., arm exercises for clients who just had a mastectomy).

The home care nurse needs to realize that the same priorities outlined in the hospital need to be outlined at home. If the client only receives four hours of home health aide service in the morning and the client's appetite is poor, the home health aide has to be instructed to make sure that the client's main meal is lunch. The home health aide can also prepare snacks and supper and leave them in the refrigerator. If the client's fluid intake is poor, the client may need to have a pitcher and glass set up to be a constant reminder to drink. Clients may be confused when they report their history or other significant facts, but they may be able to function well in all ADL activities.

A client who is recovering from hip surgery resulting from a fall may need to find a grocery store that delivers or get help from family or neighbors. The family should be involved as much as possible but only with the client's permission. Elderly clients may not realize the importance of hiring someone to assist them. The nurse can determine what a private aide can help with and realistically plan how many hours of assistance is needed and how it may impact the client's budget. If the nurse compares the cost of a private aide with the cost of a month in an extended care facility, the client will have something with which to compare the cost favorably. Remaining independent at home with this additional help may be more welcomed after the comparison.

The key to client education is to fit in the teaching that impacts the client immediately. Medication compliance, understanding and following diet restrictions, safety, and complications to observe for are the most important goals to achieve. If the client is unable to be taught and there is no significant other available for teaching, the agency supervisor has to be made aware as the client cannot be left alone at home and other arrangements need to be made.

The nurse involves the client and, if possible, the family in every aspect of the visit. The goal is to ensure that the teaching is incorporated immediately into the client's routine and that the client continues with these practices when discharged from the home care program. The nurse needs to document what was taught and the client's and family's response to the teaching. If the client has any condition that affects or limits the amount of teaching that can be done at each visit, it must be documented. For example, if a client has limited vision, arthritis, or poor manual dexterity, this needs to be documented when teaching a client how to fill an insulin syringe.

V: VERBAL COORDINATION AND CASE MANAGEMENT

The home care nurse coordinates care with the primary care provider who has signed the plan of care. At times it may be the surgeon and at other times it may be the client's medical primary care provider. The surgeon may verify the medication or refer the home care nurse to the primary care provider who prescribed the medication. The nurse needs to coordinate care when: a case is newly opened, there is a change in the client's condition, there is a need for increased or decreased visits, or a new treatment or medication is indicated or ordered. The nurse is also responsible for coordinating with the other interprofessional team members involved in the care of the client.

In addition, the home care nurse follows up and coordinates care with case managers if the client's health insurance company requires prior approval for visits. The nurse calls the case manager with the initial visit report, before more home care visits are approved, and at the time of discharge. The nurse usually has to inform the case manager of any change in the client's condition. The home care nurse gives the case manager a detailed assessment of the client's living situation, support systems, and available caregivers. The nurse reports the client's vital signs and significant clinical findings that support the need for skilled nursing visits. The client's functional status and limitations that justify the need for a home health aide or any other services or devices are also reported. The nurse is responsible for planning realistic goals and times frames. When discussing the elderly postoperative client, the nurse gives specific details about the surgical procedure and postoperative findings. The nurse justifies all the interventions that are needed with a detailed report of the client's clinical status. The nurse needs to document very carefully who was spoken to, the outcome of the conversation, and when an updated report is due. Documentation about care coordinated with family members, primary care providers, professionals in other disciplines, and community agencies is vital and a significant part of home care nursing.

E: EVALUATION OF PLAN OF CARE

Field 22 on Form 485 is where the nurse answers the question, "What goals will be achieved by the client receiving home care services?" The emphasis in home care is directed to an outcome-oriented model of service. The home care nurse outlines a plan of care for each individual client based on the client's diagnosis and the nursing assessment. The nurse writes short-term goals that are time framed and realistic based on the client's diagnosis. Long-term goals are also realistic and measurable and help the nurse describe the anticipated outcome for the client based on the plan of care and teaching. These goals direct the nurse and plan the length of service in response to the client's needs.

At the initial visit and assessment, the nurse identifies the client's needs that require intervention. The most important thing the nurse does is determine the factors that will help or hinder the client in accomplishing the goals. As the home care nurse continues to visit, the assessment of the client is ongoing. At times, the goals have to be reevaluated. The nurse may realize that certain goals or outcomes may be unachievable for some clients, regardless of the interventions planned.

As an example, one elderly client was referred for home care services for abdominal wound care as a result of surgery. The client's daughter was very involved and stated that she would learn to do the wound care. On the initial visit, the nurse instructed the client and daughter on the signs and symptoms of infection and complications. The nurse instructed the daughter how to set up a sterile field and remove the old dressing. When the daughter saw the wound, she was overwhelmed. She had not seen the wound in the hospital and was unaware of how big it was. The daughter was very anxious and fearful and said she did not want to touch it and was not willing to learn the wound care at this time. The client could not do the wound care herself due to the location of the wound and her poor manual dexterity. The nurse carefully documented the daughter's response and supported the need for the nurse to continue visiting daily to provide the wound care while slowly reintroducing the idea of caring for the wound with the daughter. When the daughter noticed the wound was getting smaller and the client could assist somewhat, she was more willing to participate and eventually was proud of her ability to assist her mother.

On every revisit, the nurse assesses the client's progress toward goals according to the plan outlined on the initial visit. The nurse always has to question if the interventions are appropriate. If the client is not progressing toward independence and goal achievement, the nurse has to assess the factors that prevent progression. The nurse has to identify actions that must be taken and implement corrective actions.

At the time of being discharged from the home care program, goals should have been achieved and the client should be able to incorporate all the teaching into the daily routine. A client is discharged when the condition has improved or stabilized and services are no longer medically necessary or the client's maximum rehabilitation potential has been met. There are certain situations in which a client is discharged when the anticipated goals have not been met. A client may refuse home care or request that services be discontinued, or the client may refuse to obtain needed medical care when such care is considered essential for continuation of the treatment plan. The nurse needs to coordinate with the primary care provider when this occurs and inform the primary care provider that the client is being discharged.

The home care nurse always thinks in terms of goals and discharge plans and recognizes that certain goals or outcomes may not be realistic for some clients, regardless of the amount or type of intervention planned.

SUMMARY

When delivering home care services to elderly postoperative clients, the nurse must consider the special needs that older adults bring to the surgical arena. Preparing for surgery often needs more time, teaching postoperative care takes longer, healing may be complicated by other medical conditions, and recovery time is prolonged. All the areas that are important to cover when caring for the older surgical client have been shared in this chapter with the help of a mnemonic device, the word "postoperative." The information is arranged to assist the home care nurse with completing an important form (Form 485) that is essential to documentation of care of elders receiving Medicare reimbursement.

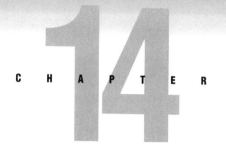

CARING FOR THE ELDERLY CLIENT WITH RHEUMATIC DISEASE

Eileen Garry

◆   ◆   ◆

Rheumatism is a common name for many aches and pains that have no peculiar identification, though owing to different causes. Most forms of arthritis are chronic, meaning they can last a lifetime, and with age the symptoms worsen. Arthritis is accompanied by both physical and psychological effects. The pain and limited movement can make ordinary daily tasks nearly impossible for the elderly client. Simply getting out of bed, dressing, bathing, walking, or opening doors can all become major chores. Psychologically, the daily pain can lead to increased stress and fatigue. This pain, stress, and fatigue can lead to anger and depression. There are also strains on the interrelationships between the person with arthritis and family, friends, and caretakers. The home care nurse, with current information on rheumatic diseases, can significantly impact the quality of life for arthritic clients and their families.

REVIEW OF RHEUMATIC DISEASE (RD): PREVALENCE, PROCESS, AND CAUSE

Rheumatic disease is composed of more than 199 different diseases that cause pain, swelling, and limited movement in joints and connective tissue throughout the body. The disease is usually chronic and specific causes are not yet known for most forms. The disease process also varies depending on the form of arthritis. Joint problems are the number one recognized cause of occupational disability, and cause suffering comparable in prevalence and severity to a major illness.

Nearly 40 million Americans (one in seven) have arthritis. According to the Arthritis Foundation as many as half of the people who have arthritis do not know what form of arthritis they have, which means they cannot make informed decisions about their own care because treatment options vary among the different forms of arthritis. Clients depend upon the home care nurse to help them understand the differences and develop an individual healthcare plan.

Most rheumatic diseases are chronic, characterized by exacerbation and remission. Rarely is there a cure, but present day research has made great strides in the areas of pain management and treatment. It is important that the client and family understand that the disease is often cyclic in nature, and they should expect both good and bad days. Clients should also understand that their actions on any given day can cause a flare up or exacerbation of the disease.

Although many forms of arthritis occur in both men and women, some of the most common and most damaging attack women more often than men. A few of the more common forms of arthritis include:

Osteoarthritis (OA): Affects 11.7 million women, representing 74% of all cases; causes the breakdown of joint cartilage, which leads to joint pain and stiffness.

Fibromyalgia: Affects 3.7 million people and seven times more women than men. Fibromyalgia is a complex disorder characterized by widespread pain and decreased pain threshold.

Rheumatoid arthritis (RA): Affects 1.5 million women, representing 71% of all cases; as an autoimmune disease, the immune system, which normally protects the body from disease, turns against healthy parts of the body, especially the joints.

Systemic lupus erythematosus (SLE): Affects 117,000 women representing 89% of all cases; also an autoimmune disease, can cause damage to the skin, kidneys, blood vessels, nervous system, heart, and other internal organs.

NONINFLAMMATORY OSTEOARTHRITIS

Osteoarthritis (OA) is not caused by the immune system; it is generally considered to be due to wear and tear of the joint surfaces that give pain on movement. Osteoarthritis is also known as a degenerative musculoskeletal condition in which the cartilage that covers the ends of bones in the joint deteriorates, causing pain and loss of movement as bone begins to rub against bone. This condition is common among elderly clients. There are many factors influencing its development, including a family history of OA and previous damage to the joint through injury or surgery, joint overuse, and obesity.

It is essential that clients and their family or caretaker understand the progression of OA so that they may begin controlling the disease through treatments and compliance with care goals. They need to know about treatments and medications to relieve symptoms.

Helping the client to understand the how and why of the diagnosis of OA is vitally important. Clients who have self-diagnosed and possibly self-treated OA may have done so for a number of reasons, including the inability to get to or pay for a primary care provider's care. If the client is self-diagnosed they may be putting themselves at risk in several ways. They may end up enduring more pain and loss of function than necessary. More importantly, an undiagnosed and untreated or improperly treated condition may progress, possibly bringing on greater loss of quality of life, joint or organ damage, and, in extreme cases, death.

Complications of OA are ankylosis (immobility and fixation) and deformity of one or more joints, with loss of sensation and decreased mobility. It may be confirmed by a primary care provider during a physical examination that includes gait analysis, laboratory analysis of synovial fluid, family history of the disease, radiological studies (x-ray, computed tomography [CT], magnetic resonance imaging [MRI]), bone scan, and by ruling out other types of arthritis. Because OA is so common, the condition may be present simultaneously with other types of arthritis.

The home care nurse needs to make the client aware that many types of arthritis reveal themselves slowly and alerting the doctor to new or changed symptoms will give enough pieces for the doctor to put the puzzle together. Every clue can help. For example, details concerning the character of the pain, such as location, its time of onset, and factors that make it better or worse are important clues. See Box 14-1 for information about conducting a client assessment for OA.

INFLAMMATORY RHEUMATOID ARTHRITIS

Rheumatoid arthritis (RA) is caused by the immune system, which normally protects the body from disease, but in this condition seems to turn against the body, especially the joints. This autoimmune reaction leads to the destruction of cartilage and connective tissue, resulting in deformity of the joints. RA is a systemic disease, meaning that it affects the entire body. Although it is not directly inherited, there is a familial association with the disease. In RA, the joint lining becomes inflamed as a result of the body's immune system activity. The chronic inflammation causes deterioration of the joint, pain, and limited motion. RA may also be caused by an infectious agent.

Rheumatoid arthritis affects children 8–15 years old, adults 25–55 years old, and more women than men. However, onset of RA can occur throughout life. It is a chronic, systemic, autoimmune inflammatory disease of the connective tissue of the body. Due to the long-term nature of the disease, however, there is a higher prevalence among the elderly population. RA is not race specific. RA affects the hands, wrists, feet, and ankles. The disease is bilateral, meaning that it affects the same joints on both sides of the body. It also affects the synovium, which becomes inflamed (red, swollen, painful, and warm). Systemic manifestations of RA may be noted in the heart, lungs, kidneys, and the skin. The change in functions of these organs is related to the degree or severity of the particular organ's involvement.

It is essential that clients and their family or caretaker understand the progression of RA so that they may begin controlling the disease through treatment modalities and compliance with care goals. They need to know about treatments and medications to relieve symptoms, exer-

BOX 14-1 • CLIENT ASSESSMENT FOR OSTEOARTHRITIS

MUSCULOSKELETAL

Signs and symptoms are usually local, as is stiffness and tenderness of the joint. Clients may complain of pain becoming worse as the day progresses. There may be swelling of the joints and a moderate degree of limitation with movement. The pain may be relieved with rest or non-weight bearing. When range of motion (ROM) of joints is incorporated, guarding (limiting movement to protect a joint) may take place. Occasionally the pain will move around and sometimes appear for a couple of seconds and disappear again. Referred pain in local muscle surrounding the joint is not uncommon.

HANDS

Spurs formed at the dorsolateral and medial aspects of the distal interphalangeal joints of the fingers are termed *Heberden's nodes*. Flexor and lateral deviations of the distal phalanx are common and similar changes at the proximal interphalangeal joints are called *Bouchard's nodes*.

KNEES

Characterized by localized tenderness over various components of the joint and pain on passive or active motion. Crepitus can often be detected and muscle atrophy is seen secondary to disuse.

HIPS

Osteoarthritic changes in the hip lead to an insidious onset of pain, often followed by a limp. Pain is usually localized to the groin or along the inner thigh, although clients often complain of pain in the buttocks, sciatic region, or the knee due to pain referral along contiguous nerves. The hip will appear deformed, enlarged, and slightly edematous, warm to touch, with skin thinner and redder than normal.

FEET

OA of the first metatarsophalangeal joint is irritated by tight shoes. Irregularities in joint contour can be palpated. Tenderness is common, particularly when the overlying bursa at the medial aspect of the joint is inflamed.

SPINE

Involvement of the lumbar spine is seen most commonly at the L3–L4 area. Associated symptoms include local pain and stiffness and radicular pain due to compression of contiguous nerve roots. Muscle spasms of the lower back and cervical posterior muscles occur periodically with use and position changes.

cise, rest, and nutritional needs. They must be aware of possible surgical alternatives: the first surgical treatment is removal of the synovium. Total joint replacement is a later alternative.

Central to controlling pain is planning activities and rest periods. Some evidence suggests that emotional highs and lows play a part in exacerbating RA. Clients and their families must understand the need for planning virtually every activity of their lives. This planning is necessary because a client with this disease can cause a flare-up by overworking or by increasing physical activity or emotional stress. Rest is important for the client with RA and cannot be overemphasized. Clients should be encouraged to change their position frequently during the course of the day, ideally at least every 2 h.

RA is confirmed by a primary care provider based on a physical examination, family history of the disease, radiological studies (x-ray, CT, MRI), bone scan, and by ruling out other types of arthritis. Several blood tests can help in confirming the diagnosis. One is Rheumatoid factor, an abnormal antibody found in the blood of about 80% of adults with RA. Another is erythrocyte sedimentation rate or a plasma viscosity, which can give an indication of how active the arthritis is and is useful for measuring the effectiveness of treatment. The diagnosis of RA may require several visits over a period of time, but if left untreated, the condition can result in progressive joint destruction, deformity, disability, and premature death. Box 14-2 provides information for conducting a client assessment for RA.

Clients may exhibit symptoms of pain and loss of function in the joints, morning stiffness in one or more joints, warmth and swelling in the joint, and a tingling or pricking sensation in the hands or feet, tiredness, weight loss, and a feeling of ill health.

Complications of RA are cardiac degenerative conditions, including cardiomyopathy and congestive heart failure or pericarditis, chronic renal failure, chronic restrictive pulmonary diseases, loss of range of motion (ROM) of joints, anemia, repeated infections, ankylosis of joints, muscle wasting and atrophy, septic arthritis, and avascular necrosis of hip joints.

FEATURES OF OTHER FORMS OF ARTHRITIS

As mentioned earlier, RD comprises more than 199 different diseases. The following are other frequently seen types of RA and specific clinical findings:

BOX 14-2 • CLIENT ASSESSMENT FOR RHEUMATOID ARTHRITIS (RA)

MUSCULOSKELETAL

Hand, wrist, knee, and foot joints are the most commonly involved, but RA can affect any diarthrodial joint, e.g., the temporomandibular joints. Assess fingers and toes for Raynaud's phenomenon (color changes). Bilateral joints should be observed for symmetry; signs of inflammation, angulation or deviation, and limpness.

HANDS AND WRISTS

A typical early sign of RA is a fusiform or spindle-shaped appearance of the fingers and subcutaneous nodules with ulnar drift due to swelling of the proximal interphalangeal (PIP) joints. Assess for loss of strength in the hands and loss of the ability to maintain a good pinch. Frequently, one of the first limitations of motion in RA is of dorsiflexion of the wrist.

ELBOWS AND SHOULDERS

Appraise for flexion contractures and swelling of the elbows, as they are among the more common early manifestations of RA. Typical signs of shoulder involvement are limitation of motion and tenderness just below and lateral to the coracoid process.

NECK

Pain and stiffness are common in RA and may be associated with significant erosion in the cervical vertebra. Headache, particularly occipital, is common and may spread over the top of the cranium to behind the eye. Assess for overall weakness or tiredness.

HIPS

Abnormal gait and limitation of joint motion may be the only manifestations, as swelling and tenderness is difficult to observe. Discomfort in the groin is a frequent complaint.

KNEES

Synovial hypertrophy and effusion in the knee is common, placing these weight-bearing joints among those more frequently affected in RA. Destruction of bone and soft tissue about the knee can also result in marked joint instability.

FEET

Arthritis is frequent in the feet and may involve changes analogous to those described in the hands.

SPINE

Clinically significant spinal involvement is generally limited to the upper cervical area.

Gout: Diagnosed by taking a small amount of fluid from the joint and examining for crystals of uric acid.

Psoriatic arthritis: This diagnosis is suspected if the client has psoriasis, but sometimes arthritis can precede the rash. It can mimic many other kinds of arthritis. Sometimes pitting of the nails is a clue. The nail looks a bit like the surface of a thimble with little indentations.

Reactive arthritis: Sometimes arthritis starts after an infection such as gastroenteritis or a sexually transmitted disease. It usually involves only one or two large joints such as knees or ankles, and may also involve the lower back.

Viral and postviral: Some viral infections can result in a transitory arthritis. Examples are mumps, Rubella, or parvovirus infection.

Spondylarthritis: This condition involves the spine, usually the lower back, causing extreme back stiffness and inflexibility. It may be associated with arthritis of other joints, usually large joints such as knees and ankles. It includes a condition called *ankylosing spondylitis* and tends to run in families. There are other conditions associated with this type of arthritis including uveitis (painful, red eyes) and colitis (inflammation of the large bowel).

HELPING CLIENTS AND FAMILIES DEAL WITH THE CHALLENGES

All chronic diseases have strong effects on the emotional lives of those who have them. There may be changes in appearance, in leisure-time activities, or in relationships. People with arthritis often are caught in a cycle of stress, depression, and pain. These uncomfortable feelings are all related and therefore it may be hard to break the cycle. That is why an arthritis treatment plan often includes learning to manage stress and depression.

The National Institute of Arthritis and Musculoskeletal and Skin Diseases and The Arthritis Foundation can help in many ways, with referral lists for arthritis specialists and information on different types of arthritis and their treatment. The Arthritis Foundation offers a variety of programs that can help people with arthritis make life easier and less painful. These services include:

Self-help courses.
Water- and land-based exercise classes.
Support groups.
Home study courses.
Instructional video tapes.
Public forums.
Educational brochures and booklets for the lay public.
A bimonthly consumer magazine called *Arthritis Today*.
Continuing education courses and publications for health
   professionals.

Prevention of Disability and Preservation of Function

Another major goal in the treatment of the elderly client with RD is to
prevent disability and preserve bodily function. One way to achieve this
goal is to develop an exercise routine based on the specific needs of
each client that preserves motion, strength, functional activities, and
lifestyle. These are some general rules that home care clients and families need to be aware of before beginning any type of exercise plan.

- Apply heat to sore joints before beginning.
- Stretch and warm up with ROM exercises.
- Start strengthening exercises slowly with small weights
  (a 1- or 2-pound weight can make a big difference), but
  only use weights if advised to by the primary care
  provider or physical therapist.
- Progress slowly.
- Take pain medication as necessary before exercising.
- Use cold packs on sore or swollen joints after exercising.
- Add aerobic exercise.
- Ease off if joints become painful or red and work with the
  primary care provider to find the cause and eliminate it.
- Choose an exercise program that's most enjoyable and
  make it a habit.

Benefits of Heat and Cold Applications

Heat or cold can offer short-term, temporary relief of pain and stiffness.
Heat helps relax aching muscles and cold helps to numb the area so the
client will not feel as much pain. Ask the primary care provider or

therapist which type is best for the client. Do not use heat or cold for longer than 15–20 min each time. Let the skin return to normal temperature before using it again. Heat or cold application can also be used to prepare for exercise.

Moist heat is supplied by warm towels, hot packs, a bath, or a shower. It can be used at home for 15–20 min before the beginning of the exercise routine. Cold can be supplied by a bag of ice or frozen vegetables that have been wrapped in a towel. The cold stops pain and reduces swelling when used for 10–15 min at a time. It is often used for acutely inflamed joints.

Exercises Recommended for the Elderly

Several exercises can be recommended for the elderly client with arthritis:

- Range of motion exercises help maintain normal joint movement and relieve stiffness. These types of exercises help maintain or increase flexibility and can be done daily.
- Strengthening exercises help keep or increase muscle strength. Strong muscles help support and protect joints affected by arthritis. They can be done daily but should be done at least every other day unless the client has severe pain or swelling of the joints. One form of exercise practiced by older Chinese for more than 3 centuries is the ancient art of Tai Chi. There is a growing body of evidence showing that Tai Chi can help preserve strength and balance. The exercise involves slow, graceful, and precise body movements. Strength training can be done with elastic bands, isometrics and resistive water exercises.
- Aerobic or endurance exercises improve cardiovascular fitness, help control weight, and improve overall function. It should be done for 20–30 min three times a week unless the client has severe pain or swelling of the joints.

The home care nurse can help the client start on a fitness and exercise plan by first consulting with the primary care provider and physical therapist as to the best form of exercise for that particular client. Clients with hip disease will usually suffer from aggravated hip pain from walking on a treadmill or jogging. The best all-around exercise for such clients is swimming. Lap swimming is excellent, involving the use of most body muscles. Water aerobics cause less impact on the joints than aerobics on land because water relieves the stress on hips during exercise. Bicycling (stationary or mobile) is also well tolerated. If the client does not have access to any of the above, encourage him or her to walk as much as possible.

This advice is not at all true for the client with knee disease; the more they walk, the more the knee will hurt. Clients with knee involvement should avoid using stairs and use the escalator or elevator instead. They should also avoid long walks. However, saving the joint by becoming totally sedentary will not slow down the arthritis but will lead to a loss of muscle and bone strength. The Arthritis Foundation offers exercise programs, one of which is called "Joint Effort." These series of six to eight exercise classes are for people with very little movement or are older and less active. Most of these gentle exercises are done while seated in a chair.

Basic Teaching Guidelines

Clients should be taught to protect their joints from becoming bent or stiff. The longer joints stay bent, the more likely they are to stay that way. Clients should not sleep on their back with a pillow under their knees at night. This practice may make the knees more comfortable but may speed up the development of permanently bent knee joints, which will make walking difficult. To help avoid these problems, splints are sometimes used at night or during the day. The splints rest joints and hold them in proper positions, and keep the muscles and ligaments around the joints from becoming too tight.

There are many safety and comfort tips the home care nurse can share with clients and family members. The following are guidelines that are helpful for all elders, but especially important for those with arthritic diseases. Clients should use large joints whenever possible to do a task. For example, to open a door use a whole arm instead of a hand, or use a whole hand instead of a few fingers to open a jar. If elders use larger, stronger joints to carry loads, such as carrying a purse on a shoulder instead of with the fingers, the joints receive less stress.

Clients should spread their weight over several joints, such as using both arms to lift a book instead of one. Joints work best in their most "natural" or correct positions and clients should be encouraged not to bend them awkwardly if they do not have to. Shoes should be well designed and properly fitted. Older adults should pace themselves by listening to their body and change tasks often. They should alternate heavy or repeated tasks with easy tasks or breaks in their daily schedule.

There are helpful devices to make activities of daily living (ADL) more manageable. Using a chair with arms, straight back, and high seat, and pushing on the arms of the chair helps clients get out of chairs safely and more easily. Items with larger handles, such as extra thick pens, make holding them easier. Using a cart that can be pushed or pulled, instead of carrying heavy items is a better choice. Lifting and storing lightweight items, such as plastic or Corelle dishes instead of ceramic or stoneware dishes relieves stress on joints. Canes, crutches, or walkers can protect joints by helping to lighten the load on the knees and make ambulation more safe.

The client and family should understand the need to carry out the exercise program routinely (usually twice per day) and indefinitely. There may be days when clients note significant joint pain or swelling and will not feel much like exercising. It is important for them to understand that even on "bad" days the exercise program should continue, although it is advisable to decrease the number of repetitions to a minimum number. Likewise, when clients have a good day, they must not engage in too much exercise activity because of the potential to initiate a flare up. Therefore, the exercise program must have limits established so that the individual does not under- or overexercise.

To minimize joint destruction, splints may be used for a limited period of time. A splint can be utilized to support a joint that is inflamed, thereby reducing pain and the inflammatory process. Splints can be used to assist the placement of joints in functional positions and to support unstable joints. Caution must be used with any client utilizing a splint. The client's skin should be checked at least daily for signs of skin irritation from the splint. Splints should be removed periodically for gentle ROM activities.

Frequently, the client or family will ask the home care nurse about a variety of treatments for the pain and stiffness associated with arthritis. Sometimes the treatments are ordered by the primary care provider or physical therapist. At other times clients may seek out symptomatic treatments on their own. Several treatments that have been found to be effective are outlined in Box 14-3.

Diet and Arthritis

Careful weight control can help people with arthritis manage the pain, inflammation, and loss of movement caused by arthritis.

Maintaining a healthy diet with adequate protein and calcium is important. It is also believed that vitamin C may be helpful. Fish oils,

---

BOX 14-3 • EFFECTIVE SYMPTOMATIC TREATMENTS

HYDROTHERAPY (WATER THERAPY)

Exercising in a pool can decrease pain and stiffness. This method may be easy because water takes some weight off painful joints. Community centers, YMCAs, and YWCAs have water exercise classes developed for people with arthritis. Some clients also find relief from the heat and movement provided by a whirlpool.

MOBILIZATION THERAPIES

These therapies include traction (gentle, steady pulling), massage, and manipulation (using the hands to restore normal movement to stiff joints). When done by a trained professional, these methods can help control pain and increase joint motion and muscle and tendon flexibility. If the home care nurse is recommending massage therapy for the client and wishes to locate a reputable massage therapist, contact a local chiropractor, as they very often have a massage therapist on staff who will even make house calls. Be careful to question the person's background and knowledge of working with elderly clients and RD.

RELAXATION THERAPY

Relaxation therapy helps to relieve pain. Clients can learn to release the tension in their muscles to relieve pain. The Arthritis Foundation has a self-help course that includes relaxation therapy and also sells relaxation tapes. Health spas and vacation resorts sometimes have special relaxation courses.

ACUPUNCTURE

Acupuncture is a traditional Chinese method of pain relief. A medically qualified acupuncturist places needles through the skin and at times twirls them. They are placed in certain sites on the body based on a chart of pathways or Meridians. Researchers believe that the needles stimulate deep sensory nerves that tell the brain to release natural painkillers (endorphins). Acupressure is similar to acupuncture, but pressure is applied to the acupuncture sites instead of using needles.

---

especially tuna, salmon, and mackerel help arthritis pain by reducing levels of leukotriene B4, a substance produced by the immune system that inflames joint tissues. Diet supplements may be obtained from fish oil capsules or liquids such as cod liver oil. Clients should take no more than 1 teaspoon of cod liver oil a day to avoid a buildup of excess vitamin A that may cause liver damage.

Encourage clients to keep their weight down by reducing fats, cholesterol, and sugar. Cutting back on vegetable oils and products containing oil, like salad dressings, fried food, and margarine, saves "hidden fat calories" in addition to reducing the intake of omega-6 fatty acids that have been shown to worsen inflammation. Clients may use canola or olive oil, as they are low in omega-6 fatty acids. For clients with RA, encourage them to avoid foods from the nightshade plant family such as white potatoes, tomatoes, eggplant, and all peppers except for black pepper.

SELF-HELP AND ASSISTIVE DEVICES

Home modification and repair includes adaptations to homes that can make it easier and safer for clients with RA to carry out activities such as bathing, cooking, and climbing stairs. Alterations to the physical structure of the home can be made to improve its overall safety and condition for an elderly client with arthritis. Some of the typical problems older RA clients experience include:

Difficulty getting in and out of the shower.
Slipping in the tub or shower.
Difficulty turning faucet handles/doorknobs.
Physical access to the home.
Problems climbing stairs.

Possible solutions include:

Install grab bars, shower stools, or transfer benches.
Place nonskid strips or decals in the tub or shower.
Replace knobs with lever handles.
Install a ramp to the front or back door.
Install handrails for support, especially in long hallways.

Box 14-4 identifies 25 suggestions and modifications for making life easier when a person has a disability. These are ideal pieces of information home care nurses can share with RA clients and their families.

CHRONIC PAIN AND MEDICATION NEEDS

The home care nurse needs to recognize the reality of the problems of chronic pain. The pain of arthritis can be annoying to some sufferers while being crippling to others. There are different classifications of drugs clients may chose to use, or have prescribed for them, based on symptoms and response to the available medication choices. Primary care providers will always select the most effective drug that eliminates the pain and inflammation while causing the lowest intensity of side effects.

BOX 14-4 • ACTIVITIES OF DAILY LIVING MADE EASIER

AT HOME

1. Keep a small wastebasket lined with a plastic bag close by when doing odd jobs around the house and use it to throw things away without bending. When finished with the task, lift the plastic bag out for easy disposal. Also, store extra bags in the bottom of the basket.
2. Hang a plastic shopping bag on the outside handle of the front door and ask the newspaper carrier to put the daily paper in it so the client will not have to bend to retrieve the paper.
3. Wear rubber gloves to improve grip and to protect hands from hot and cold water as well as from household cleaning products.
4. Sprinkle cornstarch or baby powder inside plastic or rubber gloves to make them easier to put on and take off.
5. Slip an old cotton sock over one hand and use it as a dust cloth.
6. Use the hooked end of an opened wire hanger to "hook" clothing and pull it out of the washer or dryer. Cover the hook with heavy tape so it does not catch on clothes.
7. Use a dust ruffle and comforter instead of a bedspread. The comforter serves as both a blanket and a bedspread.
8. Take a full trash bag out to the curb by pulling the bag on a child's disk sled.
9. Use long barbecue tongs to pick up twigs, branches, and other debris in the yard.
10. Have someone wind a few rubber bands around the largest part of a doorknob so it is easier to grasp and turn. Or replace regular household doorknobs with lever handles.
11. Install a dimmer switch in the room where the client regularly rests. If someone must enter the room while the client is resting, the lights can be turned on dim and will not disturb the client.
12. Purchase "touch lamps" that turn on when lightly touched.
13. Loop a towel through the handle of the refrigerator door and pin or tie the ends together. Put an arm through the loop and pull to make opening the door easier.
14. Roll a cart with a basket on it in front of the dryer to load and unload clothes.

(continued)

Classes of Drugs Used

Topical Pain Relievers/Over the Counter (OTC) External Analgesics

Topical pain relievers such as OTC external analgesics are available in creams, rubs, or sprays. Most contain counterirritants, substances that make the skin feel hot, cold, or itchy. Some scientists believe these work by distracting attention from arthritis pain. Common counterirritants include camphor, capsaicin (from hot peppers), menthol, and salicylates.

BOX 14-4 • Continued

AT THE DINNER TABLE

15. Encourage the client to drink from a glass with a bumpy exterior rather than from one that is smooth so it can be grasped better.
16. Eat with an iced tea spoon—it has a smaller bowl than a regular spoon so the client will not have to open his or her mouth as wide; the longer handle is also easier to use if elbows are stiff.
17. Ask the server to bring water in a wine goblet when dining out—it is light-weight and the stem makes it easier to hold.
18. Request that food be cut up in the kitchen before it is brought to the table when dining out.

OUT AND ABOUT

19. Ask bookstore salespeople to open and break the binding on new books purchased so they will open more easily.
20. Purchase and use a personal self-inking address stamp on all order forms, questionnaires, prescription blanks, etc., to avoid extra writing.
21. Make two grocery lists—one with things absolutely needed and the other with items that can wait. If too tired to finish shopping, at least the essentials will have been bought. If someone else can stop and pick up a few things for the client the essential list will be prepared. Also, make lists in the order of the store aisles.
22. Use a large plastic bag or a piece of lining fabric on upholstered car seats to make sliding into the car easier.
23. Keep a pair of kitchen tongs in the car to use when mailing letters in drive up mailboxes.
24. Make reservations at a restaurant and request a table near the entrance so the client does not have to walk as far.
25. Use a seam ripper to make clipping coupons easier.

Adapted from Shelley Peterman Schwarz. (1997). 250 Tips for Making Life with Arthritis Easier. Longstreet.

Nonsteroidal Antiinflammatory Drugs (NSAIDs)

Some of the most common NSAIDs are ibuprofen, fenoprofen (Nalfon), tolmetin (Tolectin), and naproxen (EC-Naprosyn). These drugs should be taken with food or antacids and with a full glass of water to protect the stomach as they can cause irritation to the gastrointestinal system. There are at least 20 of these drugs on the market and all are related to aspirin. They have similar effects but with different duration of action and side effects. NSAIDs reduce the swelling, pain, and stiffness in arthritis and other rheumatic complaints. However, they treat only symptoms and do not change the progression of the disease. Therefore, if the disease is likely to be long term, other additional treatment may be required. The main problem with all NSAIDs is the risk of stomach irritation, which can sometimes lead to ulcers.

Nonacetylated Salicylates

For clients with only mild joint pain and inflammation, nonacetylated salicylates are the drugs of choice. These drugs are chemically similar to aspirin but specially formulated to be easier on the stomach and are a safe alternative.

Analgesic–Antipyretic Agents

The first line of drug treatment for any type of arthritis is usually analgesic–antipyretic agents that come in many types and strengths. This group of drugs includes aspirin and acetaminophen and is useful for its pain- and fever-relieving properties.

Disease-Modifying Antirheumatic Drugs (DMARDs)

Unlike NSAIDs, the DMARDs are thought to have some effect on altering the progression of RA. Further, in contrast to NSAIDs, DMARDs are slower acting and it may take weeks or months for benefits of the drugs to be noted. It is essential for the home care nurse to reinforce this delayed action concept to clients with RA so that clients do not stop the drug prematurely because it is "not working."

The DMARDs are further divided into the following major classes: antimalarial drugs, such as gold thiomalate and penicillamine, and gold injections, which are used mainly in the treatment of RA. The injections contain real gold, but in the form of a dissolved salt. They are usually given on a weekly basis initially, but the frequency may then be reduced. It is not known how gold injections work in treating RA and they do not work for everybody. The injections can take 6–12 weeks before taking effect and, once established, it may be necessary to take them for many years. Their main side effects are skin rashes and mouth ulcers; it is also necessary to check the blood and urine, as the injections can sometimes affect kidney function.

Penicillamine tablets are used in more severe RA situations. Similar to other second line drugs, they may take several weeks to work and minor side effects such as taste disturbance or skin rashes can occur.

Penicillamine can also affect kidney function, which must be checked during treatment.

Immunosuppressive and Antineoplastic Agents: Methotrexate and Azathioprine

Both methotrexate and azathioprine seem to work by suppressing the immune system, thereby reducing the inflammation and slowing progression of the arthritis. They are used in low doses so that the immune system can still work to fight infection. The main side effects are related to this immune suppression.

Corticosteroids: Cortisone, Prednisone, and Dexamethasone (Decadron)

There are many types of steroids used to treat arthritis and related rheumatic conditions. Usually tablets are given, but steroids may also be injected into the vein, muscle, or directly into the joint. This class of drugs provides good relief of pain and swelling in the joints and, in a client's experience, excellent relief from the symptoms of arthritis. However, low doses of steroids are used whenever possible so that the side effects associated with steroid treatment are kept to a minimum. These side effects include osteoporosis, fluid retention, weight gain, diabetes, bruising, depression, and infections. Because steroidal side effects are serious, use of these drugs must be monitored closely, kept to as short a period of time as possible, and eliminated if other categories of drugs provide the needed relief.

In general, the primary care provider will start the client with progressive disease on a DMARD prior to destructive changes in the bones or joints. These drugs have been shown to suppress symptoms in the average client with RA. In some instances, complete remission of RA may occur while the medications are continued.

Because of the toxicity of DMARDs, clients need to be reevaluated carefully and frequently by the primary care provider. The rate of discontinuation of these drugs, because of toxicity, ranges from 20% in sulfasalazine up to 60% in penicillamine. The elderly client may be more vulnerable to toxicity caused by drug interactions and should be monitored for reactions during home visits.

"Cures" for Arthritis

Occasionally the general public will read about or hear of potential "cures" for a variety of maladies. Arthritis cures are also touted. Some of the claims support dietary supplement for osteoarthritis. Recently the supplements glucosamine and chondroitin sulfate, which are readily available at health food stores, have been associated with "curing" arthritis. These supplements are not regulated by the United States Food and Drug Administration. These are just two of many products people associate with curing arthritis. The home care nurse may come across many elderly clients who are using OTC treatments, home remedies, or folk medicine practices to treat their arthritis. The nurse must research the safety and usefulness of the treatment practice to ensure client well-being. Pharmacists and the client's primary care provider are good resources. If the treatment practice is deemed safe the nurse can incorporate the practice in the primary care provider-directed medication plan. If the practice is contraindicated or harmful to the client's health, the nurse must take an approach that focuses on client education. With factual information about their choices, clients can make informed decisions.

SURGICAL INTERVENTIONS

Relieving pain, reducing disability, and preventing deformity are the main treatment goals for clients with RDs. If a client's pain continues unabated, the client may experience a loss of function, weakness, and psychological problems. The ability to function is an ongoing goal that can be addressed through physical therapy, medications, surgical intervention, or a combination of all three. Preventing deformities is not always possible even with therapy. But prevention of deformities should, nevertheless, remain a long-term treatment goal.

Home care nurses play a critical role in giving clients with RDs useful information. Being knowledgeable of the latest facts and research about the disease permits the nurse to educate clients about their conditions, medications, and disease-specific interventions. Home care nurses can improve the quality of their clients' lives significantly. The key to helping clients make an educated decision is to be an informed healthcare practitioner with facts about all treatment options and to discuss them with the client, client family, and the primary care provider.

Most people with arthritis will never need surgery. As discussed earlier, the management of arthritis in many situations can be achieved by nonsurgical treatments, including proper medication, physical therapy, exercise, rest, and joint protection. For most people these treatments are sufficient to ease pain and improve or maintain mobility.

Before recommending surgery, the primary care provider will consider the client's physical and medical status, and the reasons for considering the surgery. The decision to have surgery is a major one and can only be made after weighing all options.

Joints that can benefit from surgery are those in the feet and toes, ankles, knees, hips, hands, fingers, shoulders, and wrists. Among the types of surgery available are arthrodesis (bone fusion), arthroplasty (rebuilding of joints), osteotomy (correction of deformity by cutting and then resetting the bone), resection (removal of a bone or bone part), or synovectomy (removal of the diseased synovium that surrounds the joint area).

Considerations for joint surgery are the type of arthritis, the location of the joint affected, and the degree of involvement by arthritis. The risks associated with surgery include infection following surgery and breakdown of an implant after months or years of use. Nonetheless, the benefits associated with surgery such as relief of pain, improved movement, and improvement in the alignment of deformed joints may outweigh the risks. The decision to undergo surgery is something the client and primary care provider must seriously consider, especially if other treatment choices do not sufficiently improve the client's quality of life.

ARTHRITIS RESOURCES FOR CLIENTS

Arthritis Today is an excellent source of information for people who have arthritis and for those who care about people who do. It is published six times a year by the Arthritis Foundation and is available on newsstands or may be ordered by contacting:

The Arthritis Foundation
P.O. Box 19000
Atlanta, GA 30326
1-800-283-7800

For basic information about arthritis or to find the nearest Arthritis Foundation local offices, the public may call toll free 1-800-283-7800. Chapter addresses include:

Arthritis Foundation
Southwestern Ohio Chapter
7811 Laurel Avenue Cincinnati, OH 45243
(513) 271-4545; FAX (513) 271-4703

or:

Arthritis Foundation
P.O. Box 19000
Atlanta, GA 30326
1-800-283-7800

At times the home care nurse may desire additional information for the client. Frequently there are articles in nursing journals and there are many medical textbooks available on arthritis. Public and university libraries can do online searches for additional and very current information.

The local Area Agency on Aging or Title VI Program may have information helpful to the nurse, client, or family members and can be contacted by referring to the telephone directory in the Blue Pages or government listings and/or in the Yellow Pages under aging, senior citizens, community services, or social services. The Yellow Pages of many telephone books have a special section in the front of the book with the names and addresses of various service organizations.

The Eldercare Locator is a nationwide service to help families and friends find information about community services for older people. The Eldercare Locator provides access to an extensive network of organizations serving older people at state and local community levels. Their toll free telephone number is 1-800-677-1116.

An additional service that may be helpful to clients needing transportation is the National Transit Hotline. It can provide the names of local transit providers who receive federal money to provide transportation to the elderly and people with disabilities. Their toll free telephone number is 1-800-527-8279.

SUMMARY

Arthritis diseases affect millions of people, especially the elderly. There are several types of arthritis, causing varying degrees of inflammation, discomfort, pain, and deformity. These disease effects hinder the day-to-day activities and quality of life of older adults who are frequently suffering from other maladies as well. For the home care nurse to be an effective healthcare practitioner, the nurse must understand how this chronic disease affects the client's life. There are different types of arthritis, each of which require different treatment modalities and medication choices. All clients with arthritis can benefit by helpful home management tips and community resources that are available, some of which have been shared in this chapter.

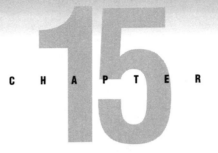

CARING FOR THE ELDERLY CLIENT WITH DIABETES

Elaine Edelstein

◆ ◆ ◆

Diabetes care has changed dramatically in the last decade and will continue to change. As the third millennium approaches, keeping up with the advances in technology, pharmacological interventions, and research findings which impact diabetes management becomes an ongoing challenge for all healthcare providers. As increasing numbers of clients receive care at home, the client with diabetes becomes more visible in the home care nurse's case mix. In order for the home care agency to provide state of the art care for the homebound person with diabetes, all staff, most importantly the licensed nursing staff, must remain current in their knowledge of diabetes home management.

The ability of the home care nurse to be an effective partner in the care of the client with diabetes is paramount in the successful management of the disease. The importance of various aspects of this role including assessing, teaching, counseling, monitoring, collaborating with other professionals, and providing hands-on care cannot be overemphasized. Consequently, this chapter addresses these roles to prepare home care nurses in the timely detection and current management of diabetes in older adults.

◆ ◆ ◆

PROFILE OF DIABETES

There are approximately 16 million Americans with diabetes, and the fastest growing population with diabetes is the elderly. It is estimated that 18.5% of the older adult population has diabetes, or almost 20% of people aged 65–74 years. About 50% of those with diabetes do not know that they have the disease. Symptoms can be subtle and often confused with a myriad of other common ailments, especially among the elderly. Often people are diagnosed by their healthcare provider only after experiencing complications of the disease.

Statistics show that diabetes is a disease that has extreme costs related to it. Costs that exceed $98 billion per year are incurred due to the loss of productive work years for clients, along with the long-term medical (medications and supplies) and surgical management (American Diabetes Association, 1998). Nondollar costs are measured in the dependency and loss of quality of life occurring for some clients who have mismanaged their diabetes, either by choice, misinformation, or ignorance.

Diabetes, among the elderly, is the seventh leading cause of death and tends to occur more frequently among minority groups. The prevalence of people diagnosed with diabetes is almost 6% among non-Hispanic Whites and Cuban Americans, over 10% among non-Hispanic African Americans, and close to 15% among Mexican Americans and Puerto Rican Americans, whereas among Native Americans the prevalence is more than 20%. Asian population groups have growing incidences of diabetes that is of concern to healthcare practitioners.

Diabetes is a chronic disease in which there is an inability to metabolize carbohydrates, proteins, and fats. It is characterized by glucose intolerance with hyperglycemia present at time of diagnosis. There are several clinical classifications of diabetes, including insulin-dependent diabetes mellitus (IDDM) (Type 1), non-insulin-dependent diabetes mellitus (NIDDM) (Type 2), gestational diabetes, and secondary diabetes.

Type 1 diabetes is diagnosed among approximately 10% of the population with diabetes. These individuals are insulin dependent, with the disease occurring at a younger age, usually before age 30. It has been identified as an autoimmune disorder in which the beta cells in the pancreas are destroyed and there is no insulin production. Susceptibility to Type 1 diabetes is linked to a Chromosome 6 abnormality involving the DR3 gene in the human leukocyte antigen (HLA). People with Type 1 diabetes are dependent on exogenous insulin for life. (See Table 15-1 for comparison between Type 1 and Type 2 diabetes.)

Type 2 diabetes is the most prevalent form of diabetes, with almost 90% of persons with diabetes having this diagnosis. It is associated with aging, usually occurring after the age of 40 years. In Type 2 diabetes, most people are able to produce insulin but are unable to use it efficiently or are resistant to the effects of insulin. Hyperglycemia found in Type 2 diabetes is a result of insulin resistance and glucose toxicity. People with Type 2 diabetes tend to be hyperinsulinemic because of the large amount of insulin needed to overcome the insulin resistance. Factors that put people at risk for this disease include obesity, family history, ethnicity, inactivity, and history of gestational diabetes. Type 2 diabetes has a strong genetic link. This finding is based on research in monozygotic twins. It was found that if one twin developed diabetes there was almost a 100% chance that the other twin would also develop diabetes.

Gestational diabetes mellitus (GDM) occurs among women during pregnancy as a result of normal changes that cause insulin resistance leading to glucose intolerance. It is associated with older age, obesity, and family history of diabetes. GDM occurs in 2–5% of pregnant women.

TABLE 15-1 • COMPARISON OF DIABETES, TYPE 1 AND TYPE 2		
	Type 1	**Type 2**
Age of onset	Usually under 30 years	Usually over 40 years
Type of onset	Sudden	Gradual
Body weight	Normal	Obese in 80%
HLA association	Positive	Negative
Insulin in blood	Little to none	Some usually present
Islet cell antibodies	Present at onset	Absent
Prevalence	0.2–0.3%	2–4%
Symptoms	Polyuria, polydipsia, polyphagia, weight loss, ketoacidosis	Polyuria, polydipsia, pruritus, peripheral neuropathy
Vascular and neural changes	Eventually develop	Will usually develop
Stability of condition	Fluctuates, difficult to control	Fairly stable, usually easy to control

Adapted from Thomas, C. L. (1993). Taber's cyclopedic medical dictionary (ed. 17). Philadelphia: F. A. Davis.

Women who have experienced GDM are at increased risk for the development of diabetes later in life.

Secondary diabetes is diabetes that occurs as a result of other medical conditions. Endocrine disorders such as Cushing's disease, thyrotoxicosis, and acromegaly can cause diabetes. Other conditions such as pancreatic disease (pancreatitis, cystic fibrosis, and pancreatectomy) and conditions requiring certain pharmacological agents (glucocorticoid, thiazide diuretics, estrogen, nicotinic acid, phenytoin, and catecholamine) can also cause a secondary diabetes.

HOME CARE PROFILE OF DIABETES

Most diabetes clients today receiving home care have Type 2 diabetes and are the elderly. Among the home care population, people with diabetes account for 8% of all clients. Of those, 11% are 85 years or older and 22% are younger than 65 years of age. Diabetes is one of the leading diagnoses among home healthcare recipients aged 45–64 years, which are often the years of onset, when clients are newly diagnosed with Type 2 diabetes. Home care services help the client adjust to the care and management of their health with the new diagnosis.

It is important for the home care nurse to understand the differences between the two types of diabetes and to be able to identify the classification of diabetes among their caseload. The clinical types of diabetes may not be clear on the home care referral form (HCFA 485). The ICD-9 code and diagnosis on the referral usually reflects the client's medication treatment. For example, if a client with Type 2 diabetes is being treated with insulin and is referred for home care, the ICD-9 and diagnosis states the client is insulin dependent (because the client is being treated with insulin), but the diagnosis may be incorrect. There are many Type 2 clients treated with insulin. The ICD-9 diagnosis code is not a clinical diabetes classification but rather a treatment statement. As part of the initial nursing assessment, it is important to find out the client's type of diabetes. If the client can not identify his or her type of diabetes, the presence of the common characteristics of the two types (see Table 15-1) can be confirmed with the client's primary care provider.

DIAGNOSTIC CRITERIA

The latest recommendations, endorsed by the Centers of Disease Control and Prevention and the National Institute of Diabetes and Digestive and Kidney Diseases (NIDDK), have changed the diagnostic diabetes criterion of the fasting blood glucose (FBG) and reduced it to 126 mg/dL or higher. This criterion is based on research that revealed that people with FBG readings in the 120s developed complications of diabetes (American Diabetes Association, 1997). Conducting a FBG on two separate occasions or a frank increase in blood glucose level (Bglu) with classic signs are used to diagnose diabetes.

Symptoms of Diabetes

The symptoms of diabetes commonly referred to as the three Ps are polyuria, polydipsia, and polyphagia. Clients also experience lethargy and blurred vision. Clients can present to the primary care provider with signs and symptoms of infection such as a vaginal infection or a urinary tract infection, or with slow healing wounds. Some people experience a rapid unexplainable weight loss. In older adults some of these symptoms may be mistaken for age-related changes and the diagnosis of diabetes is delayed. Home care nurses, who visit clients for other health problems, can screen for signs and symptoms of diabetes as they provide comprehensive client care.

COMPLICATIONS OF DIABETES

The complications of diabetes can be separated into two categories, microvascular and macrovascular complications. The microvascular complications associated with diabetes include retinopathy, neuropathy, and nephropathy. The macrovascular complications include coronary artery disease, cerebrovascular disease, and peripheral vascular disease.

The results of a 10-year landmark study called the Diabetes Control and Complications Trial (DCCT) has direct implications on the risk and progression of diabetes microvascular complications among people with Type 1 diabetes. This study was done to determine if blood glucose control slows or prevents diabetes complications. The DCCT supported that clients who received "intensive" therapy (multiple daily insulin injections, frequent blood glucose monitoring, and frequent contact with their healthcare providers), thereby controlling their blood glucose, had a slower progression and lower risk of retinopathy by 76%, neuropathy by 60%, and nephropathy by 54% (DCCT, 1993). As a result of this study, primary care providers have been more aggressive in their diabetes management approaches and together with their clients, have set the goal for better blood glucose management.

Microvascular Complications

Retinopathy

Diabetes retinopathy is the leading cause of new cases of blindness in the United States. Retinopathy is the most common eye disorder in people with diabetes. This disorder involves changes to the retina, which is found in the back of the eye. The retina records images and converts them to electrical signals for the brain to interpret. Retinopathy is diagnosed in clients frequently after 5-years' duration of diabetes Type 1; retinopathy can be a presenting symptom in clients with Type 2 diabetes. Clients with hypertension or nephropathy are at increased risk for retinopathy. There are three stages of diabetic retinopathy: nonproliferative, preproliferative, and proliferative.

Nonproliferative retinopathy is the earliest stage of the disease. The capillaries around the retina become dilated, can be damaged, and develop microaneurysms and intraretinal hemorrhages. The client may experience some blurred vision or may be asymptomatic.

In *preproliferative* retinopathy there is further destruction of the retinal blood vessels, diminished circulation, and infarction can occur.

Proliferative retinopathy has continued retinal ischemia and neovascularization networks develop that tend to be fragile. The fragility and proliferation of this vessel growth lead to hemorrhage into the vitreous fluid, which then diminishes the client's vision.

Retinopathy treatment modalities. All clients with diabetes must have an annual dilated eye examination. Only through pupil dilation and direct examination of the retina can changes be identified. Prevention of retinal disease progression through early detection is the best way to prevent blindness. The home care nurse, as the coordinator of care, needs to determine if and when a dilated eye examination was done and to schedule, arrange, and encourage the client to have this eye test done yearly. Working together with the client to control blood glucose levels and blood pressure is essential in maintaining vision. The quality of life is enhanced with the preservation of vision.

Treatment for proliferative retinopathy involves photocoagulation (laser treatments). Scatter photocoagulation, which is hundreds of small flashes of laser, is used across the retina. It requires several treatments for completion. The laser treatments dry up and slow down new blood vessel formation. A vitrectomy may be performed when bleeding from the new blood vessels clouds the vitreous or for a detached retina. This procedure involves the removal of the vitreous fluid and scar tissue from the retina and the replacement of vitreous fluid with saline. The goal of this procedure is to restore vision.

Neuropathy

Diabetic neuropathy occurs in 60–70% of all people with diabetes. Neuropathy is a condition characterized by damage to the nerves, and its effects are felt all over the body. There are two types of diabetes neuropathy, peripheral and autonomic neuropathy.

Peripheral neuropathy is most common and its effects are experienced in the legs, feet, and hands. This condition involves the sensory motor nerves. Clients experience numbness, tingling, stabbing or deep bone pain, burning, paresthesia, impaired balance, and sensory incoordination. Along with these sensory impairments, motor neuropathy is found. Motor neuropathy is experienced as muscle weakness, atrophy in the feet, and foot deformities, such as claw toes, hammer toes, Charcot's joint, loss of fat pads, callus formation, metatarsal head prominence, and foot drop.

Peripheral neuropathy is primarily responsible for foot ulcers due to sensory and motor losses. Fifteen percent of all people with diabetes will develop foot ulcers. Loss of sensation leads to traumas such as mechanical injuries due to pressure, friction or sharp objects (glass, nails, or tacks), chemical burns, and thermal injuries from exposure to heat and cold. Home care referrals for the treatment of foot ulcers and wounds are frequently seen, many of which could have been prevented. If a client has a foot ulcer, the home care nurse should include a wound care specialist, podiatrist, and pedorthist whenever possible to assist in the development and implementation of the plan of care.

Along with angiopathy and infection, neuropathy is responsible for the high rates of lower extremity amputations among clients with diabetes. There are 54,000 lower extremity amputations performed on persons with diabetes annually. It is estimated that 50% of these amputations can be prevented (American Diabetes Association, 1996).

Treatment for the pain of peripheral neuropathy is generally palliative and supportive. The nonpharmacological treatments can include relaxation, biofeedback, and transcutaneous electrical nerve stimulation (TENS) therapy. Pharmacological therapy can include the use of nonnarcotic analgesics (ibuprofen and sulindac) or anticonvulsants (phenytoin and carbamazepine) or antidepressants (amitriptyline and fluphenazine) or topical capsaicin. Research has also found aldose reductase inhibitors (tolrestat) may limit the progression of nerve damage.

Foot care and foot injury prevention education is critical in preventing the development and progression of severe problems such as foot ulcers, foot injury, and amputation. The United States Public Health Service, Department of Health and Human Services created a nationally recognized foot prevention program called Lower Extremity Amputation Prevention (LEAP) Program. The program has a superb foot care education component and also includes a new foot sensation screen. The sensory screening program is important in order to identify sensory loss early, prevent injury, and counsel clients appropriately. The program stratifies clients in risk categories with recommendations for care, treatment, and follow-up screening. The foot sensation assessment is done with a monofilament, which is a tool developed at the Hansen Disease Center in Carville, Louisiana. The monofilament is a nylon bristle on a plastic handle; it is depressed against the client's foot in 10 check areas and the client reports whether the touch of the filament can be felt. If the filament is not felt, there is sensory loss.

Autonomic neuropathy involves autonomic nerve damage to multiple body systems. It can involve the bladder, the intestinal tract, genital organs, and the vagus nerve (see Table 15-2).

TABLE 15-2 • AUTONOMIC NEUROPATHY

Body System	Complications	Client Education and Treatment
Gastrointestinal	Gastroparesis Nocturnal diarrhea Fecal incontinence	Eat small, frequent meals Low fat and low fiber diet Medications
Genitourinary	Neurogenic bladder	Bladder training, antibiotic therapy for infections, drugs to improve nerve contraction
	Sexual dysfunction	Counseling for client and partner
	Male: Impotence, retrograde ejaculation	Vacuum device, vasoactive drugs (Viagra), penile prosthesis
	Female: Vaginitis, decreased lubrication	Lubricant vaginal creams, prevention of vaginitis
Cardiovascular	Postural hypotension Neuropathy of the vagus nerve	Gradual position changes Elastic stockings Medications Avoiding heavy exercise
Impaired insulin counter-regulation	Hypoglycemia unawareness	Avoidance of hypoglycemia Blood glucose monitoring Wearing medical identification Glucagon
Sudomotor dysfunction	Anhydrosis (absent sweating) in lower extremities	Foot care and lubrication of feet
Pupillary	Slow dilation of the pupils	Avoid night driving Safety in the home

Autonomic neuropathy is a complication of diabetes that is difficult to manage because it may involve different systems. It is important for the home care nurse to provide information, encourage clients to seek support from family and friends, and to assist them to continue with their normal daily activities.

Nephropathy

Diabetic nephropathy is a serious condition that can lead to end stage renal disease (ESRD) requiring dialysis or kidney transplantation.

Nephropathy is characterized by albuminuria, hypertension, and renal insufficiency. About 21% of people with diabetes have nephropathy. Clients with diabetes are considered to have nephropathy if their urine protein is >30 mg/dL. The use of a convenient dipstick to screen for microalbumin is now available, making early diagnosis and treatment possible. One third of ESRD clients have diabetes and renal failure occurs in 5–15% of clients with Type 2 diabetes. African Americans and Native Americans with diabetes have twice the risk for ESRD.

Nephropathy treatment modalities. Prevention of renal complications is linked to tight blood glucose control, as demonstrated in the Diabetes Control and Complications Trial (1993). The home care nurse needs to teach the client strategies that can limit the progression of the disease. These strategies include limiting the client's protein intake, maintaining good glycemic control, controlling hypertension with angiotensin converting enzyme (ACE) inhibitors, preventing and promptly treating urinary tract infections, and avoiding nephrotoxic medications and radiographic dyes.

Clients with ESRD can be treated with hemodialysis, peritoneal dialysis, or kidney transplantation. Clients who are being treated with continuous ambulatory peritoneal dialysis (CAPD) are provided home care as necessary. Nurses should be aware that there are specific dietary restrictions such as limited fluid intake, sodium limitations, potassium limitations, phosphorus restrictions, and increased allowance in fat. Dietary modifications are made based on the client's individual needs and are dependent on the mode of ESRD treatment. Renal diets are complex and need coordination with registered dietitians (RD). All dialysis centers have RDs and should be contacted by the home care nurse if the client is also seen in a dialysis center.

Macrovascular Complications

Coronary Artery Disease

The leading cause of mortality among persons with diabetes is cardiovascular disease. People with diabetes have a two- to four-time higher risk for the development of heart disease than the general population.

The risk factors associated with cardiovascular disease are obesity, hypertension, lipid abnormalities, physical inactivity, and smoking.

Cerebral Vascular Disease

Clients with diabetes are two to four times more likely to have a stroke than persons without diabetes. The mortality rate as a result of a stroke is also higher among persons with diabetes. The nurse must monitor the client's blood pressure and assess the client's adherence to prescribed antihypertensive agents.

Peripheral Vascular Disease

Peripheral vascular disease (PVD) causes a decrease in the blood flow to the legs and feet, resulting in reduced oxygenation. It is characterized by intermittent claudication. The client experiences pain in the thigh or calf that is relieved at rest. The prevalence of PVD in clients with diabetes is 10% higher than the general population.

◆   ◆   ◆

MANAGEMENT OF DIABETES

Diabetes is a chronic illness with no present cure. This disease can be successfully managed through meal planning, medications as necessary, and exercise and activity. In addition, blood glucose monitoring and the use of adaptive equipment is important in the management of diabetes. The home care nurse needs to assess and evaluate that these essential diabetes management components are included in the plan of care.

NUTRITIONAL MANAGEMENT FOR TYPE 2 DIABETES

Meal Planning

Medical nutrition therapy is an important component for successful diabetes management. The purpose of meal planning is to assist clients to improve their overall health. The goals of medical nutrition therapy include:

> Controlling blood glucose levels through the balance of nutrition, activity, and medication.

Achieving optimal lipid levels by decreasing saturated fat and cholesterol in the diet.

To provide appropriate calories to maintain reasonable weight. Weight issues in the elderly can cross the spectrum. Forty percent of the elderly clients with diabetes are considered overweight. On the other hand, it is known that poor appetite, poor dentition, depression, diminished taste and smell sensations, and other chronic conditions can lead to weight loss below the ideal range.

To prevent and treat acute and chronic complications of diabetes.

The American Diabetes Association (1997) recommends that all clients with diabetes receive a nutritional assessment and nutritional management direction from an RD. Many home care agencies have RDs available for consultation or for home visits to the complex client. Traditionally, nutritionist services were not reimbursed by Medicare. This practice may be changing with new Medicare laws in which care provided by state-certified professionals can be reimbursed by Medicare. In most cases the home care nurse works with the client to plan appropriate meals following the prescribed caloric regimen.

Weight Loss

If a client is overweight, a moderate caloric restriction (a decrease in 250–500 calories daily) will lead to a gradual weight loss. Research indicates that a moderate weight loss can improve glycemic control, reduce cholesterol levels, and assist in controlling hypertension.

Meal Composition and Assessment

Daily meal plans should include between 45–55% of daily total calories as carbohydrate sources. Carbohydrate sources are starches, fiber, and sugars. Protein should make up 12–20% of the daily total calories. Proteins come from animal and vegetable sources. Clients with renal complications are placed on protein-restricted diets. Fats make up 30% of the daily calories. Saturated fats should be limited to less than 10% of the total fat calories, and cholesterol should be less than 300 mg daily. Meals should be spaced 4–6 h apart, with the daily calories divided accordingly.

The common belief that simple sugars should be limited and the use of complex carbohydrates be used instead is not supported by the latest nutritional research (American Diabetes Association, 1997). The premise that simple sugars are quickly digested and can cause hyperglycemia has not been supported in the current literature. Therefore, the latest nutritional recommendations focus on the total amount of carbohydrates consumed rather than the type of carbohydrates (American Diabetes Association, 1997).

It is important to assess the nutritional status and learning needs of the person with diabetes. The assessment should include: food history, weight, laboratory data (glucose levels, cholesterol, lipid profile), medical history, nutritional prescription, cultural heritage, learning style, and socioeconomic issues.

Strategies for Teaching Meal Planning

Deciding on an appropriate strategy for educating the client with diabetes about a meal plan is an important part of the home care nurse's role. No single educational tool works in every situation. Each client is different and each educational situation is unique. Based on the assessment of the client's learning abilities, educational level, language and literacy issues, visual abilities, and physical condition, an educational strategy should be identified and implemented. There are a variety of educational tools and approaches available to assist the home care nurse in this process.

The *Exchange System* is made up of six food group lists to be used as an ideal guide to identify for people the foods to eat in the right balance and variety. The foods within a group are alike in terms of the amount of carbohydrate, protein, and fat they contain. The six food groups are: bread/starch, fruit, milk, vegetable, meat/meat substitute, and fat. Each food group has a list of choices with their serving sizes. The exchange system is often used with clients placed on a calorie-restricted diet such as a 1,200, 1,500, or 1,800 calorie American Diabetes Association (ADA) diet. New ADA guidelines allow meals to be planned so that carbohydrates can be interchanged.

Carbohydrate counting could be one approach used by clients with diabetes. Foods such as fruits and milk can be exchanged for a starch, thereby allowing clients to select foods to their liking. When using the lists of foods in the Food Group (see Box 15-1) the client participating in carbohydrate counting can substitute items in the bread/starch, milk, vegetable, or fruit categories. The diet is then supplemented with foods from the meat and substitutes and fat categories.

BOX 15-1 • FOOD GROUPS

Each serving size shown represents one exchange.

BREAD/STARCH

Dry cereal, unsweetened, 3/4 cup
Cooked cereal, 1/2 cup
Bread, 1 slice
Whole grain crackers, 4–6
Rice cakes, 2
Rice, 1/3 cup
Dried beans, cooked, 1/3 cup
Dried peas, 1/3 cup
Corn, 1/2 cup
Lima beans, 1/2 cup
Potato (baked), 3 oz
Potato (mashed), 1/2 cup
Winter squash, 1 cup
Popcorn, 3 cups (popped without fat added)
Pretzels, 3/4 oz
Pasta (cooked), 1/2 cup

MILK

Milk (skim), 1 cup
Yogurt (non-fat), 1 cup

VEGETABLES

Servings for the following are 1 cup raw, 1/2 cup cooked.

Asparagus
Beans (green, wax)
Beets
Broccoli
Brussel sprouts
Cabbage
Cauliflower
Green pepper
Mushrooms (cooked)
Onions
Sauerkraut
Spinach
Tomatoes
Turnips
V-8, tomato juice

FRUIT

Apple (2"), 1
Apricot, 1/2 cup
Banana (9"), 1/2
Cantaloupe (cubed), 1 cup
Cherries, 1/2 cup
Grapefruit (medium), 1/2
Grapes, 1/2 cup
Orange (2 1/2"), 1
Peach (2 3/4"), 1
Pear (small), 1
Pineapple, 1/3 cup
Raspberries, 1 cup
Strawberries, 1 1/4 cup
Watermelon, 1 1/4 cup

MEAT AND SUBSTITUTES

Use lean cuts.

Beef
Round steak, 1 oz
Sirloin steak, 1 oz
Flank steak, 1 oz
Tenderloin, 1 oz
Pork
Tenderloin, 1 oz
Ham, 1 oz
Canadian bacon, 1 oz
Veal, 1 oz
Poultry (no skin)
Chicken, 1 oz
Turkey, 1 oz
Fish
Fresh, 1 oz
Frozen, 1 oz
Canned (in water), 2 oz
Cheese
Cottage, 1/4 cup
Parmesan (grated), 2 Tbsp
Lowfat, 1 oz (less than 55 calories/oz)
Peanut butter, 1 Tbsp
Lunch meat (95% fat free), 1 oz
Egg whites, 2

FATS

Unsaturated
Margarine, 1 tsp
Mayonnaise, 1 tsp
Cashews, dry roasted, 1 Tbsp
Peanuts, 20
Olives, 5
Salad dressing, 1 Tbsp
Oils, 1 tsp
Corn
Cottonseed
Safflower
Soybean
Sunflower
Olive
Peanut

American Association of Diabetes Educators. (1995). Guide to teaching diabetes survival skills. Chicago, IL: Author.

The *Food Guide Pyramid* is another tool that can be used to teach healthy meal planning. This is a general guide of what types of foods to eat each day. It is a visual tool that calls for eating a variety of foods daily. The Food Guide Pyramid can be reviewed in the chapter on nutrition, Chapter 6. It is also incorporated in ADA material called, "First Steps in Diabetes Meal Planning," which may be ordered from the American Diabetes Association or the American Dietetic Association.

In cases in which the learner is having difficulty understanding food exchanges or carbohydrate counting, an alternative approach may be to use a "No Concentrated Sweets" diet. This diet is designed to be a simple guide on foods to be avoided. It is a one-page tool created by the American Dietetic Association to highlight sugar-dense foods. It provides suggested substitutions for concentrated sugar foods.

An effective tool to assist with a nutritional assessment and eating pattern is for the client to keep a food diary. Food diaries are helpful in identifying foods that cause elevations in blood glucose levels, eating patterns, food portions, and progress made toward short-term goals.

Teaching clients how to read food labels assists them in identifying several important factors that should influence their food choices. All of today's packaged foods have labels that provide nutrition information specific to that food based on the serving size. The home care nurse may teach the client to look at the total calories per serving along with the calories from fat. Any food that has more than one third of the calories per serving from fat is a fat- and calorie-dense food and should be avoided.

If the client cannot comprehend nutritional labels, an alternative would be to instruct the client to read ingredients on prepared foods. The purpose of reading ingredients would be to identify foods with concentrated sugar. Clients should be instructed about sugar words that are frequently included in ingredients and mean sugar. Sugar words include: corn syrup, maltose, lactose, sucrose, corn sweeteners, modified food starch, dextrose, levulose, honey, molasses, and natural sweeteners. Clients are taught that if any of the above sugar words are among the first three ingredients in a food, the food should not be included in their meal plan.

Another important consideration is the client's use of alcohol. Because hidden alcohol use can be a problem among the elderly, assessing for signs of alcohol use or abuse, followed by some discussion of alcohol use, should be included in the home care nurse's teaching plan. Alcohol and insulin with no food intake can lead to severe hypoglycemia. The home care nurse should look at total carbohydrates in a client's diet.

It is important and knowing how to substitute carbohydrates in a meal plan may be a way to work with clients who use alcohol.

Nutrition Education Tips

The home care nurse should assess the home environment for safety and food storage, preparation, cooking facilities, and shopping practices. To assist with dietary compliance the home care nurse should suggest not buying foods the client has a hard time eating in small portions or infrequently. When storing foods, if they are out of sight they may be easier to resist, so keeping foods in closed cupboards or in the refrigerator helps. Safe and low fat cooking choices should be encouraged. The use of a microwave oven is safer than frying in an open pan where fat can splatter and burn the client. It also will reduce the fats consumed. If clients receive senior meal delivery they need to be reminded these meals are not part of a special diabetic diet but can be used by adjusting other foods eaten. Also, many frozen meals such as Lean Cuisine or Weight Watcher Smart Ones can be purchased in the grocery store. They are relatively inexpensive, avoid the preparation of a hot meal, which may be difficult for some clients with diabetes, and have nutritional or food exchange information on the box.

MEDICATIONS

The use of medications in the treatment and management of diabetes remains a critical component for most clients. There have been several recent advances in the pharmacological arena with new insulin and new classes of oral medications. In addition, the use of combination therapy, several diabetes medications used together, has become widely accepted and successful in controlling blood glucose.

Insulin Therapy

Insulin is a hormone naturally produced in the beta cells of the pancreas. Insulin acts to stimulate the entry of glucose into cells to be used for energy. It also stimulates the entry of amino acids into cells and enhances fat storage. When referring to insulin made by the pancreas, it is called endogenous insulin. Exogenous insulin is pharmaceutical insulin used for injection.

Indications for Insulin

- All clients with Type 1 diabetes (IDDM).
- Clients with Type 2 diabetes (NIDDM) whose blood glucose has not been adequately controlled with diet, exercise, and oral agents.
- Clients with gestational diabetes who could not be managed with diet alone.
- Clients with secondary diabetes.

Insulin Sources

Insulin was discovered in 1921 by Frederick Banting and Charles Best. The first animal source of insulin used was beef. Over the years pork, beef–pork, and human insulin were developed. Animal sources of insulin differ from human insulin at one to three amino acid sites on the insulin chain. Beef insulin is no longer available in the United States. Currently there is pork, beef–pork, and human insulin available. Human insulin is manufactured by using recombinant DNA technology using *Escherichia coli* or bakers' yeast. Human insulin has lower antigenicity than the animal sources of insulin. Human insulin is preferred for newly insulin-treated clients and for clients being treated temporarily with insulin.

Insulin Types

Four types of insulin are available: rapid acting, intermediate acting, long acting, and insulin analog. Insulin types are classified into these groups based on their onset, peak (maximum effect), and duration of action.

Rapid-acting insulin is regular insulin. Regular insulin begins to work 30–60 min after it is injected. Its peak of action is 2–4 h and its duration of action is 6–12 h. Intermediate insulins are NPH and Lente. The onset of intermediate-acting insulin is 1–4 h, with a peak at 8 h and duration of action of 10–24 h. The long-acting insulin is Ultralente. This insulin lasts 24–36 h. Ultralente's onset of action is 4–6 h and it peaks at 18 h.

The newest type of insulin is the insulin analog, lispro. Lispro is a very rapid-acting insulin; it begins to work in 15–30 min after injecting. Lispro peaks between 1–2 h and its duration of action is 3–4 h. The benefits of this insulin include a reduction in post-meal hyperglycemia and potentially reduced incidences of nocturnal hypoglycemia. Meals are to be consumed at the time of injection and not 30 min after with this type of insulin.

There are two mixed insulin combinations currently available in the United States. Fixed combinations of mixed insulin, such as 70/30 and 50/50, contain a premixed combination of NPH and regular insulin in a set ratio. The onset, peak, and duration of action of both insulin types remains unchanged. The nurse must remember that there is regular insulin in each mixture and the insulin should be administered 30 min prior to a meal.

Insulin Concentration

Today, insulin is available in U-100 and U-500 concentrations. Other countries continue to have U-40 insulin, so if clients travel abroad they should be instructed to bring their own insulin. The U-500 insulin is very concentrated and is available for those rare situations when a large dose of insulin is required.

Insulin can be administered via a pump, known as continuous subcutaneous insulin infusion (CSII). Some elderly clients may receive insulin by this method. The home care nurse must contact the patient's primary care provider or diabetes educator for specific information and protocols.

Insulin Injection Sites

The preferred insulin injection site is the abdomen (above and below the umbilicus). The abdomen provides the steadiest and most rapid absorption. Other insulin injection sites include the outer aspects of the arms, the lateral aspects of the thighs, and the buttocks. Older clients may be more familiar with using these alternative sites and should be encouraged to use their abdomen. Absorption depends on the site used and the extent to which the site is exercised. Differences in Bglu may occur because of the site used.

Insulin injections should be inserted into the subcutaneous (SQ) tissue at a 90° angle. The home care nurse should be aware that when injecting clients who are extremely thin, with minimal SQ tissue, that the angle of the injection should be reduced so as not to inject the insulin into muscle.

Rotation of insulin injections is recommended within one site up to a month at a time. This practice minimizes the variability of the insulin absorption rate. Each injection should be spaced at least 1 inch apart within the site to avoid atrophy and hypertrophy of the tissue.

Morning insulin should be given prior to breakfast. Clients requiring twice a day insulin should receive their first dose prior to breakfast and the second injection before dinner (unless otherwise ordered by the primary care provider). There should be at least 8 h between AM and PM injections when using an intermediate-acting insulin. The home care nurse should check the insulin vial for its expiration date and be certain that the insulin is free of precipitate, frosting, or crystals. Insulin that the client is currently using may be kept at room temperature (59–68°F) for 1 month. Room temperature insulin does not sting as much upon administration. However, some clients keep their home temperatures much warmer and for those clients it is recommended that the insulin be kept in the refrigerator. Clients should be instructed to date the insulin vial when it is first started. All extra insulin vials should be stored in the refrigerator (36–46°F).

Many clients are prescribed two different types of insulin, most commonly rapid-acting and intermediate-acting, to be administered at the same time. NPH and regular insulin can be mixed together in the same syringe. If the home care nurse is prefilling syringes for the client to use, they may be kept in the refrigerator for 21–30 days. Timing of mixed insulin prior to the meal is important. For example, if the nurse is administering NPH and regular insulin at 8:00 AM, the client must eat breakfast at 8:30 AM (with the one exception, lispro). The regular insulin is always drawn up first, remember the phrase "clear before cloudy."

The literature explains that when mixing Lente and regular insulin in the same syringe there is a binding of the regular insulin. This binding continues for 24 h and blunts the activity of the regular insulin. It is recommended that when mixing Lente and regular insulin in the same syringe that the patient or home care nurse keep the time between mixing and injecting consistent each day.

Lispro (Humalog) insulin can be mixed with intermediate- and long-acting insulin such as Humulin NPH, Humulin Lente, and Humulin Ultralente. To maximize the rapid absorption rate, the insulin should be mixed and injected immediately. The effects of lispro with animal sources of insulin or insulin from other manufacturers have not been studied.

When prefilling syringes for clients, the syringes should be stored in the refrigerator in a horizontal position. The nurse should mark the prefilled syringes with the prefill date, dose, and type(s) of insulin. If the client is taking two daily injections, the morning and evening syringes should be stored in separate containers that are clearly marked.

Although there are many insulin regimens used, some common mixed regimens are:

- Rapid- and intermediate-acting insulin once a day (before breakfast).
- Rapid- and intermediate-acting insulin twice a day (before breakfast and dinner).
- Rapid- and long-acting insulin before breakfast and rapid-acting before lunch and dinner.

Insulin Syringes

Insulin syringes are manufactured in several different cc and unit capacities. There are 25-unit ($1/4$ cc), 30-unit ($1/3$ cc), 50-unit ($1/2$ cc), and 100-unit (1 cc) syringes. One syringe manufacturer produces a 200-unit syringe for those clients taking more than 100 units of insulin in a single injection. There is a wide assortment of needle gauges available to provide clients with comfortable injections, with needle lengths between $1/2$ and $5/16$ inch.

Manufacturers of insulin syringes recommend that the syringes be used only once to maintain sterility. However, there are some clients (never the home care nurse) who reuse their syringes because of the economic constraints. This practice is controversial and reuse of insulin syringes may increase the client's risk of infection. According to the ADA, if the client can demonstrate that he or she can recap the syringe safely without contaminating the needle, then it is safe. The ADA position statement elaborates that "Patients with poor personal hygiene, an acute concurrent illness, open wounds on the hands, or a decreased resistance to infections for any reason should not reuse a syringe" (American Diabetes Association, 1997).

Diabetes Oral Agents

Oral medications are used in Type 2 diabetes as an adjunct to diet and exercise. In the past few years three new classes of oral agents have been introduced, giving a total of four classifications available. The four classifications are sulfonylureas, biguanides, alpha-glucosidase inhibitors, and thiazolidinediones.

Sulfonylureas

Sulfonylureas are oral agents that lower the blood glucose by stimulating the pancreatic release of insulin and increasing insulin sensitivity of peripheral tissue. The sulfonylureas are divided into first- and second-generation agents. Table 15-3 has a complete list of oral agents.

Sulfonylureas are contraindicated in clients with known allergies to the drug, diabetic ketoacidosis, pregnancy, and in children with Type 1 diabetes. Adverse reactions include hypoglycemia, gastrointestinal reactions, allergic skin reactions, and hematologic reactions (leukopenia, agranulocytosis, thrombocytopenia, hemolytic anemia, aplastic anemia, and pancytopenia). These agents should be used cautiously in clients with renal or hepatic dysfunction. Only one sulfonylurea should be prescribed to the client at any one time. The oral agent is initiated at a low dose and can be increased as necessary to control the blood glucose.

Special caution needs to be taken when chlorpropamide is used in the elderly because of its long duration of action (up to 72 h). This prolonged duration of action can cause a delayed hypoglycemic reaction up to 72 h after the medication was administered. With chlorpropamide, clients also run the risk of a disulfiram (antabuse-like) reaction with alcohol.

Biguanides

Metformin (Glucophage) is a biguanide agent whose mode of action is to reduce hepatic glucose production and enhance glucose transport in skeletal muscle. This medication can be used alone, in combination with insulin, or with other classes of oral diabetes agents. Adverse reactions include: anorexia, abdominal bloating, flatulence, diarrhea, nausea, vomiting, and having a metallic taste in the mouth. To minimize the gastrointestinal (GI) symptoms, it is advised to start this medication with a low dose and increase it slowly. A rare but dangerous reaction associated with biguanides is lactic acidosis. The nurse must be aware that Metformin should not be administered if there is any liver or renal disease, metabolic acidosis, or history of alcohol abuse. The signs and symptoms of lactic acidosis are: lethargy, weakness, muscle pain, dyspnea, abdominal pain, feeling cold, dizziness, lightheaded, or a slow or irregular heart rate.

Metformin is contraindicated in clients described above, clients who have Type 1 diabetes, pregnant women, children, and clients with congestive heart failure (CHF) or unstable cardiac conditions. There is a potential drug interaction with Metformin and cimetidine. Metformin has been shown to reduce triglyceride, low-density lipoprotein (LDL), and total cholesterol levels.

(text continues on p. 324)

TABLE 15-3 • ORAL AGENTS

Drug	Recommended Dose	Maximum Dose	Half-Life (h)	Onset (h)	Duration (h)	Metabolism and Excretion	Comments
FIRST-GENERATION SULFONYLUREAS							
Tolbutamide (Orinase)	0.5–3.0 g divided doses	2–3 g	5.6	1	6–12	Totally metabolized to inactive form; inactive metabolite excreted in kidney	Most benign; least potent; short half-life; especially useful in kidney disease
Acetohexamide (Dymelor)	0.25–1.5 g single or divided doses	1.5 g	5	1	10–14	Metabolite's activity equal to or greater than parent compound; metabolite is excreted via kidney	Essentially no advantage over tolbutamide, although a few patients who fail on tolbutamide are controlled
Tolazamide (Tolinase)	0.1–1.0 g single or divided doses	0.75–1.0 g	7	4–6	10–14	Absorbed slowly; metabolite active but less potent than parent compound; excreted via kidney	Essentially no advantage over tolbutamide; said to be equipotent with less severe side effects
Chlorpropamide (Diabinese)	0.1–0.5 g single dose	0.5 g	35	1	72	Previously thought not to be metabolized, but recently found that metabolism may be quite extensive; significant percentage excreted unchanged	Longest duration; caution in elderly patients and those with kidney disease; disulfiram-like reactions may occur with alcohol; hyponatremia may be a problem

(continued)

TABLE 15-3 • Continued

Drug	Recommended Dose	Maximum Dose	Half-Life (h)	Onset (h)	Duration (h)	Metabolism and Excretion	Comments
SECOND-GENERATION SULFONYLUREAS							
Glyburide (DiaBeta, Micronase, Glynase Prestabs)	1.25–10 mg single or divided dose (0.75–12 mg Glynase)	20 mg (12 mg Glynase)	Biphasic 3.2 + 10	1.5	24	24% absorbed; completely metabolized in liver to inactive derivatives; excreted in urine and bile 1:1	50–200 times more potent than other agents; no disulfiram-like reaction; low toxicity; caution in the elderly
Glipizide (Glucotrol/ Glucotrol XL)	2.5–20 mg single or divided dose (Glucotrol XL once per day dose)	40 mg (Glucotrol XL 20 mg)	3.5–6	1	12–16	Metabolized in liver to inactive metabolites; excreted primarily in urine	Needs to be taken on an empty stomach (Glucotrol XL: no need to take on an empty stomach); no disulfiram-like reaction; low toxicity; caution in the elderly
Glimepiride (Amaryl)	1–4 mg single dose	8 mg	2.5 ± 1.2	2–3	24	Completely metabolized via oxidative biotransformation to two major metabolites. Metabolites are excreted 60% via renal and 40% via hepatic elimination	Take with first main meal: once daily dosing. Indicated for monotherapy and second-line combination use with insulin

(continued)

TABLE 15-3 • Continued

Drug	Recommended Dose	Maximum Dose	Half-Life (h)	Onset (h)	Duration (h)	Metabolism and Excretion	Comments
BIGUANIDE							
Metformin (Glucophage)	500–850 mg t.i.d.	2,550 mg/day	6	Not related to dose	Approx. 6	Excreted unchanged in urine	Do not use in patients with renal or hepatic dysfunction, or in patients with active alcoholic disease
ALPHA-GLUCOSIDASE INHIBITOR							
Acarbose (Precose)	25–100 mg t.i.d.	300 mg/day (150 mg/day if patient weighs less than 60 kg)	2	Immediate	Approx. 6	<2% absorbed, metabolized in GI tract	Take with first bite of meal for maximum effectiveness

Note: Adapted from Campbell, R. K. (1987). How oral agents are used in the treatment of type II diabetes. Pharmacotherapy Times, 53(10), 32–40; Stenman, S., et al. (1993). What is the benefit of increasing the sulfonylurea dose? Annals of Internal Medicine, 118, 169–172; Santeusanio, F. & Compagnucci, P. (1994). A risk-benefit appraisal of acarbose in the management of non–insulin-dependent diabetes mellitus. Drug Safety, 11, 432–444; Bayer Pharmaceuticals. (1995). Precose package insert.

Alpha-Glucosidase Inhibitors

Acarbose (Precose) is the available agent. Acarbose slows the absorption of carbohydrates in the upper GI tract by delaying the carbohydrate digestive enzyme called alpha-glucosidase. This process is useful in clients who experience a lag time in the release of insulin after meals. Acarbose can be used alone or in combination with insulin or other classes of oral agents. It is contraindicated in clients with known hypersensitivity to this drug, diabetic ketoacidosis (DKA), cirrhosis, and chronic inflammatory bowel diseases (bowel syndrome, colonic irritation, or intestinal obstruction). Adverse reactions include: abdominal distention, diarrhea, flatulence, and rare elevation of serum transaminase levels.

The home care nurse needs to instruct the client that Acarbose is to be taken with the first bite of each meal. Acarbose alone does not cause hypoglycemia but when given in combination with an oral hypoglycemic agent or insulin the client may experience a hypoglycemic reaction. The only effective method of treating a hypoglycemic reaction in clients taking Acarbose is with glucose tablets, because any form of complex carbohydrate will be absorbed at a slower rate and will not act rapidly to resolve hypoglycemia. The home care nurse needs to educate clients on the need for glucose tablets.

Thiazolidinediones

Troglitazone (Rezulin) is an insulin sensitizer. It enhances insulin action on target tissue. Troglitazone increases glucose uptake, glucose oxidation, and lipid synthesis in muscle and adipose tissue. It reduces insulin resistance associated with Type 2 diabetes. Troglitazone can be used alone or in combination with insulin. Many clients taking insulin are able to reduce their insulin doses when Troglitazone is added to their regimen. Troglitazone is contraindicated in clients with known sensitivity to the drug, pregnancy, or DKA, and should be used with caution in clients with liver disease. Adverse reactions include: hematological changes (hemoglobin, hematocrit, and neutrophil counts) and liver enzyme elevation.

EXERCISE AND ACTIVITY

Exercise is the third mode of treatment for diabetes. Exercise and physical activity have benefits for blood glucose control and for general health. The benefits of exercise include: improved cardiovascular functioning, improved cardiac and skeletal muscle efficiency, improved glucose tolerance, improved insulin resistance, reduced weight and fat, control of hypertension, and reduced stress. Prior to beginning an exercise program, a client should undergo a thorough medical examination.

The elderly home care client is usually homebound. It is often inappropriate to involve the frail, elderly, client with diabetes and multiple comorbidities, in a formal exercise program. The degree of the exercise and activity is dictated primarily by the client's physical condition. Some examples: a client with a foot ulcer should not be ambulating and placing weight on the ulcer, a client with proliferative retinopathy is prohibited from certain physical activities, and a client with heart failure may have activity restrictions. Special concerns with the elderly and exercise include: vulnerability to temperature extremes leading to heat exhaustion or frostbite, certain medications that limit their activity, and the possibility of a hypoglycemic reaction.

If the client has been given approval for an exercise program by the primary care provider, there are several components to be considered, such as what type of exercise the client should perform. There are anaerobic exercises used to build muscle strength, stretching exercises, and aerobic exercise for oxygenation and functional capacity. Clients involved in exercising need to monitor their blood glucose levels before and after exercise. They should have a snack before exercising based on their Bglu guideline and carry 15 g of rapid-acting carbohydrate in case of hypoglycemia. It would be best if the client exercised with a friend or buddy and avoided extremes in weather. Chair exercises for some clients should be considered. Many clients can do some exercise in a chair at a level determined by their condition. These exercises can be taught to the client and family members or the caregiver can reinforce them.

BLOOD GLUCOSE MONITORING

Finger stick blood glucose monitoring has revolutionized the care and management of diabetes. Today, both client and home care nurse are able to determine a blood glucose level immediately. With a finger stick and a blood glucose meter or test strip, the blood glucose results are only seconds away.

Blood glucose monitoring is recommended for all clients with diabetes whether they are treated with insulin or not. However, it is expensive, about 50 cents per strip, and for some clients not on insulin the cost may be prohibitive. Most endocrinologists recommend blood glucose monitoring for all clients with diabetes. A normal blood glucose is 70–110 mg/dL.

The main purpose for blood glucose monitoring is to evaluate blood glucose patterns and assess long-term control. The blood glucose results can be used to learn about meal planning, physical activity, and medication effectiveness. Many situations affect blood glucose levels and blood glucose monitoring can help in their identification and treatment.

There are advantages and disadvantages to blood glucose monitoring. The advantages greatly outweigh the disadvantages but it is important for the home care nurse to acknowledge both with the client. The advantages include the ability to obtain immediate accurate results, the technology is easy to use, it is useful in detecting and confirming hypoglycemia, and therapy can be adjusted based on the results. The disadvantages include the cost of the test strips, the discomfort from the finger stick, and possible false results with inaccurate use.

For the home care nurse to perform a finger stick and blood glucose monitoring in the home, a primary care provider's order is necessary. The primary care provider's order should include the frequency of testing and the parameters for notification. It would be ideal to obtain from the primary care provider the client's target range, to assess overall diabetes control. The frequency of blood glucose monitoring should be individualized to include how well controlled the client's blood glucose level is and what the client is willing and able to do. Finger sticks are usually performed before a meal; however, they can be done after a meal. The values after a meal can give more useful information.

When evaluating the client's blood glucose control, the home care nurse needs to assess the several factors that may affect the blood glucose results: When did the client last eat or drink? What did the client eat and drink? What medications does the client take? When were the medications last taken? What signs and symptoms are reported and observed?

Blood glucose monitoring can be performed using visual test strips or meters. Both methods are accurate when performed correctly, but visual test strips give blood glucose ranges, not exact results. The nurse needs to be aware that whether the client is using visual or meter testing, accuracy of the test is dependent on several factors. The test strips must be stored in their original container and the container should remain covered all the times. Blood glucose test strips are extremely sensitive to moisture and heat and when exposed they are ineffective. The home care nurse should teach the client to check the expiration date of the vial of test strips before purchasing them and intermittently at home. Other factors affecting the accuracy of the results are the skill of the tester, whether the directions are being followed, if enough blood was used, and how the blood was applied (dropped on test strip or smeared on).

There are many home blood glucose meters on the market. The home care nurse may be unfamiliar with the client's meter when first making a home visit. For quick assistance with the use of an unfamiliar meter, the nurse can review the manufacturer's direction manual. If an instruction manual is unavailable, the nurse can call the toll-free telephone number on the back of the meter for assistance. If the client's meter is not functioning, the toll-free number can be used to obtain a replacement meter.

When the home care nurse is instructing the client on the use of a blood glucose meter, there are some basic quality assurance steps to be included in the teaching plan. The quality assurance principles can be taught to the client using a simple 4 Cs approach. The 4 Cs stand for Code, Check test, Control test, and Cleaning. The *code* is a calibration procedure to match the code on the meter to the code number on the test strip vial. The *check test* is done to determine the functioning of the inner components of the test meter. If the check test indicates that the meter is not functioning the nurse should repeat the test. If the second check test confirms this information, the blood glucose meter should *not* be used. The *control test* is performed to assess that the test strips are in working condition. Control testing is done with control solution provided with the meter. Control solution is good for 30 days after opening the bottle (the bottle should be dated upon opening). A control test is performed in the same manner as a blood test but instead of applying the blood sample to the strip, control solution is applied. The manufacturer will provide the correct test range results usually on the vial of strips. If the control test does not fall within the manufacturer's designated range, repeat a second test. If the second test is also out of range, the nurse needs to obtain a new vial of strips. *Cleaning* the meter is done to remove old blood and allow for clear readings (cleaning may be unnecessary in several newer meter designs). The cleaning procedure should follow the manufacturer's guidelines.

Home blood glucose meters utilize batteries for energy. Most meters require battery changes every 6 months. The home care nurse needs to determine from the client the age of the batteries and recommend changing them as needed. A few meters do not have replaceable batteries and need to be discarded when the life of the battery has ended.

Glycosylated Hemoglobin Test

The glycosylated hemoglobin is a laboratory blood test that should be ordered by the primary care provider and drawn every 3 months on all clients with diabetes. The measurement of the glycosylated hemoglobin test or a HbA1c is used to assess diabetes control for the preceding 9–12 weeks. Plasma glucose attaches itself to the hemoglobin in the red blood cells in a process called glycosylation. The higher the blood glucose level, the more hemoglobin will become glycosylated. This glycosylation is measured through this blood test; the higher the result, the poorer the blood glucose control. There are different types of glycosylated hemoglobin assays, so to determine the client's results the home care nurse needs the norms from the laboratory running the test. The HbA1c normal values are usually between 4% and 6%.

Urine Testing

Urine testing used to be the way a client's overall diabetes control was monitored. It is no longer the preferred method of testing for glucose. The disadvantage of urine glucose testing is that the test provides a delayed picture of the glucose levels and is dependent on the client's renal threshold, which with aging, provides false-negative results.

However, urine is used to test for ketones, which is measured to determine impending DKA. Ketone testing is recommended for clients during acute periods of illness or stress and when blood glucose levels are consistently elevated greater than 240 mg/dL. This test is especially important for clients with Type 1 diabetes.

ADAPTIVE EQUIPMENT

Diabetes self-care frequently involves several psychomotor skills and visual acuity. Insulin self-injection, filling insulin syringes, performing a finger stick, and using a blood glucose meter are common self-management activities requiring these skills. Elderly clients often have one or several obstacles to performing these types of activities independently. Visual impairments can be related to diabetic retinopathy or can be due to other ophthalmologic disorders unrelated to the diabetes. Clients with diabetes often have significant vision impairments and are considered legally blind and are able to qualify for federal government benefits.

Clients who are legally blind have visual limitations or low vision that can be minimized with the use of adaptive equipment. A visual assessment must be performed by the home care nurse to evaluate the client's ability to participate in self-care activities.

Aside from the visual limitations, there are also fine motor issues that can be obstacles in diabetes self-care. Fine motor issues may relate to diabetic neuropathy but often can be due to other medical conditions such as rheumatoid arthritis, Parkinson's disease, stroke, or amputations. These impairments can make it difficult to fill insulin syringes, push down on the plunger, self-inject, handle the syringe, and use blood glucose meters.

In addition to visual and dexterity limitations, the home care nurse needs to assess the client's cognitive abilities. The nurse evaluates a client's ability to comprehend and follow multiple-stepped directions and short-term memory. Adaptive devices require these cognitive abilities for successful use. Some clients have limited abilities due to their fears, especially when it involves the insulin syringe and injection. These limitations must be assessed in order to intervene appropriately and to achieve the desired outcome.

To promote independence in diabetes management and maximize the client's abilities, the use of adaptive devices are recommended. There are a large variety of devices specifically designed for persons with diabetes and other tools that can be found in rehabilitation/independence aids catalogs that can be used creatively to meet the needs of the client. There are devices that can assist with visual limitations such as magnifiers and devices that can assist with motor issues such as injection devices. Clients with low vision, legal blindness, or who are blind should be referred to community resources such as the "Lighthouse" or to rehabilitation centers for assistance with home safety, mobility, communication, counseling, and education.

◆　　◆　　◆

HYPOGLYCEMIA

Hypoglycemia is generally defined as a blood glucose level of 60 mg/dL or below. Persons may have blood glucose levels of 60 mg/dL or below without experiencing symptoms of hypoglycemia and others may experience hypoglycemic symptoms with a blood glucose above 60 mg/dL. Hypoglycemia usually occurs as a result of treatment with insulin or an oral agent. Hypoglycemia is classified as mild, moderate, or severe. The classifications are based on the client's symptoms and the ability to self-treat or the need for the assistance from others.

Causes of hypoglycemia vary, but the most common cause is insulin excess (from insulin injections or the effects of the oral agent). Inadequate food intake, late or skipped meals, and poor timing of meals with medication often precipitate hypoglycemia. Other causes of hypoglycemia can include exercise, alcohol ingestion, drug interactions, and intensive management. Some clients may not experience warning symptoms of hypoglycemia. This phenomenon is called hypoglycemia unawareness. Hypoglycemia unawareness is due to the normal aging process, repeated past episodes of hypoglycemia, autonomic neuropathy, use of beta blockers, or other disease processes. Clients with hypoglycemic unawareness will be safer with less stringent blood glucose control. (See Box 15-2 for symptoms of hypoglycemia.)

TREATMENT

The treatment of hypoglycemia is initiated when the client's blood glucose is 60 mg/dL or below or if the blood glucose is 60–100 mg/dL and the client is experiencing hypoglycemic symptoms. In the conscious client, the treatment is 15 g of a rapidly acting carbohydrate. This may include 4 ounces of fruit juice or regular soda, 4 teaspoons of sugar in water, 7–10 Lifesavers, or 3 glucose tablets (remember clients who take Acarbose [Precose] can only be treated with glucose tablets).

Once the treatment of hypoglycemia has been initiated the client's blood glucose should be reassessed 15–30 min later. If the client's blood glucose did not rise above 80 mg/dL they should be retreated with 15 g of rapid-acting carbohydrate. If the client's blood glucose has returned to 80 mg/dL or above the client should eat the next meal. If the next meal is not prepared and will be more than 1 h away, a protein and carbohydrate snack should be eaten, that is, bread with meat or cheese.

If the client is unconscious, the family or caregiver should be instructed to call 911 and not to give any treatment by mouth. If the client has frequent severe hypoglycemic reactions, the family or caregiver (if available) can be taught to administer Glucagon I.M. A primary care provider's prescription is required for Glucagon, which can be purchased as an emergency kit.

It is critical that hypoglycemia be avoided in the elderly client. Many home care elderly persons with diabetes have cardiac comorbidities and

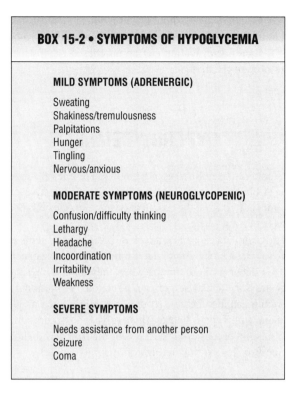

BOX 15-2 • SYMPTOMS OF HYPOGLYCEMIA

MILD SYMPTOMS (ADRENERGIC)

Sweating
Shakiness/tremulousness
Palpitations
Hunger
Tingling
Nervous/anxious

MODERATE SYMPTOMS (NEUROGLYCOPENIC)

Confusion/difficulty thinking
Lethargy
Headache
Incoordination
Irritability
Weakness

SEVERE SYMPTOMS

Needs assistance from another person
Seizure
Coma

hypoglycemic reactions can be mistaken for other medical problems or can lead to life-threatening problems.

PREVENTION

The home care nurse must educate the client on the signs and symptoms, treatments, and prevention of hypoglycemia. The client needs to be instructed to monitor blood glucose and treat at the first indication of hypoglycemia. The client should monitor blood glucose more frequently when there are changes in the treatment regimen. Clients who are treated with insulin therapy need to be instructed to eat a snack when their prescribed type of insulin is scheduled to peak in order to prevent hypoglycemia. When exercising, the client should monitor blood glucose before and after and carry a quick-acting source of carbohydrate in case of a reaction.

All people with diabetes should wear medical identification to alert others about their condition in case of an emergency (i.e., hypoglycemic reaction). Medical identification can be purchased at most pharmacies or ordered through the mail.

◆　　◆　　◆

HYPERGLYCEMIA

Hyperglycemia can be defined as any blood glucose level above the normal range. A blood glucose above 240 mg/dL is indicative of glucose not being transported from the vascular system into the cells and that catabolism is occurring.

Hyperglycemia is caused by a lack of insulin. For clients with Type 2 diabetes, this lack of insulin is due to their insulin resistance. Hyperglycemia can occur in these clients when they have a physical or psychological stressor, such as surgery, an infection, or emotional problem. Hyperglycemia can also be caused by medications such as glucocorticoid. In clients with Type 1 diabetes, hyperglycemia occurs similarly due to a lack of insulin because the beta cells of the pancreas do not produce insulin. (See Box 15-3 for symptoms of hyperglycemia.)

HYPERGLYCEMIC HYPEROSMOLAR NONKETOTIC SYNDROME (HHNKS)

HHNKS occurs in clients with Type 2 diabetes. It is characterized by extremely elevated blood glucose levels, electrolyte imbalance, and severe dehydration due to prolonged osmotic diuresis. This condition occurs frequently in the elderly, may go unrecognized, and is life threatening.

HHNKS can be precipitated by hyperglycemia, infection, diarrhea, GI hemorrhage, burns, dialysis, hypertonic feeds, and diminished thirst sensation in the elderly. The blood glucose levels can climb to 800 mg/dL and higher. The blood serum osmolality is >350 mOsm/kg.

The signs and symptoms of HHNKS begin with the signs of hyperglycemia and weakness. The hyperglycemia continues and dehydration occurs leading to decreased mentation, neurological signs such as hemiparesis or aphasia, appearing CVA-like, and coma.

The main treatment of HHNKS is rehydration to restore the fluids and to correct the electrolyte imbalances. Insulin is used to restore nor-

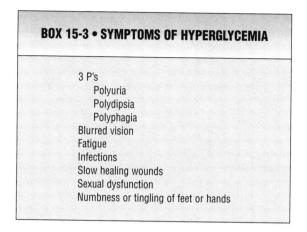

BOX 15-3 • SYMPTOMS OF HYPERGLYCEMIA

3 P's
   Polyuria
   Polydipsia
   Polyphagia
Blurred vision
Fatigue
Infections
Slow healing wounds
Sexual dysfunction
Numbness or tingling of feet or hands

mal blood glucose levels. The key in the treatment of HHNKS is to identify and treat the underlying stressor that precipitated the HHNKS. It is important to understand that the precipitating stressors can include a myocardial infarction, stroke, or infection.

The home care nurse, having frequent contact with the client, should be alert to the signs and symptoms of HHNKS. HHNKS develops over the course of 5 or more days, allowing the nurse to assess elevations in blood glucose that are not related to therapy changes and to other signs of HHNKS. The nurse should be suspicious of this condition and assess the client for other possible medical or psychological problems that may precipitate the condition.

It is important to prevent HHNKS. The home care nurse should educate clients that when they feel ill they should monitor the blood glucose more often and to call the primary care provider if the blood glucose is above the expected range. The nurse should encourage the elderly client to drink adequate amounts of water especially when ill.

❖ ❖ ❖

DIABETIC KETOACIDOSIS (DKA)

DKA occurs in clients with Type 1 diabetes due to a lack of insulin. This lack of insulin usually occurs as a result of missing an insulin dose or illness. Because persons with Type 1 diabetes do not produce insulin, they must always inject exogenous insulin. The lack of insulin may be precipitated by an increase in counter-regulatory hormones (epinephrine, growth hormone, and cortisol), which are secreted due to a stressor.

When there is a lack of insulin, the glucose cannot be transported from the blood into the cells for energy. The body then looks to another source of fuel for energy, which is fat. The liver produces fuel from fatty acids, which break down into ketoacids. The liver also breaks down glycogen into glucose. The glucose and ketoacids are released into the blood stream and are excreted in the urine. Because they are large molecules they pull volumes of water, sodium, and potassium with them, causing an osmotic diuresis. Acidosis occurs from the ketoacids and the body tries to compensate through the respiratory and renal systems.

The diagnosis of DKA is made based on the client's history of Type 1 diabetes, blood glucose level greater than 250 mg/dL, pH < 7.35, low HCO_3 (bicarbonate), and positive ketones in blood and urine. The symptoms of DKA include hyperglycemia symptoms, weakness and lethargy, headache, nausea and vomiting, abdominal pain, Kussmaul respirations, and fruity odor to the breath.

Treatment of DKA involves providing insulin (usually intravenously via a continuous drip) and the restoration of fluid and electrolyte balance. Efforts are made to determine the precipitating events of DKA.

The client and family need to understand that insulin must always be taken as prescribed and that people with Type 1 diabetes do not produce their own insulin. They should be instructed that when illness occurs to monitor blood glucose levels closely. If the blood glucose level is more than 250 mg/dL, they should check their urine for ketones, drink plenty of water, and contact their primary care provider.

◆　　◆　　◆

DIABETES EDUCATION WITH THE ELDERLY CLIENT

Diabetes is a life-long illness that is controlled through self-management behaviors. Education is one key to clients' managing their disease. Cognitive and psychomotor skills are necessary to self-manage diabetes. In the elderly client, it is important to recognize that the educational approach and curriculum used with the adult may have to be modified. Some methods that can be used to enhance the education process are speaking slowly and clearly, focusing education on only two or three points, augmenting interaction with visual aids, relating learning to past and present experiences, setting mutually established goals, encouraging participation in decisions, considering comfort and available energy, and providing opportunities for recall and practice.

When using written educational materials with the elderly client, special modifications should be considered. Written materials should have large font sizes to allow for easier reading. The materials should be written in an appropriate reading level with clear, nontechnical language. The materials should consider cultural dietary patterns. There should be clear illustrations that depict people from their age and of similar ethnicity.

PROMOTING POSITIVE BEHAVIOR CHANGES

The key to successful diabetes disease management is directly attributable to the client's ability to modify certain behaviors and maintain these changes. The client needs to be assessed for readiness for change. The readiness for change model (1993) developed by James Prochaska, PhD, explains that there are five stages of readiness. The five levels are:

Precontemplation—The client has no intention of changing.
Contemplation—The client is aware of the need to change
  and is thinking about it.
Preparation—The client is in the decision-making phase.
Action—The client is making the change.
Maintenance—The client is maintaining this change.

The client should be assessed for the stage of readiness to change a particular behavior. Based on this assessment, actions can be directed to progress the client through these stages. For example, smoking cessation is an important issue in diabetes and for general well being. The client can be assessed for feelings about smoking behaviors. If the client states "I know it is bad for my health, I'm thinking of cutting back," this client is in the contemplation phase and the home care nurse should provide support networks, give positive feedback about the client's ability to change this behavior, and highlight the benefits.

Setting goals with the client is a critical component for successful behavior change. Goals should be measurable, achievable, specific, and mutually agreed upon.

Intervention is the third part of the behavior change process. The client implements the action plan and the nurse provides the needed information, and counsels and supports the client.

Evaluating whether the client has achieved the desired behavior change is critical to success. The home care nurse needs to take on a "coaching" role and encourage and support success always using a nonjudgmental approach. If the desired change was made, then the home care nurse needs to provide support focused on sustaining the behavior and assisting in the maintenance. If outcomes were not achieved, then modifications to the plan need to be made. The home care nurse and the client must realize that behavior change is an ongoing, long-term process.

◆ ◆ ◆

SUMMARY

Diabetes mellitus is a life-long disease once diagnosed. Because there have been many advances in the care of the person with diabetes, many clients live a longer life and are older. These clients make up a large portion of the home care nurse's case load and with recent changes in the management of the client with diabetes it is important for the nurse to remain current in information about diabetes care.

This chapter reviewed the latest diabetes classifications in use, the newest and most common oral medications, and types of insulins currently in use. Signs and symptoms of medications and disease complications were shared so the home care nurse can deliver safe and effective care to clients with diabetes. Even with changes in medications and treatment, there are teaching guidelines that have remained unchanged but when combined with a population that is aging some modifications in teaching and use of community resources are needed, and these were also highlighted.

Diabetes remains a major disease entity among America's elderly population and their care is primarily delivered at home with the expectation that the client will be able to manage self-care. The home care nurse, who is current with caregiving for clients with diabetes, can help make this a reality.

REFERENCES

American Diabetes Association. (1996). *Diabetes 1996 vital statistics*. Alexandria, VA: Author.

American Diabetes Association. (1997). Clinical practice recommendations. *Diabetes Care, 20*, s50–s53.

American Diabetes Association. (1998). Economic consequences of diabetes mellitus in the U.S. in 1997. *Diabetes Care, 21*, 296–309.

Diabetes Control and Complications Trial Research Group. (1993). The effect of intensive management of diabetes on the development and progression of long-term complications in insulin-dependent diabetes mellitus. *The New England Journal of Medicine, 329*, 977–986.

Expert Committee on the Diagnosis and Classification of Diabetes Mellitus. (1997). Report of the expert committee on the diagnosis of diabetes mellitus. *Diabetes Care, 20*, 1183–1195.

Prochaska, J. O., DiClemente, C. C., & Norcross, J. C. (1993). In search of how people change: applications to addictive behaviors. *Diabetes Spectrum, 6*, 2.

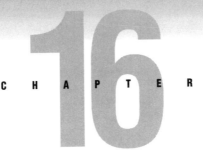

CARING FOR THE ELDERLY CARDIAC CLIENT

Patrice Kenneally Nicholas
Alexandra Paul-Simon

◆   ◆   ◆

Hypertension
Coronary Artery Disease, Angina Pectoris, and Myocardial Infarction
Congestive Heart Failure
Summary

As clients age, many encounter problems related to the cardiac system. Heart disease is the number one killer of adults in the United States and the elderly have cardiac diagnoses along with other diagnoses, many of which are covered in this book. The home care nursing management of the client with cardiac disease is discussed in this chapter. As the heart grows older, efficiency of the heart muscle diminishes resulting in a variety of possible health problems. The home care nurse is in a unique position to intervene early if signs and symptoms of cardiac insufficiency exist. Catching early manifestations of an impending crisis can save the client's life.

HYPERTENSION

Hypertension is diagnosed in more than 1,800,000 people annually, with the prevalence of hypertension increasing with age. The diagnosis is frequent among the elderly client visited by home care nursing services. The overall prevalence of hypertension in adults has decreased over the past 10 years, primarily due to lifestyle modifications, increased levels of awareness of the problem, and status of treatment. Heart-healthy diet and exercise practices are topics most adults have heard in the media and from their primary care providers. Foods professing to be low in fat or cholesterol-free are increasing on the market shelves. People in general are much more aware of what should be done to maintain heart health.

Classifications of Hypertension

Hypertension does, however, remain a serious health condition for the aging client. In particular, isolated systolic hypertension is a disease mainly of older persons affecting nearly 20% of clients aged 80 and older. Systolic and diastolic hypertension are more common among men under age 55, women older than 55 years, in African Americans at all ages, and in individuals in lower socioeconomic groups. Approximately 75% of individuals with hypertension have stage I hypertension (systolic blood pressure [BP] from 140 to 159; diastolic BP from 90 to 99). Recently the Sixth Report of the Joint National Committee on Detection, Evaluation, and Treatment of High Blood Pressure (1997) at the National Institutes of Health (NIH), National Heart Lung and Blood Institute addressed the classification of BP for adults (Table 16-1).

TABLE 16-1 • CLASSIFICATION OF BLOOD PRESSURE FOR ADULTS AGED 18 YEARS AND OLDER

Category	Systolic (mmHg)		Diastolic (mmHg)
Optimal	<120	and	<80
Normal	<130	and	<85
High normal	130–139	or	85–89
Hypertension			
Stage 1	140–159	or	90–99
Stage 2	160–179	or	100–109
Stage 3	≥180	or	≥110

Note: Adapted from The Sixth Report of the Joint National Committee on Detection, Evaluation, and Treatment of High Blood Pressure—1997. Archives of Internal Medicine, volume 157, Nov 24, 1997, pp 2413–2446.

The classification is based on an average of two or more readings taken at each of two or more visits after an initial screening. When systolic and diastolic pressures fall into different categories, the higher category should be selected to classify the individual's BP stage. For example, an elderly client with a BP of 182/100 on an initial visit and 190/100 on two or more visits would be classified as stage 3 (severe) hypertension.

History and Risk Factors

Target organ disease is another complication related to disease progression in hypertension, and is particularly prevalent in the elderly population. Although most clients with hypertension are asymptomatic, potential complications frequently occur after one to two decades of disease. These complications include:

1. Cardiac problems: coronary artery disease (CAD), left ventricular hypertrophy, or cardiac failure;
2. Cerebrovascular system: transient ischemic attacks (TIAs) or stroke;
3. Peripheral vascular disease (PVD): absence of pulses, aneurysm;
4. Renal system: proteinuria, microalbuminuria, elevated serum creatinine;
5. Eyes: hemorrhages or exudates with or without papilledema.

What should the nurse consider at the visit for a client with cardiovascular disease, particularly hypertension? First, the nonmodifiable and modifiable risk factors should be considered, particularly that the annual risk of major cardiovascular events is higher for older patients. The history should address these nonmodifiable and modifiable risk factors. Nonmodifiable risk factors include heredity, race, sex, and age.

Heredity is a risk factor because clients with one or both parents with cardiovascular disease are at increased risk of disease. Regarding race, African American clients have a higher risk of cardiac disease. Although males are at a higher risk of cardiac disease, the incidence among females increases after menopause and nearly equals men as the women age.

Modifiable risk factors are those that can be reduced or eliminated to decrease the risks of cardiovascular disease. These risk factors include sedentary lifestyle, smoking, high BP, and blood cholesterol. On home visits with all clients, regardless of diagnosis, the home care nurse can reinforce the health benefits of making positive lifestyle changes.

After obtaining the history related to these risk factors, the nurse should ask about high BP, including medications, side effects of previous treatment regimes, and successes or failures with treatment regimes. Inquire about symptoms of cardiovascular disease, cerebrovascular disease, renal disease, diabetes, hyperlipidemia, or gout. Discuss weight control, physical activity patterns, and tobacco use. When examining dietary patterns the home care nurse should include questions about sodium intake, alcohol use, and a diet high in cholesterol and saturated fats. A thorough exploration of the family history for hypertension, CAD, stroke, vascular disease, diabetes, and hyperlipidemia should be conducted. A complete medication history needs to include prescription and over-the-counter medications, steroid use, nonsteroidal antiinflammatory drugs (NSAIDs), decongestants, and antidepressants. The nurse must also examine psychosocial and environmental factors that may affect BP control and cardiovascular status. In the home care setting, factors such as stress and diet are easier to assess.

The Physical Examination

The physical examination should be a focused cardiovascular examination with the home care nurse considering all of the following for the client with hypertension:

- Obtaining two or more BP measurements separated by 2 min with client supine or sitting and after standing for 2 min. BP should be obtained in both arms to verify measurement.
- Measure height and weight, noting any recent changes in weight.
- Assess neck veins for distention. Check for carotid bruits and thyromegaly.
- Examine the heart. Check heart rate and rhythm especially noting bradycardia or tachycardia, shift in the point of maximal impulse (PMI), and clicks or murmurs. The nurse should note any arrhythmias and extra heart sounds (S3, S4).
- Perform a thorough abdominal examination, especially looking for an abdominal aortic aneurysm, which would be apparent with a pulsation palpated to the left of the umbilicus. Examine for enlarged kidneys.
- Assess the extremities for peripheral arterial pulses and bruits. Assess for symmetry of pulses, color of extremities, hair loss, and edema.

Another important nursing responsibility is to check the Osler Maneuver. In elderly clients with increased BP measurements, the Osler Maneuver should be performed because the elderly may have pseudohypertension due to excessively sclerosed large arteries. The technique for the Osler Maneuver is to palpate the radial or brachial artery. Inflate the BP cuff above the systolic pressure (at this point no pulsations can be palpated). Determine whether the artery is palpable even though it is pulseless. The Osler Maneuver is considered positive when the artery is palpable and is indicative of a sclerosed artery; an Osler maneuver is negative when the artery is nonpalpable.

BP ranges for the individual client should be determined by the primary care provider. The home care nurse should always be aware of the BP range that the primary care provider would like the client to maintain and when the primary care provider wants to be notified. The goals of treatment for the client with hypertension are aimed at maintaining arterial BP below 140 mmHg systolic (SBP) and 90 mmHg diastolic (DBP). The Sixth Report of the Joint National Commission recommends a specific treatment algorithm (see Figure 16-1). Elderly clients should have the goal to reduce SBP to less than 160 mmHg for individuals with a pretreatment SBP greater than 180 mmHg and to reduce SBP by 20 mmHg for persons with pretreatment SBP between 160 and 179 mmHg. The goals for DBP treatment are similar to those for other adults, but the nurse must keep in mind that in the elderly, pharmacologic treatment for hypertension should always involve lower doses of drugs and to increase (titrate) doses of antihypertensive agents in smaller increments.

Nonpharmacologic Management

Nonpharmacologic management is known to be as effective in lowering BP as pharmacologic measures. The best known measures for nonpharmacologic management of hypertension are reducing salt intake in the diet, weight reduction, limiting alcohol intake, and increasing physical activity. A 2-g sodium diet is frequently a mainstay of therapy for the client with hypertension. One of the most important facts to discuss with the client is that in the United States, individuals eat 20 times more salt than they need. Sodium acts like a sponge in the body to hold water and often the body has difficulty getting rid of sodium. Using no salt in cooking, no table salt, and avoiding high salt foods will result in a sodium intake of 2 g per day. The home care nurse can introduce the use of herbs and spices to flavor food instead of using added salt and a consultation with an agency (acute care setting or home care agency) dietitian can assist the client with meal planning.

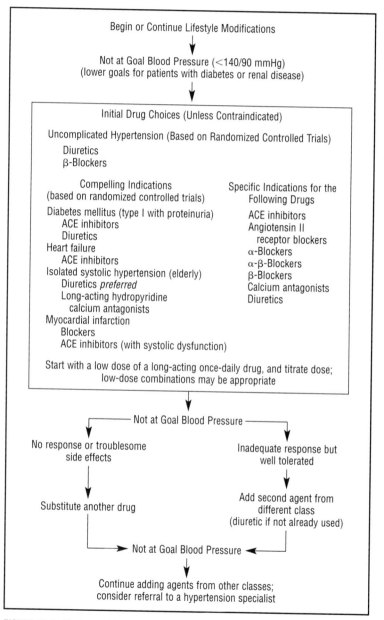

FIGURE 16-1 • Treatment Algorithm for Hypertension. Adapted from The Sixth Report of the Joint National Committee on Detection, Evaluation, and Treatment of High Blood Pressure—1997. Archives of Internal Medicine, volume 157, Nov 24, 1997, pp 2413–2446.

Specific lifestyle changes may lower BP and/or reduce cardiovascular risk factors. Moderation of alcohol consumption can reduce hypertension. Clients should be advised to limit their total daily intake of alcohol to 4 ounces of wine, 1 ounce of whisky, or 8 ounces of beer. Physical activity is a major factor in reduction of hypertension. For healthy clients, the nurse should suggest moderate physical activity (e.g., walking) from three to five times per week for 30 to 45 min, however for homebound elderly clients, exercise may be limited to walking in the home or active range of motion exercises such as leg lifts. If the client has other cardiac disease, an exercise tolerance test may need to be obtained in consultation with the primary care provider. Sodium reduction and following a 2-g sodium diet is an important element of antihypertensive management especially for African-American clients, who are frequently salt sensitive. Finally, reducing saturated fat and cholesterol in the diet will decrease the risk of cardiovascular disease. Specific suggestions regarding limiting salt in the diet are discussed at the end of this chapter and in Chapter 6.

Pharmacologic Management

When evaluating the goals of treatment in pharmacologic management of hypertension, the home care nurse considers several issues. Drug therapy is needed in clients whose BP remains at or above 140/90 after a 3- to 6-month period of lifestyle modification. The first drugs initiated are usually diuretics or beta blockers because of their association with a reduction in morbidity and mortality. Angiotensin-converting enzyme (ACE) inhibitors, calcium antagonists, and alpha receptor blockers are helpful antihypertensive drugs, but do not have controlled clinical trials to demonstrate long-term success in management of hypertension. Also, African Americans are usually more responsive to diuretics and calcium antagonists than to beta blockers or ACE inhibitors. Beta blockers can also worsen other chronic health problems, particularly asthma, diabetes, and peripheral ischemia. However, beta blockers improve angina pectoris, some cardiac dysrhythmias, and migraine headaches. Beta blockers have also been found to prolong life after myocardial infarction. If the elderly client has hypertension and has a history of myocardial infarction, then beta blockers are an excellent option for medications.

Other facts to consider with medications for hypertension are that loop diuretics (including furosemide, bumetanide), metolazone, or indapamide are needed when serum creatinine is high, especially in clients with renal disease. ACE inhibitors are particularly helpful for diabetic clients because of their effect on proteinuria and renal function although serum potassium may become elevated. Alpha receptor blockers and central adrenergic agonists may decrease serum cholesterol levels. Finally, clients with gout should avoid diuretics because of the potential for gout exacerbations. When administering medications, the expert home care nurse reviews all possible side effects and considers drug–drug interactions. Cost of medications and using possible less expensive alternatives should also be explored.

If antihypertensive therapy is initiated, the client should be started with the lowest dosage possible of a particular drug. If after 1–3 months there is inadequate lowering of BP or if side effects or adherence are a problem, then the nurse needs to consult with the primary care provider. The client may need to:

- Increase the drug dose.
- Substitute a drug from another class.
- Add a second agent from a different class (for example, if a beta blocker was chosen as the first drug, adding a diuretic may enhance the effect of the beta blocker).

The nurse caring for the elderly hypertensive client in the home should notify the primary care provider immediately when a BP reading is higher than the established parameters. Appropriate drug regimens for resistant BP should include a diuretic plus two of the following classes of drugs: beta adrenergic blockers or another antiadrenergic agent, or direct vasodilator, calcium antagonist, or ACE inhibitors. Resistant BP is defined as pressure that cannot be reduced to less than 140/100 mmHg by appropriate treatment when pretreatment BP was 170/100.

For clients with Stage 3 hypertension, who are being followed through a home care agency, drug treatment is generally needed for those with SBP of 180 mmHg and/or DBP of 110 mmHg. Often a second or third drug needs to be considered after a short interval if the BP remains elevated greater than 140/90. In the elderly, two or three drugs may be used to control hypertension, but this protocol should be monitored closely by the nurse. The nurse should consult with the client's primary care provider if the BP remains elevated despite therapy.

For the elderly client with sustained diastolic pressures of 90 mmHg or higher, reduction of the diastolic BP to less than 90 is recommended. If the systolic BP is higher than 180 mmHg, the initial goal is to reduce SBP to less than 160 mmHg. The home care nurse should be aware that a trial of up to 1 year of nonpharmacologic measures is suggested for older patients with Stage I hypertension (SBP of 140–159 mmHg and/or DBP of 90–99 mmHg).

CORONARY ARTERY DISEASE, ANGINA PECTORIS, AND MYOCARDIAL INFARCTION

Coronary artery disease (CAD) occurs secondary to deposition of atheromas in the large- and medium-sized arteries serving the heart. Cholesterol and other material can collect on artery walls causing plaque build-up, which narrows the arteries. This process, known as atherosclerosis, limits the amount of blood that can pass through the arteries. Two cardiac events may then occur: (1) atherosclerotic plaques build up over time until an angina attack or a myocardial infarction (MI) occur; or (2) blood cells cling to the atherosclerotic deposits forming a clot (thrombus). When the thrombus grows, complete blockage of the coronary artery can occur or the thrombus can break away and travel to a smaller artery, lodge in the smaller artery, and severely compromise circulation.

Both angina pectoris and MI are potential complications of CAD. Angina pectoris occurs due to myocardial ischemia, which occurs when oxygen demand exceeds oxygen supply to the heart. Most frequently, oxygen demand exceeds supply because of narrowing of the coronary arteries due to atherosclerosis. MI occurs when an atherosclerotic plaque ruptures with a thrombus extending out from the plaque subsequently occluding the coronary vessel and resulting in irreversible necrosis and death of segments of the heart muscle.

The risk factors in CAD, angina, and MI are hypertension, hyperlipidemia, diabetes mellitus, cigarette smoking, family history of premature CAD (for example, individual whose father died of CAD before age 60 is at higher risk), and certain other factors including sedentary lifestyle, oral contraceptives, personality type, and obesity. The clinical presentation for CAD varies from silent to dramatic because symptoms may be absent until critical stenosis, thrombosis, aneurysm, or embolism develops. Angina frequently presents as tightness, pressure, or aching, most frequently in the substernal area, radiating down one or both arms for 5 min or less and often precipitated by exercise or emotional stress and relieved by rest and nitroglycerin. Other symptoms include dyspnea, nausea, gas, sweating, weakness, and palpitations.

Angina is often categorized as stable, progressive, or unstable. Stable angina is characterized by no change in frequency, severity, or duration of angina over the past 6 weeks. Progressive angina occurs with increased frequency, severity, or duration of anginal episodes over the past 6 weeks, but not requiring hospitalization. Unstable angina occurs with increasing severity, frequency, or duration and often occurring at rest.

The nurse should be knowledgeable about the differences between the symptoms of angina and MI. Distinguishing between angina and an acute MI is often difficult; however, clients with acute MI often have severe ischemic discomfort that lasts more than 20–30 min and is not relieved by rest or sublingual nitroglycerin. Many MIs are considered silent MIs and are unrecognized clinically because the client has few symptoms or has an atypical presentation such as discomfort in the arm, neck, back, or jaw without chest pain. Complications after MI include arterial embolus, angina, congestive heart failure (CHF), and arrhythmias.

At-Home Assessment and Evaluation

For the nurse in home care, the elderly client should have evaluation of angina attacks and the potential for MI. A careful cardiac history, physical examination, and a 12-lead electrocardiogram (EKG) should be obtained for the client experiencing angina pectoris and especially to rule out an MI. The history should be directed toward a symptom analysis for pain focusing on the eight features of the pain symptom:

1. What is the quality of discomfort?
2. Where is the pain located?
3. How long does the pain last?
4. On a scale of 0 (being no pain) to 10 (severe pain), how would you describe the severity of the pain?
5. What precipitates the pain (e.g., exercise, sexual activity)?
6. What factors relieve the pain?
7. How long does the pain last?
8. What associated symptoms occur with the pain (e.g., nausea, vomiting, sweating, shortness of breath, etc.)?

It is helpful for the nurse to inquire about other symptoms such as orthopnea, nocturnal dyspnea, and edema to eliminate other possible etiologies such as congestive heart failure.

The history should include questions about previous cardiac disease, particularly prior MI and other risk factors: smoking, diabetes mellitus, hypertension, hyperlipidemia, and family history. Finally, the client should be instructed to keep a record of angina attacks. An example of an angina record, the Angina Journal, is shown in Figure 16-2.

The physical examination conducted by the home care nurse should be aimed at observing general appearance, noting signs of distress, specifically dyspnea, pallor, diaphoresis, weakness, and mental status changes. Vital signs should be obtained, comparing them with the client's normal vital sign pattern. Either hypotension or hypertension may signify an impending cardiac problem. Neck veins may show evidence of jugular venous distention (JVD). The cardiac examination may indicate a third (S3) or fourth (S4) heart sound or murmur. Examine peripheral pulses and the extremities for edema. Finally, a complete lung examination should be performed, especially checking for rales or rhonchi, which may indicate evidence of heart failure.

Frequently Ordered Tests

An EKG is appropriate for clients with CAD, angina, or suspected MI. A chest x-ray is needed if impending heart failure is considered and the client may need to be transported to the hospital after consultation with the primary care provider.

The most frequently ordered tests for the client with ischemic heart disease are exercise tolerance stress tests (ETT) and cardiac catheterization. Although not performed in the home, these tests may be included in the discharge summary record of the home care client. Sometimes these tests may need to be ordered after the client is home. ETT involves riding a stationary bicycle or walking a treadmill while an EKG is performed (often a dye is injected as well). The accuracy of ETT is approximately 90%; however, the test can only detail blood flow but cannot determine where or how severely the cardiac vessels are blocked.

Cardiac catheterization indicates the location and severity of blocked coronary arteries. The elderly client should understand whether he or she has single-, two-, or three-vessel disease and the percentage of blockage in the vessel(s). Cardiac catheterization and/or angioplasty may be helpful for both evaluation and improved vascularization of blocked vessels.

The elderly client in the home care setting affected by CAD and angina may require frequent monitoring by the home care nurse. The nurse should monitor symptoms of CAD:

ANGINA JOURNAL

Medication name and dose:

Describe your angina attack:

    Date:

    Time:

    Activity at time of angina attack:

    How did it feel?

    How long was the angina attack?

    How many nitroglycerin pills did you take?

        1st pill   How did you feel after the 1st nitro pill?

        2nd pill   How did you feel after the 2nd nitro pill?

        3rd pill   How did you feel after the 3rd nitro pill?

    Rate your chest pain on a scale with 0 being "no pain" to 10 being "worst possible pain".

        The pain of my angina attack was: 0 1 2 3 4 5 6 7 8 9 10

FIGURE 16-2 • Angina Journal

1. The frequency of symptoms.
2. Severity of the symptoms.
3. Is the client's condition worsening?
4. Are medications improving the client's ischemic symptoms?
5. If the client has had an ETT and cardiac catheterization in the past, does the client need a referral to the primary care provider for reevaluation of symptoms?

The client should be made aware that ischemic heart episodes may worsen with a reevaluation of the cardiac status, ETT, cardiac catheterization, or angioplasty.

Educating the client about reporting worrisome angina symptoms is one of the most important roles of the home care nurse. The nurse should convey the following signs that indicate that the client should be transported immediately to the hospital. The four specific signs are:

- Pain or discomfort that is very bad, gets worse, and lasts longer than 20 min.

- Pain or discomfort along with weakness, feeling nauseous, or fainting.
- Pain or discomfort that does not go away after 3 nitroglycerin tablets.
- Pain or discomfort that is worse than the client has ever had before.

The Teaching Role and Pharmacologic Management

For the elderly client with CAD, angina, or MI, prevention addresses several issues. Smoking cessation and reduction in serum cholesterol are two important mainstays of care. Regular exercise and maintenance of ideal body weight should be incorporated into the client's lifestyle. Treatment of hypertension is necessary to prevent complications. Low dose aspirin (75–325 mg/day) has been shown to be beneficial for clients with CAD and angina. The risks and benefits of hormone replacement therapy in postmenopausal women should be discussed with all women because cardiac disease is the leading cause of death for women in the United States.

For the elderly client with stable angina, the nurse should teach regarding the correct administration of nitrate therapy. Nitroglycerin can be administered as one tablet (0.3–0.4 mg) sublingually for attacks that occur infrequently (one to three times per month). The nurse should offer specific instructions on nitroglycerin storage and administration. The medication should be kept in the original container, kept in a cool, dry, and dark place, and discarded after 6 months. The client should be instructed to sit down before taking the nitroglycerin tablet. The client should wait 5 min before taking a second nitroglycerin tablet. If the discomfort does not go away after 5 more min, instruct the client to take a third tablet. If the discomfort has not gone away after three tablets in 15 min, the client should be transported immediately to the hospital because this pain could be a warning signal of an impending heart attack.

When educating the client about nitrate therapy, it is important for the nurse to discuss the purpose of these medications. Nitrates, nitroglycerin, and isorbide (oral therapy) are used to increase the blood flow to the heart muscle and the blood vessels while decreasing the workload of the heart. These medications are usually able to decrease the pain of angina.

The different methods of administration of nitrates are important for clients to understand. Nitrate creams or patches are used to provide maintenance therapy. Isorbide tablets are administered for maintenance therapy and prevention of anginal discomfort. Sublingual nitroglycerin should still be used even if the client uses isorbide or nitroglycerin creams or patches. Side effects of the medication include dizziness or light headedness and headache due to vasodilation of cerebral blood vessels.

Beta blockers are a third mainstay of therapy for clients with CAD and angina. These medications work by decreasing the amount of work that the heart has to do by decreasing the oxygen requirements of the heart. Side effects of beta blockers are dizziness, tiredness, depression, diarrhea, and skin rash. Occasionally some clients experience confusion, shortness of breath (SOB), headache, or heartburn. Clients should be instructed to take their medications as ordered, for example, if medications are prescribed four times per day, then they should be administered as close to every 6 h as possible within the lifestyle of the client.

Nonpharmacologic Treatment

Other treatment options include angioplasty and surgery such as coronary artery bypass grafting (CABG). Angioplasty is a procedure whereby a thin catheter is inserted into an artery in the groin and threaded to the blocked artery. When the catheter reaches the blocked artery, a balloon on the catheter can be inflated, thus reopening the area of blockage and allowing blood flow to occur. After the blood flow is restored to a blocked vessel, anginal pain may diminish or disappear completely.

CABG is a surgical intervention aimed at restoring blood flow to blocked vessels. To restore blood to the blocked vessels, grafts of vessels from the leg veins are excised and grafted to the diseased vessels. Based on the numbers of diseased cardiac vessels, clients may have single, double, triple, quadruple, or quintuple bypass surgery. CABG surgery is a great asset for selected clients with severely diseased cardiac vessels who do not respond to medical management. Benefits of CABG surgery are relief of anginal pain, prolonging life, increasing physical activities, and decreasing the need for medications. Risks of CABG surgery are intraoperative and postoperative bleeding, wound infection, blood clots and stroke, heart attack, and death.

The home care nurse's role in educating clients about medications, angioplasty, or CABG surgery is important. Often elderly home care clients require careful monitoring of medications. Techniques such as using a pillbox to ensure accurate administration of medications and a diary to evaluate the use and response to sublingual nitroglycerin tablets for anginal attacks are important nursing responsibilities. Assisting the client in decision making for medical or surgical management requires individualized evaluation of the client's symptoms, response to therapy, disease severity, and evaluation of other chronic illnesses.

Some of the most important strategies for clients to adopt to prevent further blockages or to prevent recurrences after angioplasty or CABG include: take aspirin every day, stop smoking, eat foods that are lower in fat, keep weight down, increase physical activity, control high BP, and lower stress.

Follow-up care for the elderly home care client with CAD or angina requires close monitoring for severity and frequency of angina attacks, careful BP monitoring, evaluation of the success of medications (nitroglycerin, isorbides, aspirin) in preventing angina and MI, and weighing the risks and benefits of surgical (CABG) or angioplasty interventions.

CONGESTIVE HEART FAILURE

Congestive heart failure (CHF) is the inability of the heart to pump blood efficiently enough to meet the body's needs. CHF is characterized by signs and symptoms of volume overload including SOB, rales, edema, or manifestations of inadequate tissue perfusion including fatigue and low activity tolerance. In the U.S., heart failure affects over 2 million people with 400,000 new cases diagnosed annually.

Pathophysiology of CHF

In CHF, as the heart's ability to pump is reduced, several cardiac compensatory mechanisms occur to try to overcome the signs and symptoms of the CHF syndrome. Both hemodynamic and neurohormonal mechanisms occur to try to overcome the reduced pumping ability of the heart. First, the heart may attempt to compensate by dilating to increase cardiac output. Ventricular hypertrophy may develop to handle the greatest preload and maintain cardiac output by increasing contractility. Although initially these mechanisms may improve CHF symptoms, over time, heart function is compromised.

With the decreased efficiency of the heart's pumping, neurohormonal mechanisms are triggered. Subsequently plasma renin activity, aldosterone levels, and plasma arginine vasopressin levels are increased, resulting in systemic vasoconstriction and sodium and water retention, which may lead to increased atrial pressure or pulmonary congestion. Secondly, increased sympathetic tone occurs, which initially improves cardiac output and BP; however, this mechanism eventually increases oxygen demand and accelerates myocardial cell death by causing excessive increases in ventricular preload and afterload.

Heart failure may occur for a number of reasons, most frequently because of ischemic heart disease, hypertension, or cardiomyopathy. Decompensation can occur due to lack of compliance with drugs or diet, uncontrolled hypertension, cardiac arrhythmias, infection, endocrine, disorders, anemia, stress, or liver disease.

At-Home Assessment and Evaluation

CHF signs and symptoms usually result from either left- or right-sided failure. Left ventricular failure is usually the most common type with symptoms of pulmonary congestion including dyspnea on exertion, orthopnea, paroxysmal nocturnal dyspnea, cough, and hemoptysis. On physical examination, the home care nurse may find bibasilar crackles in the lungs and an S3 gallup on cardiac examination. Right ventricular failure results in symptoms including abdominal pain, anorexia, nausea, bloating, and constipation. On physical examination, the nurse may find peripheral edema, jugular venous distention, and hepatomegaly. Nonspecific findings of CHF include exercise intolerance, fatigue, weakness, CNS symptoms, and nocturia. Physical examination often reveals pallor, cyanosis, and tachycardia.

The New York Heart Association Functional Classification for Heart Failure is an important tool for determining the client's level of disease, planning appropriate therapy, and for the home care nurse's evaluation of CHF. The functional class is rated from I to IV based on the descriptive findings and activity limitations in the client:

- Class I: No physical limitation in activity.
- Class II: Slight limitation in physical activity resulting in fatigue, palpitations, dyspnea, or angina.
- Class III: Marked limitation in activity; clients are comfortable at rest, but ordinary activity leads to symptoms.
- Class IV: Symptoms are present at rest; any activity leads to increased discomfort.

The home care nurse should elicit a careful history from the client with CHF. Ask about previous history of heart disease including MI, hypertension, valvular heart disease, and cardiac myopathies. The nurse should then ask about any problems with difficulty breathing. How far can the client walk without developing SOB? Does the client wake at night with SOB? How many pillows does the client need to sleep at night? Does the client have a cough?

The nurse should ask the client about chest pain. What is the chest pain like? Ask the client about the frequency, duration, and treatment for chest pain. Does the client require oral nitrates or sublingual nitroglycerine for chest pain? What kind of relief does the client achieve from chest pain?

Next, the home care nurse should elicit a history on risk factors including smoking history, hyperlipidemia, and diabetes. Does the client have a family history of heart disease? Finally, a thorough history of medication use should be obtained.

The physical examination in the client with CHF is important to assist the home care nurse in determining the appropriate classification. First, the nurse should observe the client's appearance during the general survey. Does the client appear to be in any distress? The nurse should determine whether activity such as walking causes any distress or if the client is in distress while resting. The client's respiratory status should be assessed for dyspnea at rest or on exertion. Examine the skin for color, moisture, and turgor. Is there evidence of circumoral pallor (white area around the mouth contrasting vividly with the color of the client's face) or cyanosis? Check the mucous membranes for evidence of cyanosis especially in dark-skinned clients.

The nurse should measure vital signs, carefully noting decreased or increased BP, tachycardia, or tachypnea. It is absolutely critical to measure the client's weight at each visit. An increase in weight of only 3 lbs can indicate a significant problem in the client with CHF. A complete cardiac and respiratory examination should be conducted because clients with CHF usually have extra heart sounds and murmurs. The point of maximal impulse (PMI) may also shift to the left and downward in the client with CHF. The lungs may show evidence of bibasilar crackles, particularly in the client with left ventricular failure. The abdomen should be examined for evidence of ascites or hepatomegaly. Finally, assess the extremities for edema and evaluate the peripheral pulses especially in the lower extremities.

Nursing Management of the Client with CHF at Home

Because CHF is a complex syndrome and not a disease process, the nurse must consider the underlying cause of the syndrome. The nurse should also be alert to other possible problems that present with signs and symptoms similar to CHF. If the client with CHF has dyspnea, the nurse should also consider the possibility of chronic obstructive pulmonary disease (COPD) or asthma, particularly in the client with a smoking history. If the client with CHF has chest pain, elicit further history and physical examination data to check for angina, MI, pulmonary embolism, or bacterial endocarditis. Does the client with CHF have edema? Then the home care nurse must determine whether the client is affected by liver or renal disease. If the client has peripheral edema, is the edema related to heart failure or venous insufficiency?

At the initial visit, the home care nurse should consider the need for diagnostic tests to evaluate the client with CHF. If the client is in acute distress (for example, experiencing SOB), the primary care provider should be notified and an EKG should be performed to rule out MI, arrhythmias, or other conduction problems. Also the client may need further evaluation in consultation with the primary care provider. A chest x-ray may be needed to determine heart size and evaluate pulmonary congestion and to rule out pneumonia. Blood tests can evaluate for anemia (hematocrit, hemoglobin) or for an infection (white blood count, differential). Both anemia and infection would compromise the client's oxygenation. Renal function should be evaluated by blood urea nitrogen, creatinine, and urinalysis. Electrolytes (sodium, potassium, chloride, carbon dioxide) should be monitored to evaluate response to therapy, especially if the client is on digoxin and diuretics. Potassium depletion may occur with diuretics and requires careful monitoring. Of course, the most important step in management of the client with CHF is to assess the level of CHF, determine the etiology of CHF, and evaluate the medication management and activity plan for the client in the home.

The nursing management of CHF is aimed at improving quality of life while maintaining optimal functioning. The home care nurse can assist the client in symptom management and increase survival. The most important role of the home care nurse is to teach the client when the symptoms are serious and when to call the nurse and primary care provider or go to the hospital. If the client is having severe dyspnea, he or she should go to the hospital immediately. However, most clients begin to develop dyspnea over days or weeks, and the dyspnea may be more apparent at night when the client is lying down. The home care nurse must educate the client about the gradual onset of symptoms and to be alert to signs of fluid overload.

Pharmacologic Management of Clients with CHF

The home care nurse should also be knowledgeable about pharmacologic therapy and that it must be individualized based on the degree of cardiac impairment and the severity of symptoms (as described in the functional classification from Class I to Class IV). Three classes of drugs are used in the management of CHF based on degree of impairment and severity of symptoms: vasodilators, diuretics, and cardiac glycosides.

A stepwise approach to the management of CHF was recently developed that (1) uses an ACE inhibitor coupled with diuretic therapy and (2) if the condition worsens, adds digoxin or a hydralazine combination. ACE inhibitors are especially recommended for the treatment of CHF because research has indicated that ACE inhibitors prolong survival, especially for clients with decreased left ventricular function. For clients on these drugs, the home care nurse should advise the client to report cough, dizziness, and skin rash, which may be side effects of the medications.

Diuretic therapy was once the mainstay of treatment in CHF, especially for clients in functional Classes I and II. Advantages of diuretics are that they reduce CHF symptoms; however, diuretics do not slow progression of CHF. Usually clients will be started on a thiazide such as hydrochlorothiazide (initial dose 25–50 mg q.d./b.i.d. and maximum dose 100–200 mg). Over time, clients may become resistant to thiazides especially with renal failure (serum creatinine greater than 2–4 mg/dL). When such resistance develops or when there is severe heart failure, metolazone (zaroxolyn, 2.5–10 mg q.d.) should be added.

A loop diuretic may be substituted for thiazide therapy when serum creatinine increases to 2–4 mg/dL or if CHF symptoms worsen. Furosemide (Lasix) can be initiated with 20 mg dose and double dose to 160–240 mg/dL. Doses higher than 240 mg/dL q.d., adding hydrochlorothiazide or metolazone may be beneficial. Spironolactone (Aldactone) may also be added to the regimen, but not if the client is on ACE inhibitors. Remember to increase potassium-rich foods in the diet (cereals, fresh meats, fresh vegetables and fruits) if the client is on thiazide or loop diuretics without a potassium-sparing diuretic.

Digitalis (Digoxin) or cardiac glycosides with positive inotropic action that increase the force of myocardial contractility are also used in the treatment of CHF. Although digitalis and cardiac glycosides do not improve survival, they are recommended for clients with atrial fibrillation (AF), dilated hearts, and those in whom symptoms of heart failure appear to be due to a decreased inotropic state of heart muscle (ejection fraction less than 40–45%), clients with diastolic dysfunction. Digoxin (Lanoxin) is recommended usually at the dose of 25 mg q.d. unless the client has renal impairment, in which case the dose should be 125 mg po q.d. If the client was recently started on digoxin and discharged home, the nurse needs to know that full digitalization occurs in 5–7 days. The home care nurse should observe for signs and symptoms of digoxin toxicity, which may be related to low electrolyte levels. These signs and symptoms include a slow heart rate; anorexia, vomiting, diarrhea; and neurological symptoms including impaired mental status. The primary care provider should be notified immediately if any of these signs or symptoms occur.

For treatment of diastolic dysfunction, beta blockers particularly propranolol (Inderal) (80 mg q.d. to maximum of 160 mg q.d.) are used. Atenolol (Tenormin) 50 mg q.d. to a maximum of 100–200 mg q.d. may also be used. Calcium channel blockers and verapamil (Calan) 80–120 mg q8h are frequently used in the treatment of diastolic dysfunction. Digoxin should be avoided in clients with diastolic dysfunction because digoxin will further increase myocardial contractility.

Client Education and CHF

Client education is essential in the successful management of the client with CHF. Frequently clients with CHF live years, even decades at home. Successful home care management is based on a partnership of the home care nurse, the client, family, and primary care provider. The client needs education about balancing activity and exercise and knowing body cues that signify a need for rest. The nurse's goal at the initial visit is to assess the client's activity/exercise limitations and to begin to formulate a teaching plan. The nurse should prepare a medication management overview to evaluate which medications the client is on, the purpose of the medications, possible side effects, and the medication schedule. The client should be able to describe the medication, its purpose, and the daily medication schedule.

Other lifestyle issues are related to smoking cessation, weight reduction, stress/anxiety relief, and minimizing alcohol intake and must be addressed in the teaching plan. Dietary modifications, especially eliminating sodium in the diet, are a cornerstone of effective management.

Some of the most important strategies in successful home care management of clients with CHF relate to diet management, balancing activity and rest, and educating the client about what CHF is and how it occurs. Teaching the client about CHF should focus on the signs and symptoms of CHF, particularly SOB with activity or at rest. The home care nurse should obtain data about the client's usual activities of daily living. Specific questions may help the nurse to focus the assessment and initiate a plan of care, such as: Do you have SOB every day? How long have you had SOB? Do your feet or legs swell? Do they swell every day?

At what time of day does the swelling occur? What are your usual daily activities? Does SOB limit your activities? What do you usually eat every day? Have you had to change any activities since you noticed your symptoms?

The effective management of heart failure is often based on the principles of conservation of energy. Some of the most important nursing interventions and client education are aimed at energy conservation:

- The home or apartment should be arranged to allow for energy conservation.
- A shower or bath stool maintains safety and energy conservation. A hand-held water spout is helpful for clients. Hand rails throughout the bathroom are very important to reduce the risk of falling.
- Keep frequently used items within reach throughout the house so that frequent walking and reaching for items is minimized.
- Sit at a table or counter while preparing foods or cooking. Of course the client must be careful to sit far enough away from the stove to prevent burns, especially if the client has decreased sensation in extremities.
- In the bedroom, keep things within easy reach of the bed. A night stand with necessary items, such as a telephone, is helpful.

Some of the most important client education is related to medication and diet. Explain the importance of taking medications every day. Clients with CHF should almost always use a pillbox to be sure that medications are taken accurately.

Educating about the balance of activity and rest is one of the most important nursing interventions for the client with CHF. When a client understands the cues that the body sends regarding the need for rest because of CHF, unnecessary hospitalizations and illnesses may be prevented. Some helpful tips for balancing activity and rest follow.

1. Teach the client to ask for help; falls and injuries can be prevented by having the assistance of others.
2. Rest during the day; the body needs additional rest to balance the extra fluid it carries.
3. Pace yourself with more strenuous activity (bathing, dressing) occurring after rest periods.

The importance of weight management in CHF is critical. Clients should know to weigh themselves every day, without clothes on, preferably in the morning, before eating, and after urinating. The home care nurse should monitor the scale for accuracy because a weight change of only a few pounds may signify a problem for the client with CHF. The client should be weighed every day at the same time and a careful record maintained. The primary care provider should be notified if a weight gain of 3 lbs or more occurs in 1 day; or a gain of 5 lbs occurs in 7 days. Teach the client that this weight gain may indicate that the heart needs additional medication to pump efficiently or to get rid of extra fluid. The client should understand that if SOB occurs more quickly than usual, then the home care nurse or primary care provider should be notified immediately.

Sometimes weight gain occurs because of excess fluid and at other times weight gain occurs because of added fat in the diet. Both types of weight gain add stress to the heart's pumping mechanism and should be avoided. Alcohol should also be avoided completely or limited to 1 ounce of alcohol, 8 ounces of beer, or 4 ounces of wine daily. For many clients, it is easier to eliminate alcohol altogether than to limit alcohol intake to these recommended amounts. Fluid intake should be monitored carefully. The primary care provider needs to order fluid restrictions if indicated and the nurse needs to instruct the client in exactly what fluid restriction means. The nurse needs to actually see the cup or glass the client uses and depending upon its size, the nurse can teach the client how to measure the fluid intake that is allowed. The client should write down everything that he or she drinks in a notebook every day. This fluid journal will help the home care nurse determine if the intake of too much fluid is responsible for the client's weight gain.

If the client starts to experience symptoms of SOB, the client should be checked for weight gain, and urine output should be monitored closely. The primary care provider should be notified as the client may be advised to cut back on fluid intake (for example, to decrease fluids from 1 L to 800 mL per day).

Smoking cessation is essential for the client with CHF. Discuss with the client that heart failure worsens because of smoking. Also, other lung problems (pneumonia, COPD) occur more frequently in the client with CHF. There are many helpful suggestions to assist in smoking cessation. The nicotine patch may help some clients and keeping a journal on how many cigarettes are smoked each day with goal setting for decreasing the number of cigarettes smoked daily is helpful for others. Having a stop-smoking buddy and a supportive family can also assist the client.

Eating a balanced diet is very important to maintaining health for the client with CHF. Encourage a diet with more fruits and vegetables as they are free of fat and cholesterol while being good sources of vitamins and minerals. Animal protein should be limited because it is high in saturated fats, which raise cholesterol levels. The home care nurse should discuss with the client the following concepts about cholesterol:

	Normal Value	Client's Value
Cholesterol	Less than 200 mg/dL	_____
LDL (bad) cholesterol	Less than 129 mg/dL	_____
HDL (good) cholesterol	35 to >55 mg/dL	_____

In general, when considering a healthy diet for the client with CHF, the following advice should be fundamental to the dietary approach:

- Eat more raw fruits and vegetables.
- Eat foods with less fat and lower cholesterol (less dairy; fewer eggs; less meat).
- Consume no visible salt or have less salt in diet.

A low salt diet may be difficult to follow at first, but by eliminating added salt (getting rid of the salt shaker) and avoiding visible and hidden salt, fluid weight gain can be avoided. In particular, clients should be counseled to avoid the following foods, which are sources of hidden salt: canned foods, processed meats (hot dogs, bologna), pickled meats, salted or smoked meats (bacon and ham), Chinese foods with MSG, tomato sauce, cheeses, frozen foods (including fruits and vegetables), seasoned salts (especially garlic salt), and snack foods (potato chips, pretzels, nuts). One of the most important aspects of teaching is to advise the client that it takes time to adjust to the taste of food without salt but after a while food will taste good again and herbs and spices can be added as flavorful substitutes for salt.

Preparing a contract with the client who has CHF is an effective way to explain aspects of the disease; clarify expectations for both the nurse and client; and evaluate the success of the nurse's teaching plan. The following figures (Figures 16-3 and 16-4) are examples of a client/nurse contract for the management of the client with CHF and a fluid and weight journal. The contract addresses the most important aspects of home care management for the client, but can be tailored for clients with other cardiac diseases or chronic illnesses. The fluid and weight journal can be used alone or with the CHF contract.

CONGESTIVE HEART FAILURE CONTRACT

I understand that I have heart failure and require certain medications, dietary changes, and lifestyle changes to make my heart work better.

Client's signature:

Nurse's signature:

Nurse's phone number:

Primary care provider's phone number:

Symptom Checklist

I understand that I must report any of the following symptoms to my home care nurse and primary care provider:

Symptom	How Long Symptom Lasted	Date and Time
Increased shortness of breath		
Cough		
Fatigue		
Increased heart rate		
Inability to do normal activities		
Waking up at night with shortness of breath		
Needing more than 1 pillow at night		
Increased swelling in legs/feet		

FIGURE 16-3 • Contract for the Client With Congestive Heart Failure

SUMMARY

This chapter details the pathophysiology, assessment, and at-home management of clients with cardiac diagnoses. The chapter also includes nonpharmacologic and pharmacologic treatment and client teaching specific to five major categories of cardiac disease. The diagnoses discussed are hypertension, coronary artery disease, angina pectoris, myocardial infarction, and congestive heart failure. Elderly clients have a high incidence of

---

FLUID/WEIGHT JOURNAL

Write in your daily weight every day. Weigh yourself before breakfast and after you go to the bathroom (urinate). Call the home care nurse if you have a weight gain of 3 pounds in 1 day or 5 pounds in 7 days.

Week	Sun	Mon	Tues	Wed	Th	Fri	Sat
1							
2							
3							
4							
5							
6							

Salt and Fluid Intake

My fluid intake is _____ ounces (or cups) each day.

_____ ounces (cups) in morning

_____ ounces (cups) in afternoon

_____ ounces (cups) in evening

I will not use a salt shaker and will avoid food with salt as described to me by my nurse.

SMOKING JOURNAL/AGREEMENT

I will stop smoking. _____

　　OR   I will cut back my cigarette smoking to _____ cigarettes per day.

I agree to stop smoking by _____.

I will try a nicotine patch. _____

I will seek out a Stop Smoking Partner. _____

FIGURE 16-4 • Fluid/Weight Journal and Smoking Journal/Agreement

cardiac maladies due to many factors, including many years of unhealthy lifestyle choices and an aged heart. It is for these reasons that home care nurses have a large number of clients with cardiac diagnoses. The successful home management of clients with cardiac diseases is essential for client safety and an improved quality of life. Both of these the home care nurse can influence through the implementation of appropriate cardiac care that is initiated from an adequate and up-to-date knowledge base.

CARING FOR THE ELDERLY CLIENT WITH RESPIRATORY PROBLEMS

Andrew J. Devlin

◆ ◆ ◆

With healthcare in a constant state of flux, the focus is changing on how clients are being cared for at home. Clients who would normally spend extended periods of time in intensive and progressive care units in the hospital are now at home and requiring highly technical intervention. This chapter is designed to assist the home care nurse who provides care for the client with respiratory problems and outlines the various basic to high technology therapies that are delivered to clients at home and the home care nurse's responsibilities.

Lung disease is a leading cause of death among the elderly. Many elders have a long history of tobacco use or years of occupational exposure to toxins and filaments, which cause a compromised lung status. Along with lifestyle issues there are the effects of the aging process, both contributing to chronic lung disorders that have profound effects on quality of life.

The home care nurse must deal with clients who have respiratory equipment, medications, and treatments to improve lung capacity and air exchange. A nurse who is well informed about current treatment modalities can educate clients, families, and caregivers, creating an environment for an improved quality of life.

MEDICARE/MEDICAID GUIDELINES FOR HOME OXYGEN USE

Oxygen therapy in the home is more popular today than in the past. The difference now is the strict guidelines that must be met to qualify for oxygen coverage under the Medicare and Medicaid programs. Many of the health maintenance organizations (HMOs) and managed care companies are also starting to adhere to similar guidelines. For the home care provider to be reimbursed for oxygen ordered for a client, the client must meet the following parameters:

PaO_2 (partial pressure of oxygen) = 55 mmHg or less
SaO_2 (percent saturation of oxygen) = 88% or less

Medicare's definition of oxygen for reimbursement is oxygen and disposable oxygen equipment such as the system for furnishing it, the system that stores the gas, the tubing, and the administration sets that allow the safe delivery of oxygen.

Oxygen therapy use is indicated only for clients with significant hypoxemia. However, there are certain diagnoses that will allow flexibility, providing the following guidelines are met:

- A primary care provider determines the client suffers a severe lung disease or hypoxia-related symptoms that may improve with oxygen therapy.
- Arterial blood gas levels indicate the need for oxygen therapy.
- PaO_2 at or below 55 mmHg or SaO_2 of 88% or less at rest.

These are considered group one coverage classifications.

Medicare/Medicaid will not cover oxygen for the following:

- Angina pectoris in the absence of hypoxemia.
- Dyspnea without cor pulmonale.

- Severe peripheral vascular disease (it has been determined that oxygen does not improve this condition).
- Terminal illness that does not affect the respiratory system.

Under group two coverage classifications, criteria may be altered somewhat due to certain classes or diagnoses. In this group, oxygen is available to clients with arterial PaO_2 of 56–59 mmHg or arterial oxygen saturations of 89% when the following criteria are met:

- Dependent edema suggestive of congestive heart failure.
- Severe pulmonary hypertension.
- Cor pulmonale by measurement of the pulmonary artery pressure, gated blood pool scan, echocardiogram, P waves greater than 3 mm in standard leads I, II, III, or atrioventricular fibrillations (AVF) in the electrocardiogram (EKG).
- Erythrocythemia with a hematocrit greater than 56%.

There may be certain situations in which the primary care provider may write lengthy medical justification. This document will go to a medical review committee for consideration.

When arterial blood gases or saturation readings are submitted to Medicare, where the testing was performed must also be included. When clients do qualify for oxygen under group two guidelines (see above), they need to be requalified between the 61st and 90th day of the initial orders. Medicare and Medicaid are in a continual state of change and guidelines and qualifications change as well. Home care nurses need to stay familiar with changing guidelines to provide the best service to clients. The people responsible for billing in the home care agency are good resources of information about Medicare and Medicaid guidelines.

Oxygen Concentrators

Oxygen concentrators are becoming more popular to deliver oxygen to clients at home. These electrical devices take room air and concentrate it. Manufacturers are constantly improving technology of the concentrators in terms of being more efficient, economical, and quiet. They are able to deliver flow rates of up to 5 L/min and are delivered, set up, and maintained by durable medical equipment (DME) companies, as are liquid oxygen systems. In some communities a company will specialize in one service and just deliver oxygen systems.

Years ago, liquid oxygen systems were the primary source of home use oxygen and that is changing. Liquid systems require frequent deliveries and are large and awkward to move. Night stand-sized concentrators can roll on wheels, and need a source of electricity. Most concentrators can deliver between 95 and 96% pure oxygen at flow rates of 1–5 L/min, depending on the size of the client's nares, their inspiratory flow rate, and respiratory rate. These variables affect the actual inspired concentration.

Concentrators contain hour meters that are checked for preventative maintenance, client usage, and compliance. Most concentrators will allow for humidifiers to be adapted to the unit. They also contain gross particle filters. These filters prevent dust and dirt particles from being pulled into the suction sieves. The filters should be cleaned daily with soap and water and allowed to air dry. If for any reason this filter were to become clogged or blocked and prevent room air from becoming entrained, the unit would not function properly. Instructions on cleaning and preventing the filter from becoming occluded are important.

Most concentrators come equipped with alarm systems that will sound a continuous loud alarm when a power failure occurs. Intermittent alarms sound when units detect lower than therapeutic levels of oxygen purity. This problem can occur due to a blocked or clogged air intake filter or interruption to the flow of electricity. Remember, a concentrator is a mechanical device that can fail for any number of reasons. Some type of portable oxygen backup should be placed in the client's home and used until the failure can be addressed.

The length of tubing, which can be adapted to allow clients to move freely about their homes, can be as long as 50 feet. This length does not affect the liter flow; however, if water were to build up in the tubing, this could affect the liter flow and percent of oxygen. Periodic checks of the tubing ensures that there is no condensation. These maintenance checks can be performed by the home care nurse and should also be taught to the client, family, or caregiver.

Liquid Oxygen Systems

In the home, small liquid systems are used. These systems are placed in client's homes and need to have periodic refills depending on the liter flow being used. Liquid systems allow for greater liter flows (1–15 L/min), and have more ease in portability. Liquid systems can be siphoned off to fill a smaller portable tank, which gives the client the ability to be mobile. It is also much quieter than a concentrator, helping to keep the client more at ease. However, a liquid system is a labor-intensive device that requires oxygen companies to make frequent deliveries. Therefore, the liquid systems tend to be more costly. Insurance companies, HMOs, and managed care companies prefer concentrators to be placed in the client's homes rather than liquid systems.

In most liquid systems used in the home, the contents are under pressure of about 20 pounds per square inch (psi) with a venting mechanism. A hissing sound may be heard, especially in warmer weather. Liquid oxygen devices will increase the amount of oxygen that can be stored in a client's home and the amount in their portable system.

Clients should be reminded that when they transfer oxygen to their portable system from the stationary set-up, liquid oxygen may evaporate. Clients should only use the portable tank prior to leaving their home so they will be guaranteed to have a full system for their activities throughout the day. Portable units can hold between 5–9 lbs depending on the system used. Stationary units can hold from 50 to 150 lbs. Clients should be advised that the oxygen or DME company will periodically change the filter on the portable liquid oxygen tank. If water is ever noted to be leaking out of the small portable canister, a clogged filter is the most likely cause and should be changed promptly. One important concern with the liquid system is that if the liquid spills, it is very cold and can cause frostbite. Always instruct the client never to touch the frost or liquid if spilled, or the metal around it.

Most of the units today have gauges or light indicators that will show the contents remaining in the system by utilizing a lighted bar scale. Each bar lights to show how much oxygen is remaining in the system. As the liquid is used or evaporates, the light bars move down. Some systems utilize the stop light approach in which green is full, yellow means the system is low—caution, and red is time to refill. Depending on the liter flow used, the client is placed on a scheduled delivery. Initially, oxygen suppliers visit a day or so early just to ensure that the system is at the appropriate level. Once the usage becomes stable, the client is placed a routine delivery schedule. As with concentrators, precautions should be in place to ensure that if there were a failure, the client would know how to contact their supplier.

MODES OF OXYGEN DELIVERY

Modes of oxygen delivery are similar in the home as in other settings. Perhaps the most preferred modes of oxygen delivery is the nasal cannula. With this low flow device, however, it is impossible to determine the exact concentration of oxygen that is delivered. Depending on the client's breathing pattern, the oxygen concentration may vary. The deeper the client breathes, the lower the fiO_2 (fractional inspired oxygen concentration) and conversely, the shallower the client breathes, the higher the fiO_2. A generally accepted rule of thumb to approximate fiO_2 delivered via nasal cannula is: 1 L = 24%, 2 L = 28%, 3 L = 32%, 4 L = 36%, and 5 L = 40%. It is OK for a client to mouth breathe while using nasal oxygen because a reservoir of oxygen is built up in the oral pharynx, providing that the nasal passages are clear. It is also recommended that a water soluble lubricant be used around the nose rather than petroleum-based lubricants if irritation is present from the nasal cannula.

The simple mask is a low flow device delivering between 35 and 55% fiO_2. The oxygen concentration cannot be guaranteed as it is also dependent on the client's breathing pattern. It is preferable to have the liter flow above 5 L/min to help prevent carbon dioxide buildup in the mask. Clients who feel claustrophobic may prefer the nasal cannula to wearing a mask.

Venturi masks are another alternative and are sometimes preferred because they can deliver an exact concentration of oxygen. Venturi masks are high flow oxygen devices and can meet the client's breathing requirements. The Venturi mask works on the Bernoulli principle, which claims that when oxygen flows through a restriction, specific amounts of air will be entrained. Each Venturi mask has windows with a different sized hole for the oxygen to flow through. The recommended liter flow is stamped on the bottom of the adapter by the manufacturer. The air entrainment ports must not be covered up as the Venturi mask (Ventimask) will not be able to entrain air and the clients will not inspire the correct amount of oxygen. The home care nurse must read the bottom of the color-coded adapter to check the liter flow.

Aerosol masks are used when the client requires humidification because of thick secretions or a tracheostomy. An aerosol mask can deliver oxygen concentrations between 21% (if the client requires only humidity and not oxygen) to 50% fiO_2. The flow should be turned up high enough so that there is always a cloud of mist around the exhalation ports. If the client breathes in and all the mist disappears, then room air is being inspired, thereby lowering the concentration of oxygen. Aerosol masks are not indicated for asthmatic clients because bronchospasm may be induced.

An aerosol mask or aerosolized tracheostomy collar can either be room air or a specified oxygen concentration with aerosol. If just room air aerosol is required in the home, then a 50-psi compressor would be adequate enough. When oxygen is required, depending on the liter flow needed, oxygen entrains via a concentrator into the aerosol delivery system. This system can only be used for up to 45% oxygen concentration. Greater concentrations would require a liquid system.

Nonrebreather masks deliver the highest percentage of oxygen of any of the delivery devices previously discussed. The nonrebreather mask provides approximately 85–100%, depending on the liter flow set, the client's inspiratory effort, and the fit of the mask on the client's face. The nonrebreather mask is a reservoir system. As long as the flow is set high enough (minimum 61%) to maintain the patency to the bag, the client's needs are met. When the flow is not set high enough, the bag will completely collapse. The nonrebreather mask should be used in rare situations when oxygen requirements have exceeded all other devices, or when percentages of oxygen required are high. Oxygen toxicity is always a possibility. There is some risk at concentrations of 50–70%, with the greatest risk for oxygen toxicity at oxygen concentrations greater than 70%.

Transtracheal oxygen therapy is a fairly new modality in which a catheter is surgically inserted directly into the trachea. Because the oxygen goes directly into the lungs, this can be an efficient way of delivering oxygen, thereby usually lowering the client's oxygen requirements. There are currently two types of transtracheal catheters. The scoop 1 is for low flows and the scoop 2 is for high liter flows. Another benefit of this type of oxygen delivery from the vanity standpoint is that the catheter is easily covered up and not obvious like the nasal cannula or mask. The drawback is that the catheter needs to be cleaned and flushed daily. Also, as with any indwelling catheter, the potential exists for infection.

TEACHING—A HOME HEALTH NURSE'S RESPONSIBILITY

Oxygen Use and Safety

Oxygen is a drug prescribed by a primary care provider. An exact flow rate in liters per minute must be ordered with a frequency of just how many hours a client must use their device. (i.e., 12 h per day, while sleeping, oxygen use should be increased during exercise, continuous, etc.). The oxygen is prescribed by a client's primary care provider to increase the amount of oxygen in the client's blood. Always keep in mind that certain client's may be sensitive to too much oxygen (i.e., chronic obstructive pulmonary disease, clients who are CO_2 retainers). But every cell in our bodies requires oxygen to function and act properly.

Oxygen is not an addictive drug, but a necessity. The more it is used, the greater the benefit (excluding CO_2 retainers). Oxygen is not flammable nor does it explode. Oxygen will, however, support combustion and allow fire to burn quicker and stronger. Oxygen should never be used near fire (candles, matches, cigarette lighters) or stoves and clients or others should absolutely never smoke with oxygen in use. The client should have a nonsmoking sign on the door to the room where the oxygen is kept or in use and one on the door to the apartment or house. The oxygen supplier can deliver these signs. Oxygen safety teaching should be a home care nursing priority.

Relaxation Breathing Exercises

It is frightening for clients when they cannot breathe, and even more so when they need to depend on equipment and healthcare personnel to do so. Many times when a client appears to be short of breath, it is anxiety that is the root of the problem and relaxation breathing exercises such as pursed lip breathing and diaphragmatic breathing may be able to help without any other intervention.

In pursed lip breathing, instruct the client to inhale slowly through the nose for a deep breath, then through pursed lips (lips in a whistle position), exhale slowly and fully. Exhalation should be longer than inspiration. Most elderly clients with a respiratory problem will automatically do this type of breathing without ever being taught the technique.

In diaphragmatic breathing(abdominal breathing), clients are instructed to place their hands on their abdomen while breathing in and out slowly, using their abdominal muscles. The hands on the abdomen will go up and down with each breath. Ultimately, this type of breathing should be practiced throughout the day until it becomes second nature. Breathing exercises are beneficial to overcome acute shortness of breath and should be a part of a daily exercise routine for the respiratory client.

Chest Physiotherapy

Chest physiotherapy (cpt) and postural drainage is a therapy in which the caregiver cups and claps over certain areas of the lungs while the client is in certain positions conducive to drain specific areas of the lung. The positions are determined by the areas of the lungs that are affected with secretions. When successful, cpt helps to literally shake secretions from the walls of the bronchial tree, thereby allowing the client to cough them up.

However, because many of the elderly clients are frail and have difficulty breathing in certain positions, many do not tolerate cpt. It is important to be properly trained in this procedure to prevent injury from occurring to the client. Also, if the client is not positioned properly, it is possible to cause secretions to move from an affected area to an unaffected area. Some contraindications to giving cpt are broken ribs, hemoptysis, active tuberculosis, aspiration precautions, and so on. One should also be familiar with all indications and hazards of this and all therapeutic modalities before administering to a client.

Importance of Exercise

The importance of an exercise routine cannot be stressed enough! Routine exercise increases muscle mass making the client stronger, more energetic, and able to use oxygen more efficiently. The other added benefit is that clients feel better about themselves and have a much more positive outlook. Of course, all exercise routines should be started only after primary care provider approval. If a client is a candidate, the primary care provider may recommend a pulmonary rehabilitation program. In this type of program, clients are monitored during structured exercise routines, including aerobics and weight training, and are taught many alternative ways to cope with their disease. There are inpatient and outpatient programs. Whatever program the client may attend, it is imperative that the exercise routine be continued after the program is completed. Using a stationary bike combined with a walking program is ideal for aerobic benefit. Using lightweight hand weights to increase chest and arm strength should also improve the client's breathing.

Assessment of Breathing

Generally, the client's initial response to difficulty breathing is to increase the respiratory rate and increase the heart rate. Assess the client's respiratory rate. More than 30 breaths per minute is high and fewer than 8 is too low. Check the pulse rate. If possible check the oxygen saturation with a pulse oximeter. It is important to make sure that the oximeter reading is accurate. The optimal range for the oximetry reading should be 91% or higher. A reading of 91–92% correlates with a PaO_2 of 60 mmHg. Hypoxia is any value lower than 60 mmHg. Below this value, the heart has to work much harder and the brain does not function as well. The heart rate displayed must correlate with the client's actual pulse rate. Also check for cyanosis by looking at the nail beds and lips for the telltale bluish tint. Listen for breath sounds. Is there air exchange in all lobes, upper and lower? Observe the client's breathing pattern. Are the accessory muscles of ventilation being used? Is the client doing pursed lip breathing? Many times a client will breathe this way automatically when short of breath. Is the client sitting up? It is difficult to lie down if you are having trouble breathing and sleep is just about impossible. Can the client talk to you in full sentences? One of the hallmarks of dyspnea is broken sentence speech pattern because the client needs to pause to breathe every few words.

Sometimes the client is anxious and worked up about something and is able to be comforted by doing some relaxation-type exercise including pursed lip breathing and diaphragmatic breathing. In certain situations, the client just needs to be heard and by listening, the client may relax without any medical intervention.

However, if the client is truly in respiratory distress and none of the above tactics have helped, it is important to contact the primary care provider to alert him or her of the client's condition. If the client is on medication nebulizer therapy, then it would be indicated at this time to give the client a treatment to try to improve the aeration to the lung fields. It is important for the client not to overmedicate by having bronchodilator treatments too frequently. Bronchodilators seem to become less effective when overused and may have severe adverse cardiac effects.

Metered dose inhalers (MDIs) are ineffective in acute respiratory distress because generally clients cannot inhale deeply at this time. They are usually upset and start to panic and often totally forget the correct procedure, thereby rendering the medication ineffective. So whereas MDIs have their place in the client's routine regime, and are favored by most clients because of portability and convenience, they really are best to use when the client is not in distress.

Pulse Oximeters

Oximeters are wonderful devices that allow the home care nurse to measure indirectly the saturation of oxygen or monitor how well clients are doing on different levels of oxygen. The home care nurse can do spot checks with new finger probe devices that are relatively inexpensive. There are also more conventional units seen in the hospital setting that can be used for spot checks, continuous monitoring, or overnight studies. Most of these units have the capability of storing information and then downloading this information, which can be sent to the primary care provider for interpretation. Most insurance companies do not reimburse for oximeters placed in the home.

Oximeters work off of a light source and a cell to read oxygen saturation of the blood. Light waves are sent through the tissue. The amount of waves absorbed will be directly related to the saturation of hemoglobin. Inside the probe, there is a tiny heater, which warms the skin surface to approximately 37–40°C. This allows for better perfusion to the area where the reading occurs.

Oximeter probes vary in size from neonatal to adult. They are either disposable or nondisposable. Most type of probes come with small round clear dots, which are placed on the light source area. This helps to prolong the life of the probe. There are also nondisposable probes, which can clip onto a finger or toe. Some probes also allow for attachment to the ear or even the nasal septum.

Most oximeters, either small or large, will give a digital display of not only saturation, but pulse rate as well. The displayed pulse rate must correlate with the client's actual pulse rate to get an accurate reading. Also, the client must have good circulation to obtain an accurate reading of the fingers or toes. At times the home care nurse can obtain a low reading on one hand and a reading several points higher on the opposite hand. Always double check a low reading. Prior to placing the probe on the client, ensure that the probe site is clean. It is possible for nail polish to prevent the sensor light from sending waves via the finger to the opposite sensor. Artificial nails will also prevent accurate readings. It is also possible for certain diseases to cause inaccurate readings such as jaundice or high carboxyhemoglobin levels. When placing the probe on the ear or nasal septum, remember to keep it away from the cartilage.

Oximeters work by batteries or batteries/electricity. The newer devices on the market today are somewhat more portable and have rechargeable internal battery sources. Remember to take safety precautions when using any type of liquid around these devices, remembering to clean and disinfect according to each manufacturer's guidelines. Oximeters should never be immersed or autoclaved.

RESPIRATORY PHARMACOLOGY AND DELIVERY DEVICES

There are two categories of devices designed to deliver inhaled medications, nebulizers and inhalers. The medications used for respiratory inhalation include bronchodilators, inhaled steroids, and miscellaneous others. For additional pharmacologic information see Chapter 8.

Compressor Nebulizers

Compressor nebulizers, also known as medication nebulizer units, are used to power the medication nebulizer kit to deliver aerosolized medications. There are many different types of units that all basically function the same way.

The unit contains a small compressor that will produce compressed air to power a handheld nebulizer. Some require electrical connections to power them, others may be portable and run by batteries. Most units are supplied with nebulizer kits and oxygen connection tubing.

The medication is placed into the handheld nebulizer (hhn). Once the unit has been plugged in and turned on, a mist will be produced from the hhn to be inhaled. There is the capability of either connecting a face mask, mouthpiece, or tracheostomy mask to the hhn. The nebulizer has the capability of making the medication particle size small enough to deposit into the lungs. The client should always inhale slowly and pause long enough to allow for the medication to deposit deep into the lungs.

The client should breathe in and out through the mouth, not through the nose, because the cilia in the nose may trap the particles. The client takes a long pause on inspiration (3–4 sec) for good deposition and exhales completely. These steps should be repeated until all the medication has been nebulized, when no mist is seen coming from the hhn. The client should breathe at a normal rate so that hyperventilation does not occur. If the client is unable to follow the above procedure, then it would be indicated to use a mask for the treatment. Treatments should last approximately 10–15 min. If a client becomes tired during a treatment or begins to feel lightheaded, he or she can stop for a few minutes but should turn the compressor unit off to prevent medication waste.

The nebulizer should be cleaned with soap and water daily and air dried, especially the small round filter contained within the compressor. This filter should be replaced when it can no longer be cleaned properly. The respiratory company provider should be able to replace this filter without charge. When all treatments have been completed for the day and after washing, the hhn should be placed into a 50/50 solution of white distilled vinegar and water for approximately 1 h. Again, rinse thoroughly with water and allow to air dry. The connection tubing between the compressor and the hhn unit need not be cleaned. If it becomes cloudy inside, discard and have it replaced. Most units have warranties. If the compressor malfunctions the home care nurse, client, or family can contact the supply company to have it replaced or repaired.

Metered Dose Inhalers (MDIs)

MDIs deliver many of the same medications to the client either by mouth, via tracheostomy, or in line with the ventilator circuit. It is important to shake the canister prior to administration to get a proper dosage of the drug. Using a spacer on the MDI canister can assist the client in correctly inhaling the medication. It is preferable to use a clear spacer with the capability of keeping medication suspended in the chamber. Without a spacer, many clients do not coordinate the technique correctly and lose the dose. The directions that come with the MDI should be referred to and the client should be instructed in inhalation and exhalation techniques needed to keep the medication suspended in the chamber. When the procedure is followed correctly, MDIs can deliver the same dose of medication as effectively as an hhn.

Respiratory Drugs

Some of the most common respiratory drugs for inhalation fall into the following categories: bronchodilators, inhaled steroids, and miscellaneous others. These drugs are discussed in Chapter 8 and are the same drugs used by clients in various healthcare settings. They are briefly mentioned here.

Bronchodilators are used to dilate the bronchial tubes. Most inhaled bronchodilators are sympathomimetic beta agonists, which work by stimulating the beta receptor sites modeling epinephrine in the body. The desired effect is smooth muscle relaxation, thus dilating the constricted bronchial tubes. The undesirable effects include increased heart rate, shakiness, and clients may complain that their heart feels like it is racing. Some of the most common beta agonists for inhalation are:

> Bronkosol (isoetharine)
> Alupent (metaproterenol)
> Proventil, ventolin (albuterol)

Clients may develop a tolerance for these drugs, which seem to be more effective at spaced intervals. Secondly, severe adverse cardiac reactions have occurred from misuse.

Atrovent (ipratropium bromide) is also an inhaled bronchodilator that works differently from sympathomimetics. This drug is an anticholinergic and works on the muscarinic receptors. Atrovent can be given alone or in conjunction with beta adrenergic bronchodilators. Inhaled atrovent should be given with a mouthpiece rather than a mask because of possible eye irritation. Some other possible side effects include dry mouth, tachycardia, urinary retention/infection, and worsening of glaucoma. As with any medications, all undesirable side effects should be reported to the primary care provider.

Inhaled steroids are given to decrease the edema in the airways. They are usually given in addition to bronchodilators on a daily basis. Some of the most common inhaled steroids are:

Vanceril (beclomethasone)
Azmacort (triamcinolone)
Aerobid (flunisolide)

When using inhaled steroids it is important to prevent oral candida from growing by having the client rinse their mouth with water, swish, and discard. Inhaled steroids maintain a level in the body and should not be discontinued abruptly.

In the miscellaneous category is Intal and Mucomyst. Intal, also known as cromolyn sodium, is used as a prophylactic drug to prevent attacks of asthma or exercise-induced asthma. Intal works by preventing the release of histamine from the mast cells and is not indicated for the acute situation. It is given on a daily basis throughout the day. Mucomyst, also known as acetylcysteine, is a mucolytic drug that works by breaking up the sulfide bonds in the mucus. It can be irritating to the lungs and should be given with care, especially with clients who have bronchospasm. The benefits should outweigh the risk for that type of client. However, Mucomyst does have its place with clients who have very thick secretions. Mucomyst should always be given with a bronchodilator to prevent any new episodes of bronchospasm from occurring.

There are many more respiratory inhaled drugs. It is the responsibility of the home care nurse to familiarize the client and caregiver with all information available on these medications.

CARING FOR THE CLIENT WITH A TRACHEOSTOMY

Today many clients are being discharged to home with tracheostomy tubes in place. Clients and caregivers must understand how to care for this new airway. The following information assists the home care nurse in caring for a client with a tracheostomy and is useful for client and family teaching.

Most acute care settings will have given the client or caregiver complete instructions on how to care for the site, remove and replace tubes, clean the inner cannulas, and maintain cuff pressures (seals). The home care nurse must ensure that these procedures are followed completely. Clients and family members may not remember the instructions given before discharge to home.

Once a client has had a tracheostomy tube placed and is discharged home, there should always be a second tracheostomy tube readily available in case of complications with the tube already in place. The care of the tracheostomy in the hospital is no different in the home. It requires an understanding of the parts of (and care of) the tracheostomy tube, suctioning through the cannula, and the necessary dressing changes. The home care nurse is well versed in tracheostomy care with clients in the acute care setting and transfers this knowledge to the home setting.

Teaching other caregivers becomes an important role when assisting them to maintain a healthy airway that stays free of infection or occlusion. There are few differences in elderly clients with tracheostomies from younger clients but they are important enough to mention here.

First, infections can be more devastating to the elder's system, so clean technique in the home must be maintained. Tracheostomy supplies should be kept in a clean and safe place, free from cross-contamination if there are other dressings or procedures the client requires, such as colostomy care, or pressure ulcer care. Caregivers should wear gloves whenever caring for the tracheostomy and be instructed in the signs and symptoms of infection. They need to be prepared to contact the home care nurse or primary care provider if they suspect an infection. A second important factor with elders is that their skin is more fragile, which makes good skin care around the stoma imperative. Finally, elders also may need more reassurance and reeducation about the purpose and function of the tracheostomy especially if they are forgetful or confused. Some clients may be unaware of the risks to health and safety if the tracheostomy tube is removed or pulled out, especially if they are cognitively impaired. Such clients need constant monitoring, distraction, or more restrictive actions taken to ensure their safety.

ASSISTIVE VENTILATION METHODS

Continuous Positive Airway Pressure (CPAP)

CPAP was first used for the treatment of obstructive sleep apnea in 1981 by Dr. Colin Sullivan in Australia. The use of CPAP is relatively new and is being used by more home care clients and is mentioned here for the home care nurse unfamiliar with the purpose or different delivery mechanisms of CPAP.

CPAP provides a continuous positive airway pressure ranging from 3 to 20 cmH$_2$O to the airway continuously. Since the advent of CPAP, many new advancements have been made in terms of the delivery device, its headgear, and the actual mask unit. CPAP can be applied using one of the many devices such as nasal pillows, nasal mask, or full face mask. Most headgear is adjustable to each individual, from small to extra large. Adjustment straps allow clients to adjust just how snug they want their mask to fit without allowing air leaks.

CPAP systems are not to be used as life support devices. When CPAP devices are prescribed by a client's primary care provider, there has usually been a sleep study performed (polysomnography), which has already predetermined what amount of pressure the client needs to overcome the obstruction. The primary care provider then calls a DME company capable of providing this therapy with the prescribed amount of pressure needed. They will in turn preset the CPAP unit and deliver it to the client's home. The client and family will be inserviced by the therapist. Home care agency staff can be inserviced if they have several clients on CPAP and the nurses collaborate with the therapist from the DME.

CPAP units come with the flow generator unit, headgear, mask, tubing, and whisper swivel valve (for exhalation). Most units come equipped with a ramping device built into them to allow the pressure to build up over a certain amount of time. The ramping device allows clients to fall asleep and makes the transition easier. This device should not be used without primary care provider approval. Ramping is usually available from 5 to 20 min.

Most clients using CPAP for the first time will note an unusual sense of pressure when breathing. They will feel a need to push out when they breathe out. This reaction is normal and will occur automatically when they sleep. Many clients state that the pressure impedes their breathing. This is not so. Home care nurses must take the time to teach the client to adapt to this new sensation. A few deep inspirations at the onset of the startup will help to minimize this sensation.

When clients use devices that do not cover their mouths, they must be encouraged to keep their mouths closed. Air will take the path of least resistance, if their mouth is open this becomes the easier path and not the airway.

Bilevel Positive Airway Pressure (BIPAP S)

As with CPAP, clients are required to have a full polysomnography to qualify for placement on BIPAP S units. Medicare/Medicaid will not reimburse a home care company or provider if a test has not been performed. The client must have a certain amount of apneas or hypopneas within a certain amount of time to qualify.

BIPAP S is intended to assist a client's breathing by providing two separate levels of pressure via either a nasal or full face mask or nasal pillows. One pressure is utilized during inspiration, while the other is for expiration, with inspiratory pressure always being greater than expiratory pressure.

As with most devices, there are certain contraindications. BIPAP S should not be used with clients who have pneumothorax, pneumomediastinum, pneumoencephalitis, hypotension due to intravascular volume depletion, or when a client has experienced severe epistaxis.

On initial setups, clients are fitted with the proper size mask and headgear to ensure client comfort and compliance. Tubing, along with a swivel adapter, is also provided. The swivel usually contains an exhalation port. The pressures that a client is placed on were determined during the sleep study. The pressures are based on what level they functioned best at and what level was most comfortable. Primary care providers must specify the inspiratory and expiratory pressures.

The inspiratory pressure, as stated earlier, must be higher than the expiratory pressure, thus allowing obstruction and resistance within the client's airway to be overcome. The expiratory pressure is less to allow the client to exhale easier but not back to zero baseline, thus improving oxygenation. Most clients have initial difficulty getting used to the pressures, but with encouragement and explanation of the benefits, most will adhere to using BIPAP S and adapt well. Such devices may be difficult for the older client to adapt to initially but they soon find that they sleep better and feel better in the daytime, so learn to use the device regularly.

If clients experience dryness either in the nose or mouth, a humidification system should be added. This system will also require a prescription from the primary care provider. If the client has sores on the bridge of the nose, it is possible to place spacers between the mask and nose, taking the pressure off of the nose. Oxygen can be entrained into the system as well. Usually an oxygen adapter is placed at the outlet of the BIPAP unit where the tubing connects.

Clients may experience stomach bloating or distention from swallowing air. They should be reinstructed on the proper use. Clients should tell the home care nurse if they experience any difficulty with breathing, compliance, or discomfort. If the nurse is unable to solve the problem, the concerns are reported to the primary care provider.

Cleaning the system is also important. The mask should not be cleaned with either alcohol or bleach. A mild detergent should be used daily, which will also help prevent skin irritation. Tubing and headgear can and should be cleaned routinely. Filters must be changed periodically, depending on the environment and frequency of use.

It has been shown that clients who use BIPAP S as prescribed tend to sleep better and have more productive daily activities and improved job performance. It has also been shown that because the heart and lungs work in conjunction with each other, as the lungs become less stressed, so does the heart.

BIPAP ST

BIPAP ST, like BIPAP S, works from the concept of two separate levels of pressure, one during inspiration and one during expiration. BIPAP ST, though, unlike BIPAP S, will also provide a backup pressure supported rate. This rate can be set between 4 and 30 breaths per minute. BIPAP ST is used to assist a client's ventilation by supplying two separate pressures along with a backup rate via either a nasal, full face mask or nasal pillows. It will sense a client's breathing effort by monitoring airflow in the client's circuit. Again as with BIPAP S, the inspiratory positive pressure is always greater than the expiratory positive pressure. Flow in the client circuit is sensed via a flow transducer.

Along with the mask, headgear, and tubing, an expiratory valve must also be included. This valve is usually located in the swivel adapter. For client comfort and prevention of occlusion, the valve should be positioned away from the client's face. If needed for client comfort, an additional 6 feet of tubing can be incorporated into the circuit without any complications. The length of the tubing, however, should never exceed 12 feet.

BIPAP ST can work in one of four modes:

- Spontaneous—The unit cycles in between the inspiratory and expiratory levels in response to the client triggering the unit.
- Spontaneous/Timed—Like the spontaneous mode, the unit cycles between the inspiratory and expiratory pressures. During this time, if the client fails to initiate an inspiration, the unit will cycle in the inspiratory pressure at the predetermined rate set.
- Timed—During this mode, the unit will cycle between the inspiratory and the expiratory pressure completely based on the time intervals set. The client can provide other spontaneous inspirations above the inspiratory and expiratory levels.
- CPAP—Both inspiratory and expiratory pressures are equal.

Clinical indications for use of the BIPAP ST are different from those for the BIPAP S. Unlike with BIPAP S, a sleep study is not required for a client to qualify for its use. Actually, Medicare/Medicaid and insurance will not reimburse for a BIPAP ST to be used on a client with obstructive sleep apnea. BIPAP ST is used to assist a client's respirations. In obstructive sleep apnea, ventilatory assistance is not what the client needs. BIPAP ST is used clinically to assist clients with ventilatory complications such as cystic fibrosis and alveolar hypoventilation syndrome. Many primary care providers do not see any benefit to using BIPAP ST for clients with chronic obstructive pulmonary disease because clinical studies have not yet proven its benefit. Like BIPAP ST, the same disease contraindications apply.

Some side effects reported are ear discomfort, conjunctivitis, and skin abrasions. The cleaning procedure for BIPAP ST should follow the same protocol as the system used for CPAP and BIPAP S units. With proper care, the nasal mask can last up to 12 months. If any part of the client circuit is damaged, it should be replaced. If equipment is continually replaced due to abuse, insurance companies may not reimburse.

Heat moisture exchangers (HMEs) should not be used with BIPAP systems because pressure changes may occur. If oxygen is to be administered to a client, the system is capable of entraining oxygen at the outlet port of the BIPAP unit or at the client mask. Administering aerosolized medications is always possible in line with BIPAP. The delivery system should be added to the client circuit on the client side of the expiration port. A mainflow bacteria filter should be placed in line at the beginning of the BIPAP unit and removed after the treatment has been finished.

Cleaning of main air inlet filter should be done on a routine basis. If this filter is not changed routinely, high operating temperatures may result, thereby reducing the flow and pressures delivered. There also exists the possibility of burning the unit out. This filter is disposable and is part of the rental system and should be replaced as needed. Manufacturers recommend replacing a filter approximately every 30 days, but it should be replaced whenever it looks dirty.

Home Ventilation

Home ventilation, supervised by family members and other caregivers, is becoming commonplace. Home care nurses experience such clients on a regular basis. These clients receive mechanical ventilation, whether it be invasively via tracheostomy tubes or by noninvasive ventilation with masks.

The home ventilator has become more sophisticated as sicker clients are being discharged home. There are a wide variety of portable home ventilators available on the market. Some of these ventilators boast the same sophisticated capabilities that hospital ventilators incorporate. Most portable ventilators have the capability of supporting any client requiring home ventilation. Today's ventilators have assist/control and synchronized intermittent mandatory ventilation (SIMV) to meet the needs of clients.

Portable ventilators have the capability of providing a wide range of tidal volumes, inspiratory times, and respiratory rates. Some will also allow for peak flow adjustments. They can and usually do have audible and visual alarms for low pressure, high pressure, setting errors, battery source, and so on.

Nurses who are new to home care will see ventilators being used as in the acute care setting. The major difference is that unskilled, lay people are supervising the functioning of these devices. The primary role of the home care nurse becomes teacher to the caregivers and client. Ventilators are used 24 h a day and at most the home care nurse visits daily for less than 1 h. The caregivers must be available, knowledgeable, and willing to take on the responsibility this amount of caregiving demands. The ability of the home care nurse to teach and support these people will make the difference in the ventilator being managed safely and the client receiving the care needed.

For older clients the difference may be in relation to the age of the caregivers. Many older adults are cared for by an aged spouse or an adult son or daughter (a 90-year-old woman on a ventilator may have a 70-year-old daughter, with almost as many health problems, caring for her). An aged person on a ventilator may be more dependent, is homebound, and possibly bedbound, making general caregiving more physically and emotionally consuming.

Home ventilation can be invasive or noninvasive. For invasive ventilation, the client is ventilated via an endotracheal tube or a tracheostomy tube. These clients usually require a tracheostomy tube for either airway maintenance in which frequent suctioning is required, or for airway protection in which a client can no longer protect his or her own airway from secretions, aspiration, prolapse, or possibly airway collapse. Invasive ventilation is usually the route taken and it has a place in caring for these clients who usually require prolonged periods on a ventilator in the hospital setting. Invasive ventilation can be and is used in the home as well.

Noninvasive ventilation is also used in the home care setting. It is being used more often today in many settings. Noninvasive ventilation is not new. Years ago it was used when clients were placed in iron lungs, chest currases, pneumobelts, and so on. Today, noninvasive ventilation is used with BIPAP ST and portable ventilators by delivering positive pressure via mask, either nasal, full face mask, or nasal pillows. Many methods, which were used in the past, are again being introduced to clients. Many hospitals are also using noninvasive ventilation techniques.

Noninvasive ventilation can be started much earlier in disease states when it is known that respiratory failure will eventually occur. Clients with neuromuscular disorders can also benefit from noninvasive ventilation by allowing the client's respiratory muscles to be strengthened. If clients can be ventilated noninvasively, whether it is for short periods during the night or day, clients actually enhance their daily activities. There are occasions in which clients who use noninvasive ventilation early in the disease may return to the active life to which they had been previously accustomed.

When first introducing clients to the concept of noninvasive ventilation, they may feel intimidated or that they are giving up control. They may feel defeated and it is the home care nurse's responsibility to reinforce that this therapy is going to enhance their lives. Clients are encouraged to look at this therapy as a move to give them back a sense of hope. Primary care providers are realizing that by implementing this therapy early, clients can increase their productivity, decrease hospitalizations, and decrease the incidence of pneumonias that usually occur with many clients who have respiratory insufficiencies. Without noninvasive ventilation, clients tend to lose lung function by not being able to ventilate lower areas of the lung. Noninvasive therapies can assist clients by allowing adequate tidal volumes to be delivered to the terminal bronchioles. This allows for improved gas exchange and often results in a decrease in the oxygen requirements. Noninvasive ventilation can provide clients with tidal volumes, respiratory rates, and flows to meet their needs the same way invasive ventilation can.

In the home, troubleshooting ventilators takes place by family members or caregivers, and it is often up to the home care nurse to teach or reinforce teaching to the family. Because of this important role, the review of basic operating instructions is included here.

Basic Operating Instructions

Assist/control mode of ventilation. When clients are placed in this mode, they can breathe at whatever rate they desire. Each breath delivered will be the amount that is set on the ventilator for tidal volume. The client needs only to trigger the machine with a very small inspiratory effort. The set volume is predetermined by the primary care provider. If for some reason the client does not initiate a breath spontaneously, the machine will deliver the tidal volume at the predetermined breath rate.

SIMV mode. During the SIMV mode, the clinician again presets the tidal volume, rate, and inspiratory flow. The client has the capability of breathing whatever spontaneous volume he or she chooses in between the machine-delivered breaths. The ventilator will automatically synchronize the machine breaths with the spontaneous breaths to ensure the client receives the preset rate. If for some reason the client does not breathe spontaneously, the machine will deliver the predetermined volume at the SIMV rate.

Tidal volume. The tidal volume is the volume of air that will be delivered with every machine-delivered breath. Usually between 100–2,000 cc can be delivered. Tidal volume is determined by the primary care provider and is usually 10–15 cc per kilogram of ideal body weight.

Respiratory rate. This rate can be set based on the primary care provider's order. The set rate will actually be the minimum amount of breaths per minute the client will receive. If desired, the client may breathe additional breaths. As discussed previously, the volume of these additional breaths would be determined by the mode of ventilation.

Inspiratory flow rate. On certain machines, this parameter can be set manually. On other machines the inspiratory flow rate is automatically based on setting a predetermined inspiratory time in conjunction with tidal volume and set rate. The inspiratory flow rate is actually how fast the tidal volume is being delivered.

Sensitivity control. This parameter is set during the assist/control mode to allow a client to generate just enough negative pressure to trigger a machine-delivered breath. A sensitivity setting of -2 is typical in the assist/control mode.

Low pressure alarm. The low pressure alarm is generally set about 10 cm H_2O below the client's peak inspiratory pressure. This alarm is set to sound during disconnection. It also may signal tube dislodgment or a leak in the circuit. If this alarm is sounding, check all connections and the client as well.

High pressure alarm. This alarm sounds if the maximum pressure allowed is reached. If this pressure is reached, the machine-delivered volume will be terminated at this pressure. This parameter is usually set at 10–15 cm H_2O above the average peak inspiratory pressure during normal machine breaths. The high pressure alarm will most often be triggered when a client needs suctioning, during mucus plugging, or any other changes in airway resistance. The culprit may also be water in the tubing or a kink in the circuit. Sometimes an overanxious client will buck the machine and possibly trigger this alarm, too. Clients have to be taught to breathe along with the machine, not against it. The client should be suctioned and the water should also be drained from the tubing at this time.

One should bear in mind that a sudden increase in high pressures that cannot be relieved by suctioning or any other measures could possibly signal a tension pneumothorax. Immediate action would need to be taken in this life-threatening situation. Signs of a tension pneumothorax are:

- Decreased blood pressure.
- Increased respiratory rate.
- Increased heart rate.
- Decreased breath sound over the affected side.

- Mediastinal shift to the unaffected side.
- Asymmetric movement of the chest.

If a tension pneumothorax is suspected, disconnect the client from the ventilator and oxygenate manually using an Ambu bag. Seek immediate emergency help and call the client's primary care provider at once.

Humidifiers on ventilators. Due to the fact that the body's natural humidification system (the nose) is bypassed during endotracheal/tracheal intubation, it is absolutely necessary to provide some type of humidification. A humidifier will be supplied and incorporated into the circuit.

An alternative humidification device is the HME. Clients like these because they do not have to bother with water, either refilling the chamber or draining the tubing. The HME should be changed daily. However, the use of HMEs is limited to shorter term ventilation. Any client who is on a ventilator for longer than 12 h should use traditional humidification systems, unless specifically ordered differently by the primary care provider.

HMEs are contraindicated for use in clients who cough up secretions into the tubing or into the HMEs. If this occurs, it is possible for the HME to become occluded and cause adverse harm to the client. If the client is using medication nebulizer treatments or MDIs in line, then the HME must be removed during the treatment and replaced after the treatment has been completed or else the medication will become trapped in the HME, rendering the treatment ineffective.

Troubleshooting the ventilator. When troubleshooting the ventilator, it is helpful to understand why certain alarms are triggered. The low pressure alarm may signify a client disconnect, a leak in the system, or a disconnect anywhere in the tubing system. The high pressure alarm sounds when the client fights the machine, or when suctioning is required, such as when the client has a mucus plug and needs to be instilled with 2–3 mL of normal saline. It is also possible that the client may be in bronchospasm and need a nebulizer treatment. Also, excess water in the tubing may be the culprit, so drain the tubing. If the above tactics do not result in the pressure returning to the normal range for the client and it is clear that the client is in distress, it is important to contact the primary care provider because sudden increases in pressures that are not relieved can signify a pneumothorax.

Portable ventilators today for the most part contain internal batteries capable of powering the ventilator if the electric supply were to fail.

Internal battery capacities usually last approximately 30 min to 1 h and are rechargeable once the unit is plugged back into an electrical outlet. Whenever a client requires ventilation for 12 h or longer per day, the home care provider should also incorporate an external battery that has the ability to last 8–12 h depending on the ventilator settings required by the client.

Studies have shown that frequent circuit changes are not necessary. Tubing changes should be done every 2 weeks to once a month, unless recommended differently by the primary care provider. However, if a lot of secretions collect in the tubing, it may be necessary to make more frequent circuit changes. The water in the humidifier needs to be changed daily. The humidifier should be bypassed during circuit changes, removed, cleaned with soap and water, and rinsed thoroughly. It then should be disinfected with a 50/50 solution of white vinegar and water, and again rinsed thoroughly.

The main bacterial outlet filter should be changed along with the circuit changes. If secretions have gotten into it, then the filter should be changed sooner. The filters in the back of the machine should be cleaned accordingly with their environment as needed. Do not clean with alcohol.

SUMMARY

Respiratory system dysfunction and possible failure affects many clients, especially as they age. These chronically ill people are often receiving a variety of respiratory therapies in the home. The therapy may have been initiated in the acute care setting but it is maintained at home by the client, family members, or other caregivers. These therapies may involve specific physical techniques, small and simply devised handheld devices, or large and complex electrical machines. Some treatments and therapies may be new to the home care nurse but all are being used in the home setting. In this chapter all mechanisms useful to perfuse the client's damaged lungs or treat diseases through inhaled medications is reviewed. Material in this chapter applies to all clients regardless of age, but the older client with respiratory problems has special emotional, skin, and infection risk issues that are addressed. The home care nurse is able to use the information for review, if already exposed to most of the modalities presented. If the nurse is new to home care the information is helpful in making the transition from acute care.

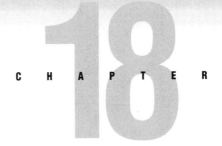

CARING FOR THE ELDERLY CLIENT WITH NEUROLOGICAL DEFICITS

Donna Diamantopulos

◆ ◆ ◆

This chapter is designed to assist the experienced nurse in home care responsibilities when caring for the aging client with different types of neurological disorders. As with other disorders in Unit IV of this book, it is noted that older clients experience some diseases more frequently than younger clients. Cancers, cardiac diseases, diabetes, and Alzheimer's disease are some of the maladies effecting older adults more frequently. Neurological disorders are seen among the elderly in greater proportions as well. This chapter reviews the steps of a neurological assessment and focuses on the specific home care needs of elderly clients with a cerebral infarction or other types of degenerative neurological disorders. The chapter also considers the nursing care information, support, and educational needs of family members and caregivers.

NEUROLOGICAL ASSESSMENT REVIEW

The purpose of the neurological assessment conducted by the home care nurse is to detect the presence or absence of neurological dysfunction. The neurological assessment allows the home care nurse to establish a baseline, which may be referred to on future home visits. This allows the home care nurse to detect life-threatening situations requiring immediate intervention, to adjust the plan of care for the client, and to determine the effects of nervous system dysfunction on activities of daily living (ADL) and independent function.

Level of Consciousness

The level of consciousness is the most important of all the parameters. The level of consciousness can almost be thought of as the barometer of the brain's functioning, in that it is the most sensitive to changes in brain functioning. The level of consciousness is the first parameter to demonstrate a change in brain functioning.

Consciousness is a state of general awareness of oneself and one's environment. Traditionally, consciousness can be divided into two components, arousal and cognition. Arousal is concerned with the person's wakefulness; whereas cognition is the sum of cerebral cortex function.

If home health clients do not have any neurological pathology, they should have an appropriate response to stimuli. Always begin an assessment of the level of consciousness with the least amount of external stimuli, that is, voice. If the client does not respond to a normal tone of voice, the next step to elicit a response would be to raise the tone of voice. Once it is established that the client responds to voice or verbal stimuli, proceed to ascertain the client's cognitive abilities. In general, three orientation questions are utilized. They include:

1. Do you know where you are?
2. Do you know what month, year, day it is?
3. Can you tell me your name?

In documenting the client's response, the home care nurse writes that the client responded to verbal stimuli appropriately and is oriented to person, place, year, and so on. It is not sufficient enough to document that the client is oriented × 2. Document specifically to what the client is oriented. Although this practice may sound trivial, when clients are becoming confused, they will first begin to lose a sense of time, then to where they are, and rarely to who they are, in that order. The nurse may also ascertain the client's cognitive abilities by asking other types of questions to assess both long-term and short-term memory problems. Common questions asked are the following:

1. Ask clients to tell you who the current president of the United States is. If they are able to the name the individual, ask them to name previous presidents in order. Example, President Clinton, President Bush. See how far back they are able to name the presidents.
2. Ask significant past historical events. Example: What happened to President John F. Kennedy? Answer: He was assassinated. Who assassinated him? Answer: Lee Harvey Oswald. Finally, what happened to Lee Harvey Oswald? Answer: He was shot by Jack Ruby.
3. For more short-term memory questions, ask clients about their medical history, what medications they are on.

These questions may seem like a game, but they provide useful pieces of information about the clients' cognitive abilities.

It is important to be cognizant of cultural differences among clients. If the client is relatively new to the United States, historical questions about the presidents may not elicit accurate neurological information, but gives information about the client's length of time in the U.S. Use questions that are culturally relevant.

If a client does not respond to the verbal stimulus, begin by providing other types of stimuli. Always begin by providing the least amount of noxious stimuli such as gentle shaking. Once again observe for an appropriate or purposeful response. If the gentle shaking does not elicit a response, then proceed to apply a more noxious stimulus. This stimulus may be accomplished by either applying deep pressure along the nail bed or pinching the Achilles's tendon. The response elicited will be one of the following:

1. Purposeful: the client immediately withdraws from the painful stimuli, and may push the examiner's hand away.
2. Nonpurposeful: the client moves the stimulated limb slightly, without any attempt to withdraw from the source of pain.
3. No response.

Document the level of consciousness as objectively as possible. When at all possible, document the stimuli provided and the response elicited. However, there is terminology that does describe the various levels of consciousness. The various terminologies used to describe the level of consciousness are briefly described:

1. Full Consciousness: The individual is found to be awake, alert, and is oriented to time, place, and person. In addition, the individual is found to be able to comprehend the spoken and written word and is able to express ideas verbally and/or in writing.
2. Confusion: This individual is disoriented first to time, then to place, and possibly person. In addition, this individual may be found to have a shortened attention span and may have difficulty with memory. The examiner may find the individual to have difficulty following commands and appear to be bewildered.
3. Lethargy: The individual found to be lethargic is oriented to time, place, and person. However, speech, thought processes, and responsiveness may be slow or sluggish.
4. Obtundation: The individual characterized as obtunded is generally arousable with stimulation and responds verbally in a word or two. The individual can follow commands appropriately when stimulated.
5. Stupor: The individual who is found to be stuporous is found lying quietly with minimal spontaneous movement. Generally is unresponsive except to vigorous and repeated stimuli to which incomprehensible sounds and/or eye opening may be noted. The individual responds to painful stimuli appropriately.
6. Coma: Persons in coma appear to be in a sleep-like state with eyes closed. They do not respond appropriately to body or environmental stimuli.

Sensory Function

The assessment of sensory function, in a noncomatose client, is accomplished by testing the function of four modalities: light touch, vibratory, pain/temperature, and position. Remember, to do an accurate assessment, all major dermatomes must be tested. This is especially true when assessing the client with acute spinal cord injury. Light touch is described here and is used in the noninjured spinal cord client. Simply get a wooden cotton-tipped swab and break it in half. With the sharp end, begin at the forehead and ask the client if he or she can feel the sharpness. The sharp end can be alternated with the cotton end to see if the client can differentiate from sharp and dull. Proceed down from the face to the arms and finally the legs. Alternate from the right to the left side of the body.

Cranial Nerve Testing

Cranial nerve testing is the second parameter measured in the neurological assessment. In general, not all 12 cranial nerves are assessed during every neurological assessment. However, for the purpose of this section a complete guide to cranial nerve testing is briefly discussed.

The function of the **olfactory nerve (cranial nerve I)** is sense of smell. It is purely a sensory nerve. To test the olfactory nerve, have the client close his or her eyes and with an aromatic nonirritating substance (such as coffee) ask the client to identify the substance. Test each nostril separately. *Normal finding:* The client will be able to accurately identify the substance. *Dysfunction:* Anosmia indicates an inability to smell. Common causes of anosmia include tumors of the base of the frontal lobe or pituitary area. In addition, fractures of the anterior fossa may also cause anosmia.

The function of the **optic nerve (cranial nerve II)** is twofold. First, the optic nerve is responsible for visual acuity. The second function of the optic nerve is visual field functioning. To test the function of the optic nerve informally, ask the client to read from printed material, for example, a newspaper. However, if the client cannot do this, the client may not know how to read (in English) or, if reading has been a skill, he or she should be formally evaluated by an ophthalmologist.

Examination of the visual fields can be accomplished in one of two ways. The nurse tests the client's visual fields against his or her own visual field. Normally the visual field extends 60° to the nasal side, 100° on the temporal side, and 130° vertically. A rough evaluation of visual field can be made using the confrontation test in which the examiner confronts or faces the client at a distance of 2 feet. The client is then asked to cover one eye lightly and look at the examiner's eye directly opposite the client. The examiner should then close one eye (the same side) thus superimposing his or her visual field on that of the client's field. A moving finger is then introduced from the periphery into the client's field of vision. Each of the client's quadrants is tested by slowing introducing the object (finger) into the client's field of vision and identifying when the object is seen. Once again the examiner uses himself or herself to establish the norm for comparison. It is important for the nurse to understand that the confrontation test is designed to reveal only gross defects of the visual field. Any question as to visual field defects must be brought to the primary care provider's attention immediately if this finding is new. *Normal finding:* Full visual field.

Visual field defects pose many safety problems. This is especially true for clients who have bitemporal hemianopsia. In this case the client has no peripheral vision. A tremendous amount of client education must be focused on many ADLs, for example, crossing the street. The client must be instructed to "look both ways" before crossing the street. A second example is the client with a right or left homonymous hemianopsia. In this case, the client has one eye with peripheral vision missing and in the second eye the nasal portion of vision is missing. Once again, the client's safety is of concern. Client education must be focused on very minute details. For example, for the male client who shaves himself, recommend that he use an electric razor and teach visual scanning techniques so that his face is completely shaven. A second example might be for the female who applies cosmetics to her face and eyes. Once again, she might need to be taught visual scanning techniques so the makeup is evenly distributed. Eating also becomes a challenge because the client may not see all the food on the plate or in his or her surroundings. Once again, by good scanning techniques, clients will be able to see what is in their immediate visual field.

Cranial nerves III (oculomotor), IV (trochlear), and VI (abducens) function both independently and in tandem. The **oculomotor nerve (cranial nerve III)** functions in three separate ways. It innervates the muscles of the eyelid to allow the eye to stay open, is responsible for pupillary constriction, and innervates the muscles for eye movement, allowing the eye to be able to look upward, inward, and downward.

When testing the oculomotor nerve, the examiner begins by first observing for symmetry and eyelid opening. The pupil and some of the iris should be able to be seen in most individuals. If the pupil is unable to be seen, the client may have a ptosis.

To assess pupillary function, begin by observing the size of the pupil. In the normal adult, pupillary size ranges from 2 to 6 mm. The pupils should be equal in size; however, approximately 20% of the population have what is known as *anisocoria* (unequal pupil size). Alone, this condition is not considered an abnormal finding as most are congenital. In addition to observing pupillary size, the examiner should observe pupillary shape. The shape of the pupil is round; however, clients who have had cataract surgery may have a keyhole appearance to their pupil.

Finally, pupillary reflex reaction is tested by both direct light reflex testing and accommodation testing. The examiner tests light reflex by first dimming the room light for maximum response; asks the client to look straight ahead while the examiner shines a light into one eye. The pupil, if functioning properly, will constrict. The examiner also may observe for consensual reaction of the opposite eye. Accommodation reflex is accomplished by holding an object from the client and moving it closer. As the object is moved closer to the client it is observed that the pupils constrict.

Cranial nerve IV, the trochlear nerve, innervates the muscles of the eye so that the eye may look inward and downward. And finally, **cranial nerve VI, the abducens nerve,** also innervates eye muscle and allows the eye to look outward. Therefore, all three nerves are assessed together by simply asking the client to look straight ahead and to follow the examiner's finger with the eyes. The examiner should ask the client to look up, to the left side, to the right side, down towards the feet, and then finally ask the client to look inward towards the nose. *Normal finding:* The client's eyes are able to follow the commands, anything else is abnormal.

The **trigeminal nerve (cranial nerve V),** has both a sensory and motor function. It provides sensation from the face, cornea, nasal and oral mucosa, tongue, external auditory canal, and the meninges. In addition, this nerve allows the jaw to open and close.

In testing for normal function of the trigeminal nerve, the examiner may begin by having the client close his or her eyes and then the examiner touches areas of the forehead, mandibular, and maxillary regions. The corneal reflex may also be tested by carefully stroking the cornea with a wisp of cotton and observing for a prompt blink.

If the client does not have a corneal blink or reflex, it is important for the nurse to instruct the client in performing frequent examinations of the eye. Because the corneal reflex is absent, small irritating particles may enter the eye and irritate the cornea, which may lead to formation of a corneal abrasion or even worse a corneal ulceration. The client should be instructed to wear sunglasses whenever he or she is outside, especially on windy days. In addition, the client should carry some type of over-the-counter lubricant eye drop. The eye drops may be used to moisten and clean the eye out. Any teaching that promotes the health of an elder's eye increases the potential for improving the quality of life.

The motor component of the trigeminal nerve may be tested by simply asking the client to open his or her jaw. The examiner then observes for any jaw deviation. If there is weakness, the jaw will deviate toward the weaker side. In addition, the examiner asks the client to bite down tightly while the examiner palpates temporal and masseter muscles for contraction. Finally, the client is asked to move the jaw laterally against pressure applied by the examiner to detect weakness or paralysis. Motor weakness from dysfunction of the trigeminal nerve is frequently seen in clients with conditions such as myasthenia gravis, Down's syndrome, and botulism. If noted, the home care nurse should bring it to the attention of the primary care provider.

Cranial nerve VII, the facial nerve, as with many other cranial nerves, has both a motor and a sensory component to it. The motor component controls muscles for facial expression allowing people to frown or smile. More importantly, the facial nerve controls eyelid closure. The sensory component of this nerve provides taste sensation to the anterior two-thirds of the tongue. In addition, it stimulates the salivary, lacrimal, nasal, oral, submaxillary, and sublingual glands.

To test the facial nerve, the examiner begins by observing the symmetry of the facial musculature. Next, clients are asked to wrinkle their forehead, frown, raise eyebrows, wink, keep eyelids closed against resistance, puff their cheeks out, and finally show their teeth. While placing a client through these various facial expressions observe for symmetry of facial movement. In addition, clients with dysfunction of the facial nerve may be observed for a decrease or loss of the nasolabial fold and or sagging of the lower eyelid on the affected side. More importantly, the examiner should observe for inability of eye closure. If this is present, it places the client at great risk for developing corneal abrasions or corneal ulceration. It is important to teach the client the importance of frequent eye examinations to check for irritation, redness, puffiness, or pain. Instruct the client to wear protective eye glasses when outside. In addition, at night the client should be instructed to use some type of eye ointment to keep the cornea from drying. Remember, this type of client is not going to have a blink response. When people blink, the cornea is bathed and lubricated. In general, it is recommended that during the day the client use an eye lubricant at least every 3–4 h and at night, it is recommended to use an eye ointment before going to sleep. Avoid use of gauze or tape to close the eye as this may cause further irritation to the cornea or to the delicate skin surrounding the eye. A cloth eye patch can be purchased in a local pharmacy. The client should also be encourage to visit the ophthalmologist every 4–6 months; however, any signs or symptoms of eye irritation should be promptly reported to the ophthalmologist.

The **acoustic nerve (cranial nerve VIII)** is primarily a sensory nerve. Anatomically, the acoustic nerve has two divisions. The cochlear division is responsible for hearing and sound conduction; the vestibular division is responsible for equilibrium.

The best and most accurate way of testing the acoustic nerve is through formal audiometric examination. To assess the function of this nerve informally, the examiner may ask the client to repeat whispered words or identify sounds such as a watch ticking or fingers rubbing together.

Dysfunction of the cochlear division of the acoustic nerve produces deafness in one ear. Dysfunction of the vestibular division of the acoustic nerve may cause the client to experience vertigo.

To assess the function of the vestibular division, the examiner can ask the client to stand with feet together, arms alongside the body. The examiner should assess the client's ability to maintain balance.

The next two nerves are the **glossopharyngeal nerve (cranial nerve IX)** and the **vagus nerve (cranial nerve X).** They are generally tested together because they function similarly. Both of these nerves have a sensory and a motor component to them.

The glossopharyngeal nerve, provides sensation to the posterior one-third of the tongue. In addition, it provides the sensation of pain, touch, and temperature to the pharynx and the throat. The afferent limb of the nerve is responsible for the gag, swallow, and carotid reflexes. The vagus nerve innervates the muscles of the larynx, inferior pharynx, and the soft palate. The carotid sinus reflex is also innervated by the vagus nerve.

To test the glossopharyngeal nerve, the examiner begins by asking the client to open his or her mouth. The soft palate and pharynx is examined and the client is asked to say "ah" and the uvula is observed for rising in the midline. The next step is to assess the client's ability to swallow oral secretions. Simply observe to see if the client is drooling, which may be a sign that the client is unable to handle secretions. Next, note the quality of speech; is it hoarse, hypophonic, or nasal in character. To differentiate areas of weakness of any of the muscles innervated by this nerve, begin by asking the client to produce the "kuh-kuh-kuh" sound. When producing this sound, the soft palate must rise, otherwise a muffled sounding "kuh-kuh-kuh" sound will be produced. To test for proper closure, ask the client to say "mi-mi-mi." The home care nurse may try this noting that the lips must be tightly closed to produce this sound. If lip closure is incomplete, this sound cannot be made. Finally, for tongue movement, ask the client to say "la-la-la." To produce this sound, the tongue must be lifted up and the tip pressed against the front teeth. To assess for the gag reflex, simply ask the client to open his or her mouth, with a tongue depressor rub up against the posterior pharyngeal wall. If the gag reflex is present the client will obviously gag or may cough. In addition to the gag reflex, assess the cough reflex or simply ask the client to give a good cough. The cough reflex is important in that the gag reflex may be absent but the client may have a good cough reflex. The cough reflex is what protects people from choking.

The vagus nerve is tested somewhat differently. The first step in the assessment is to simply listen to the client's voice. Is it hoarse, is the speech dysarthric (garbled speech); simply assess the hoarseness by asking the client to say the letter "e." Every time the letter "e" is vocalized, the vocal folds (cords) approximate.

The **spinal accessory nerve (cranial nerve XI)** is purely a motor nerve. It is responsible for innervating the sternocleidomastoid and trapezius muscles for flexion and rotation of the head. To test this nerve, the nurse begins by inspecting and palpating the sternocleidomastoid and trapezius muscles for size, contour, and tone. Next the client is asked to turn his or her head from side to side against the resistance of the examiner's hand. Then the client is asked to push the head forward against the examiner's hand. Finally the client is asked to shrug shoulders against the resistance of the examiner's hands.

The last and final nerve to be tested is the **hypoglossal nerve (cranial nerve XII).** This nerve is purely a motor nerve. To test this nerve, the nurse simply asks the client to stick his or her tongue out of the mouth and observe the midline position of the tongue. Next the client is asked to move the tongue from side to side. Dysfunction of this nerve will lead to the client experiencing dysarthric speech and difficulty chewing and swallowing food.

Clients experiencing any difficulty with cranial nerves IX, X, and XII warrant a consult from a speech/language pathologist so that the proper therapies may be instituted. In addition, to properly assess the swallowing components of these nerves, a modified barium swallow is required to ascertain which phase of the swallowing process is damaged. Of special note, clients assessed for swallowing problems should never be tested with water or other slippery substances.

MOTOR FUNCTION ASSESSMENT

Assessment of motor function can be accomplished very rapidly, in fact all of the major muscle groups can be assessed within 5 min. However, it is an important assessment, especially for the safety of the homebound client who frequently must manage ADLs independently.

To begin the motor assessment, the home care nurse inspects the major muscle groups for symmetry and for any atrophy. Muscle size and mass will be variable depending on the age, sex, physical condition, and nutritional state of the client. Begin the motor examination by asking the client which hand he or she writes with. This is the dominant hand. Test the dominant hand against the nurse's dominant hand (the dominant hand is generally stronger than the nondominant hand). The client is asked to squeeze the nurse's hands as tight as possible. Assess whether or not there is equal strength in the hand grasps.

Next, have the client lift both arms up in front, with the palms of the hands facing upward. Ask the client to close the eyes. Note if one of the hands begins to drift downward; this is known as a *pronator drift* and indicates weakness of the extremity.

To test the major muscle groups of the rest of the upper extremities, simply ask the client to lift the arms up in front and flex the arms at the elbow while the examiner applies force against the forearms toward the client. Ask the client to then bring the flexed arms in front as if holding something out in front and instruct the client to keep the arms flexed while the examiner attempts to straighten the arms out. Finally the client is asked to push against the nurse with his or her arms.

The lower extremities are assessed in a similar fashion. To begin, have the client lie flat on his or her back. First ask the client to lift one leg up while the examiner applies pressure to the leg. Next ask the client to bend a knee while the examiner attempts to straighten the leg. Ask the client then to keep the leg as straight as possible while the examiner attempts to bend the leg at the knee. Ask the client to point the toes up toward the face while the examiner applies pressure against the tops of the feet and finally ask the client to push the feet down on the examiner's hand as if applying the brakes on a car.

To document the strength of the client, a grading system is used. The optimal grade is 5 and when documenting muscle strength, it will be the grade against which the client is assessed.

Grade 5 = full range of motion against gravity and resistance; normal muscle strength.

Grade 4 = full range of motion against gravity and a moderate amount of resistance; slight weakness.

Grade 3 = full range of motion against gravity, only moderate weakness.

Grade 2 = full range of motion when gravity is eliminated; severe weakness.

Grade 1 = a weak muscle contraction is palpated, but no movement is noted, very severe weakness.

Grade 0 = no movement.

HOME CARE OF THE CLIENT WITH A CEREBRAL VASCULAR ACCIDENT (STROKE)

This section will introduce the home care nurse to the care of the post-cerebral vascular accident (CVA) or stroke client living in the home. A brief discussion regarding the types of CVAs, risk factors, and current medical management will also be discussed. CVA by definition is not a disease but rather a syndrome that is characterized by the gradual or rapid onset of nonconvulsant neurological deficits that fit a known vascular territory and lasts for more than 24 h. However, any nonconvulsive neurological deficits lasting more than 1 h would also be considered a stroke.

Risk Factors

The home care nurse is responsible for the general care of post-stroke clients; however, a discussion of risk factors is important in that post-stroke survivors are at great risk for developing subsequent strokes. Identification of risk factors is important in providing education to both the stroke survivor and to family members and caregivers. After accounting for age, sex, and race, the leading cause of a CVA is hypertension. Other common risk factors include cardiac diseases such as atrial fibrillation, valve replacements, coronary artery disease, and myocardial infarction. History of transient ischemic attacks and diabetes mellitus can also contribute to the development of a CVA. In addition, history of smoking, alcohol intake, and obesity are considered as well. It is important to recognize that no one risk factor places a client at risk, but rather it is a combination of risk factors.

Classification and Pharmacologic Management

Classifications of CVAs are based on the underlying problem created within the blood vessel and blood supply of the brain. A stroke can be classified into two categories: ischemic and hemorrhagic stroke.

Ischemic stroke can further be divided into thrombotic stroke and embolic stroke.

The goals of acute stroke management are to (1) prevent further thrombotic events or complications of stroke, (2) to ascertain the etiology of stroke so that stroke preventive management may be instituted, and (3) to initiate early rehabilitation measures.

Hypertension is the leading cause of stroke, therefore close attention must be made to the management of hypertension on a long-term basis. Careful assessment of the effects of the antihypertensive agents utilized is imperative. Other agents used in long-term stoke management may include an antiplatelet agent or long-term anticoagulation.

Aspirin decreases the risk of stroke or death from a stroke by approximately 30% (Canadian Cooperative Study Group, 1978). In general, aspirin is the drug of choice for a noncardioembolic type of stroke. It is frequently the first line treatment in the treatment of clients presenting with transient ischemic attacks. One enteric-coated aspirin daily is ordered.

Ticlopidine hydrochloride (Ticlid), a platelet aggregation inhibitor, may be prescribed. The major side effect of Ticlid is a transient neutropenia noted within the first couple of months the drug is initiated. Therefore it is imperative that the client undergo complete blood counts every 2 weeks for the first 2 months Ticlid has been initiated. Other common side effects are rashes, diarrhea, and stomach upset. In general, use of Ticlid in the management of acute stroke is the same as aspirin. However, some primary care providers utilize Ticlid when aspirin has failed.

Warfarin sodium (Coumadin), is the drug of choice and used in the prevention of further cardioembolic stroke. In addition, Coumadin is the drug of choice when the client is found to have coagulapathies such as protein C deficient or antiphospholipid antibodies, both conditions responsible for stroke. The client is initially started on heparin and once a therapeutic partial thromboplastin time is obtained (1.5 to 2 times the control), Coumadin is started. Once Coumadin is started, the international normalizing ratio (INR) is monitored. The principal danger of long-term use of Coumadin is bleeding. Client, family, and caregiver education must include observation of hematuria, melena, frequent bruising, bleeding gums, and prolonged bleeding from cuts. The home care nurse reinforces that frequent measurement of the INR is necessary. Long-term use of Coumadin carries approximately 5% chance of hemorrhage, with an average of 1% per year mortality. Refer to Chapters 8 and 16 for more specific medication and cardiac information.

Caregiving at Home

The home care nurse assigned to the client post-stroke may receive the client from the acute care hospital, acute rehabilitation hospital, subacute rehabilitation hospital, or skilled nursing home. The client post-stroke may have various neurologic deficits.

Deficits may include hemiplegia, expressive or receptive aphasia, swallowing difficulties, visual deficits, incontinence, and varied behavior problems. In addition, the home care nurse may be faced with problems related to the significant other's acceptance of the client as a result of the CVA. Many family members of stroke survivors will comment that their loved one is different; that he or she is not the same person. The home care nurse must be sensitive to the fact that caregivers need time to grieve the "loss" of the person they knew.

The goal for the home care nurse in the care of the stroke client should be directed toward achieving independence in ADLs. Secondly, the home care nurse needs to focus on the comprehensive management of the stroke survivor's environment. The role of the nurse is to aid clients and their significant others in learning lifelong strategies for coping with deficits to gain new control over their changed lives.

Management of Behavioral, Psychological, and Cognitive Changes

The CVA survivor may present with behavior problems including confusional states, delirium, depression, anxiety, or dementia. In addition, depending on which hemisphere has been affected, differences in behavior may be observed.

The left hemisphere is responsible primarily for linguistic and language-mediated tasks, calculation, and abstract reasoning. The right hemisphere in most right-handed individuals is responsible for the following four major functions:

1. Spatial distribution of attention.
2. Nonlinguistic perceptual skill.
3. Paralinguistic aspects of communication.
4. Emotions.

In general, clients who have sustained injury to the right hemisphere tend to be more impulsive and aggressive. Clients who have sustained injury to the left hemisphere may be lethargic and unmotivated. However, clients must be assessed individually and plans of care based on the subjective and objective data present.

Confusional states and delirium may be the result of either the stroke itself or from the hospitalization. Frequently these clients suffer from transitional confusion, meaning they become oriented to one setting and then are transferred to another causing a temporary confusional state or delirium. This problem can be exaggerated in the elderly client. However, the home care nurse must also focus attention on potential medications that may cause confusion. In addition, the nurse needs to assess the client for infectious states, dehydration, and electrolyte imbalance. Remember, the elderly client may not present the same signs and symptoms as the younger adult.

The first step in the management of the client presenting with confusion or delirium is to quickly ascertain the cause. Once established, the home care nurse should avoid the use of physical and chemical restraints. Often the use of physical restraints will cause greater confusion. Use of chemical restrains should be reserved for extreme cases.

There are helpful hints for the home care nurse and for others caring for the client. The client benefits from frequent reorientation, which can be frustrating to the caregivers. In addition, the nurse instructs the family to surround the client with as many familiar items as possible, such as photographs of the family and favorite mementos. Constant dialogue must occur between the home care nurse, client, family, and primary care provider for continuity of caregiving efforts.

Research has demonstrated that stoke clients suffer more depression than other individuals with comparable disabilities. In the past it has been postulated that clients who suffered right-sided strokes demonstrated more euphoric states rather than depressive states. Left hemispheric strokes tended to render the client with catastrophic, depressive responses. More recent research notes that both depression and anxiety states do occur in stoke clients with either right or left hemisphere damage and that depression in the stroke client, if left untreated, may have a negative physiologic affect on recovery. Therefore, frequent assessment of the stroke client, with early recognition of the signs and symptoms of depression, is essential. Use of antidepressants has been proven to be effective in some situations.

Positive attitudes among all those individuals caring for the post-stroke client is important to successful rehabilitation. Many clients will ask "how long will it take before my leg works or my arm works?" Or a family member may ask "How long will he be so aggressive?" The client and family needs to be informed and educated to the fact that stroke recovery varies from client to client. In general, recovery peaks at 6 months but that constant and slow recovery can still occur. An additional helpful recommendation is for the family and or the caregiver to enroll in a support group specifically for post-stroke clients, family members, and interested others. The family can call the National Stroke Association (303-771-1700) or the American Heart Association (1-800-544-3248) for the closest stroke support group.

Management of Mobility Issues

Post-stroke survivors may not be able to move an entire side of their body. They may be completely dependent on someone to meet every need, including toileting, grooming, eating, dressing or simply ambulating from one room to another. These are the challenges that post-stroke clients face on a daily basis. In addition, clients with cerebral injury associated with impaired physical mobility may not be cognitively aware of their disabilities or the prescribed treatment for maintenance, prevention, and restoration of functional loss. Goals for the elderly client with impaired physical immobility that the home care nurse can intervene with include proper positioning, range of motion exercises, balancing and sitting, transfer activities, and ambulation.

Proper positioning of the post-stroke elderly client can sometimes be a challenge. Close attention must be made to frequent assessment of skin, especially if the client has been provided with any brace or artificial fixation device (see Chapter 12). Physical therapy will provide a schedule for the amount of hours the device should remain on and off. The home care nurse should review this schedule with the client and or significant other. The home care nurse needs to assess for any skin breakdown, irritation, or swelling. If any of the above are noted, it is recommended that the home care nurse consult with the physical therapist for further adjustment.

When the client with hemiplegia sits in a chair, care should be taken to support the affected upper extremity. Care should be taken as to not allow the client's arm to hang down. If the client's limb is allowed to hang down, a subluxation may occur. The client's arm should be elevated on a pillow so that both shoulders are equal. To assess for shoulder subluxation, the nurse places a finger between the head of the humerus bone and shoulder. No more than one digit should fit in between the joint. It is also recommended that frequent passive range of motion exercise is performed at least every 2–3 h. Once again these activities can be taught to family members or other caregivers. Close attention must be given to the hand of the affected limb. Frequently, the hand becomes contracted and curls, making hygiene close to impossible. It is recommended that a soft round ball, such as a tennis ball, be placed in the hand.

Foot drop is also a common complication of immobility. To ensure proper positioning it is recommended that the client wear either a high top sneaker when out of the bed or an artificial fixation device, which is placed in the client's shoe. When the client is in bed, a boot immobilizer may be worn to maintain the foot in proper alignment. A boot immobilizer can be purchased in any surgical supply store.

When positioning the post-stroke elderly client in bed, great care must be taken to have the client assume as much of a neutral position as possible. Positioning a client on their stomach or back is less desirable. When prone, safety can be an issue. When supine, pressure is placed on the sacrum, a frequent place for skin breakdown. Positioning off the spine is preferred. The client's back may be supported with pillows or even a blanket that is rolled up into a log. In general the shoulder and the hip should be completely aligned. The shoulder that the client is lying on should not be tucked underneath the client, but rather pulled out; this will align the shoulder with the hip. The arm should be placed on a pillow. The opposite arm can be placed to rest on the hip on an additional pillow. The leg that is on the bottom should be maintained slightly bent at the knee with the upper leg resting above it; a pillow should be placed between the legs to prevent pressure ulcers. Great care should be taken to prevent pressure on the heels. The heels must be positioned so they do not rest directly on the mattress.

The client should be turned and repositioned every 2 h while in bed. The bony prominences should be massaged and the skin inspected. Remember that egg-crate type of mattresses are only for comfort measures, not prevention of skin breakdown. The home care nurse should assess the client's need for a special mattress.

When transferring the elderly stroke client, the arms of the client should never be pulled upon. This too may lead to the development of subluxation of the shoulder joint.

When dealing with problems of immobility in the elderly client with a stroke, the home care nurse needs to develop open communication with the physical therapist. Many of these clients will be discharged with assistive devices with which the home care nurse will need to be familiar.

Swallowing Deficits

Swallowing deficits are common post-CVA. Two issues are of uppermost concern: client safety and nutrition. With an understanding of the swallowing process and its management, the home care nurse can assist with client and caregiver teaching. Refer to Chapters 4 and 6 for specific information.

Bladder Dysfunction and Retraining

Urinary incontinence problems in the elderly post-CVA client can be a devastating experience. Loss of dignity and self-esteem can interfere with rehabilitation. There are several methods of managing urinary drainage. Depending on the client's level of responsiveness (unconscious versus fully ambulatory), the various methods are indwelling catheters, intermittent catheterization, condom catheter for male clients, and bladder retraining programs. Refer to Chapter 11 for detailed information about each method. Principles used to determine the choice of urinary drainage method apply to all clients, regardless of the cause of bladder dysfunction.

HOME CARE OF THE CLIENT WITH SEIZURE DISORDERS

This section introduces the home care nurse to the care of clients with seizure disorders (epilepsy) and includes a definition and description, etiology, diagnosis, and pharmacologic and nursing management.

Definition and Description

Seizures and epilepsy are terminologies commonly used interchangeably. However, by definition, epilepsy is a chronic syndrome that is peculiar to cerebral tissue and is characterized by recurrent, paroxysmal episodes in which there is a disturbance in skeletal motor function, sensation, autonomic visceral function, behavior, or consciousness. Seizures are a symptom of central nervous system (CNS) irritation, with the dysfunction being produced by excessive and abnormal neuronal discharge. In general a diagnosis of epilepsy it is considered a lifelong condition, whereas seizures may be temporary occurrences during a period of CNS irritation in a person's life. For the purpose of this discussion the term *seizure disorders* is used when referring to either state.

The prevalence of seizure disorders increases with age. Approximately 1% of the general population suffers from seizures, whereas in those older than 65 years, 2% experience seizures. Therefore, seizures become a phenomenon more apt to be seen by the home care nurse who works with the elderly.

Etiology

The etiology of seizure disorders can be divided into four categories: cerebral, biochemical, posttraumatic, and idiopathic.

Cerebral lesions account for a large category of factors that may lead to seizure activity:

1. Birth injuries, whether pre-, post-, or antenatal can contribute to the development of cerebral lesions, placing the infant at risk for developing seizures. Injuries such as trauma, anoxia, perinatal jaundice, and antenatal factors can contribute to the development of cerebral lesions.
2. Infections such as meningitis, encephalitis, abscesses, or high fever from their inflammatory processes or exudate may lead to seizure activity.
3. Sustaining an ischemic stroke, subarachnoid hemorrhage, or hypertensive encephalopathy places a client at greater risk. Seizures may also be the presenting symptom of arteriovenous malformations.
4. Head trauma that leads to the development of subdural, epidural, or intracerebral hematoma increases the risk for the development of seizure activity. In addition, neurosurgical procedures, a type of planned trauma to the brain, also places the client at risk for seizures.
5. Both primary neoplasms of the brain and metastatic lesions to the brain place the client at risk for developing seizures. As with cerebral circulatory disturbances, the seizure activity may be the presenting symptoms of the brain tumor.

It is important for the home care nurse, when dealing with the client presenting with seizures, to rule out biochemical reasons for the seizure activity. Many biochemical disorders lead to the development of seizure activity. Alcohol ingestion, drug overdoses, and ingestion of inorganic substances can place an individual at high risk for seizures. In addition, many medications such as pentylenetrazol (Metrazol) can produce seizure activity. Electrolyte imbalances such as hyponatremia or hypoglycemia must also be ruled out when clients present with seizure activity.

Posttraumatic seizures result from previously sustained cerebral trauma. Examples of posttraumatic epilepsy include craniocerebral trauma, birth injuries, cerebral infections, and neurosurgical procedures. It is also important for the home care nurse to realize that seizure activity can occur any time after a head injury.

An idiopathic seizure has no identifiable cause. It is considered an acquired seizure disorder because the cause escapes current knowledge or diagnostic methods. The basis of the chronic seizures is probably a biochemical imbalance at the neurocellular level. Much research in this area is currently being conducted. It is important for the home care nurse to have a knowledge in the precipitating factors that can lead to an increase in seizures or be the trigger for seizures in the client who has been seizure free. Common triggers for seizures include fatigue, hypoglycemia, lack of sleep, emotional stress, electrical shock, and febrile illness. Alcohol consumption, excessive intake of water, excessive constipation, menstruation, and hyperventilation may also lead to increase in seizure activity.

Diagnosis

The diagnosis of seizure disorder begins with a complete and detailed history. Included in this history is the individual's birth history, family history (maternal history during pregnancy), growth and development, childhood illnesses, questions concerning recent head injury, and exposure to chemicals. Next, a complete physical and neurological examination is performed to detect any neurological deficits. Blood work includes a complete blood count; blood chemistries, such as fasting serum glucose, calcium, potassium, blood urea nitrogen, and electrolytes; and liver function studies. A complete urinalysis is performed as well. The client will have an electroencephalogram, computed tomography (CT) scan, or magnetic resonance imaging (MRI) of the brain performed. If an infectious processes is suspected, the client may undergo a lumbar puncture. Examinations such as cerebral angiography may be performed if an arteriovenous malformation is suspected. Any or all of these tests need to be explained to the client and family members and often they are performed on an outpatient basis and instruction becomes the responsibility of the home care nurse.

Pharmacologic Management

The goal of pharmacologic management is to prevent further seizure activity and prevent side effects of the medications used. When at all possible, monotherapy is the main goal. Many antiseizure medications render the client chronically tired, feeling confused, and in some cases even changes the physical appearance of the individual. Choice of medication is dependent on the type of seizure activity the individual experiences and not the client's age, so most drugs used are familiar to the nurse regardless of the setting in which he or she works. For this reason the drugs are reviewed just briefly here. For more detailed information refer to Chapter 8.

Antiepileptic Agents

Phenytoin (Dilantin) is the primary drug of choice in the treatment of tonic–clonic seizures, focal motor, and focal sensory seizures. The dosage varies by age and weight and can be given in divided doses or one single dose using capsules, tables, a suspension, or in sprinkle form. The therapeutic serum concentration range is 10–20 μg/ml and while a client is being titrated to the correct dosage the home care nurse may be drawing blood samples monthly. Once the correct dose is established, the client may follow a 3- to 6-month treatment schedule. Dilantin can be toxic, producing behaviors that impair client safety. In some forms, Dilantin potency is affected by food consumption or other medications. Likewise, there can be severe drug interactions with some drugs. SAFETY NOTE: If the home care nurse is unfamiliar with Dilantin (or any medication), using a nurse's drug guide or a current edition of the *Physician's Desk Reference* (PDR) is recommended.

Carbamazepine (Tegretol) is an alternative agent used in the treatment of tonic–clonic, focal, and complex partial seizures. The medication is available in tablets and extended-release formulation; there is no elixir or suspension. The therapeutic serum concentration range is 4–12 μg/ml. As with phenytoin, this drug has toxic neurologic and system effects and has significant drug interactions. A serious rash can occur with carbamazepine, known as Steven Johnson's syndrome. It is an exfoliative-type rash that carries a 10% mortality rate and therefore must be reported to the primary care provider immediately. Clients with this type of rash are admitted to a burn unit.

Felbamate (Felbatol) is the first new antiepileptic drug to be approved by the U.S.Food and Drug Administration in 10 years. It received final FDA approval in 1993. The indications for use of felbamate is primary monotherapy and adjunctive therapy for intractable complex partial and secondary generalized tonic–clonic seizures. The drug is available in tablets only and begins with 1,200 mg in divided doses, increasing to 2,400–3,600 mg in divided doses every week, using increments of

600–1,200 mg. In 1994, mortality from fatal aplastic anemia and hepatotoxicity caused the drug to be restricted to severely intractable seizures. An informed signed consent is required by all clients receiving this drug. The client must have a complete blood count and liver function test monthly, which may be done by the home care nurse if the client is homebound. Any decrease in the complete blood count must be reported immediately to the primary care provider.

Gabapentin (Neurontin) was approved for use in 1993. It is indicated for adjunctive therapy in partial seizures, with and without secondary generalized tonic–clonic seizures. Dosage requires t.i.d. dosing, beginning with 300 mg t.i.d., which can be increased to 2400 mg per day. Originally, gabapentin came in a hard-to-swallow caplet, which has been replaced by a tablet. Weight gain is a significant side effect that should be discussed with the client and family and not be confused with edema associated with urinary or cardiovascular dysfunction. There is no need for routine laboratory monitoring. Antacids may decrease absorption, and drowsiness is the major adverse reaction.

Nursing Management

Nursing assessment of the client experiencing seizures is essential. Common questions that should be asked when the client does experience a seizure are the following:

1. Were there any warning signs or was there an aura?
2. Where did the seizure begin and how did it proceed?
3. What type of movement was noted and what parts of the body were involved?
4. Were there any changes in the size of the pupils or conjugate gaze position? (If the home care nurse witnesses seizure, assess for these changes.)
5. Was there any urinary or bowel incontinence?
6. What was the duration of the entire attack?
7. Was the client unconscious throughout the attack?
8. What was the behavior of the client after the attack?

These pieces of information provide a picture of the type of seizure the client experienced. When shared with the primary care provider, the correct medication choice and dosage can be prescribed. The information also gives the nurse direction to family teaching possibilities. How the caregivers react to the seizure activity provides the nurse with additional data useful when teaching. As with all clients who experience seizures, safety is most important. If an elderly client experiences a seizure in an unsafe place, the trauma to extremities or the head may cause life-threatening injury.

Education of the client with a seizure disorder can be an exhausting task. Many of these clients have experienced seizure activity for many years and have suffered the social stigmas of epilepsy, which may contribute to reluctance to discuss their disorder. Many of the antiseizure medications leave the clients feeling confused, tired, and unable to concentrate. These side effects lead to a high degree of pharmacologic mismanagement that may have caregivers mistakenly label the client as "noncompliant."

Better seizure management comes when a trusting relationship is developed between the client and caregivers, both volunteer and professional. It is vital that the client feel comfortable discussing side effects and the impact they have on ADLs.

Because seizure disorders are better understood and managed today, the younger home health nurse may not be as fully aware of the stigma people with epilepsy have lived with during their lives. Epilepsy is a chronic disease that often demonstrates itself at an early age, which (still) causes social outcasting. Many of the individuals have faced social isolation, career disappointments, and social restrictions including making marriage illegal, driving restrictions, and at times physical disfigurement.

The Epilepsy Society of America is an excellent resource for professionals, clients, and family members. They have local chapters in most communities with books, pamphlets, videos, professional speakers, and a variety of support groups for clients, family members, and for children and teens. The national headquarters can help locate local resources:

Epilepsy Foundation of America
4351 Garden City Drive
Landover, MD 20785
Telephone 1-800-332-4050

SUMMARY

Care of the elderly client after a stroke or with the diagnosis of a seizure disorder can be both challenging and rewarding for the home care nurse.

Assessment of the client's neurological functioning provides a baseline of information essential to the various caregiving roles of the nurse in the home.

Communication and a little bit of creativity can make a tremendous difference in the quality of life for the neurologically impaired client. Prior to the neurological insult, the client might have been totally independent and is now requiring assistance for the most minor tasks. Neurological changes affect the client and his or her spouse or family members and can be a devastating, even catastrophic event. These individuals require much encouragement to regain as much functioning as possible and for some to be able to successfully manage a medication regimen that has significant side effects. The teaching role of the home care nurse cannot be overemphasized when working with neurologically impaired clients.

REFERENCE

Canadian Cooperative Study Group. (1978). A randomized trial of aspirin and sulfinpyrazone in treated stroke. *The New England Journal of Medicine, 299,* 53–57.

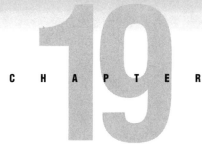

C H A P T E R

CARING FOR THE ELDERLY PSYCHIATRIC CLIENT

Mark D. Bienstock
Flora R. Bienstock

◆ ◆ ◆

Establishing a Therapeutic Relationship
Obtaining and Evaluating Medical and Psychiatric Histories
Psychiatric Diagnoses and Symptoms Common to the Elderly
Defense Mechanisms and Adaptive Behaviors
Recognizing Signs of Psychiatric Decompensation
Principles of Home Care Psychiatric Management
Family Members as Allies
Service Coordination
Summary

Mental illness does not discriminate. It knows no racial, ethnic, religious, age, or economic boundaries and no group is exempt from the devastating effects. Very few people can honestly say that they have not known, or been touched in some way, by someone suffering from mental illness. Perhaps it was a relative or a friend or a business associate who acted strangely, or withdrew from their social environment or tried to injure themselves. The ravaging effects that their illness has on them and those close to them, often leave people alienated, withdrawn, and feeling hopeless.

Many elderly, in particular, suffer from isolation, depression, hopelessness, and helplessness. When coupled with physical ailments, getting through each day feels unmanageable. The ability to perform even the simplest task appears daunting.

For the home care nurse to care successfully for the elderly psychiatric client, it is important to possess a knowledge and understanding of mental illness disorders, be able to recognize symptoms, be able to differentiate between physically and emotionally based problems, and be able to form a therapeutic relationship with the client.

ESTABLISHING A THERAPEUTIC RELATIONSHIP

It is extremely important for the nurse to feel comfortable caring for and treating the elderly psychiatric client. Similarly, it is critical that the client feel comfortable with the nurse. Success in providing care is in part determined by the quality of the therapeutic relationship that is established between the home care nurse and the client.

Home care nurses care for clients with a variety of diagnoses. If a nurse feels that he or she will look negatively upon an elderly client with a mental illness and make that client feel stigmatized, then the nurse must explore the nature of these feelings and work to overcome them before accepting the particular assignment. If the assignment is causing the nurse to feel fearful or uncomfortable, resulting in the provision of substandard care, the case should be assigned to a nurse who has more positive attitudes and experience in managing such clients. In addition, nurses with these feelings would benefit from inservice training, guided experiences with clients with psychiatric diagnoses, and any other appropriate agency support to be able to care for all clients who need service.

Physical illnesses such as heart disease and cancer usually evoke compassion. Mental illness, however, is often believed to be within the person's control and the inability to function is viewed as malingering. Additionally, individuals with mental illness usually evoke distrust and apprehension, rather than empathy and compassion. As a caregiver, it is easy to become preoccupied with concerns such as how "crazy" the client is, whether the nurse is likely to be hurt, or whether the client can be trusted. Being educated about mental illness will help home care nurses to understand what the person is struggling with, help them to feel comfortable providing treatment, and will help them to establish a therapeutic working relationship.

Years ago, before there were excellent psychotropic and mood modifying drugs, persons with the mental illness were excluded from the mainstream of society, often in large state institutions, socially isolating and ostracizing them. Older clients with psychiatric diagnoses may have lived through these years of overt prejudice and be suffering from these previous, often less than humane ways of being treated. Older home health nurses may have some of these stereotypical beliefs as well.

Many clients with mental illness are ashamed of their illness and some of them may deny it. As a result, they may refuse treatment. Some clients may experience secondary gain by using their mental illness to get sympathy or other intangible benefits, such as an excuse to depend on others or avoid socializing or taking on responsibilities. However, their psychiatric problems are nonetheless very real, as is the pain that they feel.

Most of the elderly population with mental illness are not dangerous or harmful to others. They have symptoms that are painful and debilitating; however, the symptoms are most often manifested inward toward the individual, such as depression, and not as physical assaults upon others. Although there are exceptions, clients with mental illness are more likely to be fearful and relatively passive, rather than aggressive and hostile toward others. They respond favorably to attention and kindness from others who have a genuine interest in helping them. By sharing their fears and concerns with someone else, they are able to feel less isolated and helpless. They will generally respond favorably to inquiries concerning their health, both physical and emotional, and will appreciate interest from caregivers. They can be encouraged to talk about their symptoms, thereby providing the nurse with the information needed to asses the client's problems. They are hurting inside and want to be helped.

Home care nurses may encounter clients who are hostile and do not want them in their home. The nurse must explain the reason for the visit and try to engage the client in a discussion regarding one topic at a time. By keeping the visit focused and relatively short it will help to not overwhelm the client. If these approaches do not work (i.e., the client's hostility does not abate or escalates), it may be advisable for the nurse to leave and try to engage the client later in the day or on another day. Frequently the client will be more receptive at a different time.

OBTAINING AND EVALUATING MEDICAL AND PSYCHIATRIC HISTORIES

An important prerequisite to providing good care is to obtain a complete history of the client's prior medical and psychiatric problems and previous responses to treatment. Knowledge of the client's experiences, both positive and negative, provides insights into which interventions are more likely to have desired results, and which could lead to undesired outcomes.

Historical information can come from a number of sources. The information that is included in referral documents should indicate any psychiatric and physical health problems. In addition, to the extent possible, the client can provide historical information. The nurse should ask the client about symptoms and what he or she thinks is wrong. The client may not identify mental health problems directly, however they may be brought to light through information provided by family members, other primary care professionals, or through the nurse's observations.

Family members and close friends can provide a great deal of historical information regarding the client, and therefore can be of assistance. This information can be especially important with older clients who, in addition to a history of psychiatric illness, may have age-related health problems that accentuate forgetfulness or memory problems. It is critically important that the home care nurse first obtain the client's permission prior to speaking to anyone regarding the client's health status. If the client is willing to sign a consent form for release of information, the nurse should also contact the client's medical and psychiatric caregivers to obtain firsthand information regarding current and prior problems.

If the client has recently been discharged from a hospital or other treatment facility, review the discharge instructions provided to the client to see if the client is adhering to them. Determine whether the client is complying with any medication or follow-up treatment instructions they were given. If the client is not complying, it may be by choice or simply because he or she did not understand the instructions. Another possible reason may be that what is expected of the client is too unwieldy, either due to physical or psychiatric limitations. It is important to assist the client so that he or she is able to comply with the prescribed treatment regimen. For example, if the client is easily confused, possibly as a result of a thinking disorder, and is not able to take medications reliably, set up a system to help get the client organized. Establishing a system of boxes, color-coded for time of day and labeled for the days of the week might help the person know when to take specific medications. The home health nurse may need to pre-pour medications or obtain the assistance of a family member when setting up such a system.

Evaluate the client's symptoms to determine whether new problems have emerged that need to be addressed by medical and/or psychiatric professionals. If indicated, assist the client in accessing such consultations. Additionally, it is important to monitor the client's progress to identify changes, both positive and negative, that may relate to prior treatment and signal the need for further assessment or intervention.

Prior histories provide useful information, specifically:

1. The client's previous symptoms and medical/psychiatric problems are helpful in order to become familiar with his or her needs. Additionally, reviewing previous treatment outcomes (either by speaking to previous primary care providers or by reviewing whatever written information is obtainable), assists the nurse in knowing which interventions were successful and which should be avoided.

2. A pattern of abusing medication, either purposeful or inadvertent, is helpful information. Such abuses can include taking more medication than is prescribed, taking medications at the incorrect times or in incorrect combinations, missing doses, or not taking prescribed medications at all. It is not uncommon for clients to stop taking medications because they are feeling better and no longer see the need for them. Some may put the pill in their mouth in the presence of others, "cheek" it, and remove it when others are not looking. Other clients may see more than one primary care provider for different complaints and receive medication from each provider without the others' knowledge. Still other clients may horde their medications and take them in incorrect amounts or incorrect combination. Each of these types of situations can be serious and must be addressed immediately with the client.

3. Negative reactions to prior medications or treatment modalities, in particular, serious reactions to medications must be revealed. Allergies, side effects, or otherwise undesired results related to a specific medication should be noted to ensure that the offending medication is avoided. If the nurse notes that such medication or treatment modality has been prescribed, the prescribing practitioner should be alerted immediately.

4. The client has a history of failing to adhere to treatment recommendations. This problem may relate to treatment resistance on the part of the client or be a result of the client's inability to comply. Perhaps the client did not have access to suitable transportation or was overwhelmed by the demands placed upon him or her. It is often hard for elderly people to cope with the burden of medical or psychiatric illnesses. Adding the demands of

coordinating treatment appointments can result in mistakes or even inertia.

5. Information about past incidences of violent behavior is significant, but does not necessarily mean that the client will act in such a manner now. Treatment interventions may have already addressed the underlying precipitants to aggression and the home care nurse may only need to assess for signs of decompensation that may lead to the onset of renewed violent behaviors. In the event these behaviors are observed and it is believed that the client is beginning to act in an aggressive manner, immediately alert the primary care provider or psychiatrist who has been providing psychiatric follow-up.

6. A past history of suicide attempts constitutes essential information. Prior suicide attempts should be taken seriously and may indicate an increased risk of future attempts.

A thorough knowledge of the client's medical and psychiatric history provides invaluable information. It allows the nurse to be sensitive to the individual's needs and helps to establish a strong caregiving relationship with the person.

Underlying Physical Conditions

When faced with a client who is exhibiting psychiatric symptoms, it is critical that the home care nurse consider whether the symptoms are caused by an emotional problem or an underlying physical complication or illness. Many medical problems can manifest in ways that mimic mental illness symptoms and elderly clients may have other diagnoses. Untreated diabetes, for example, can result in psychosis. Additionally, some people can have a negative reaction to the medication they are taking. It is possible that the medication that has been prescribed to address a physical problem can cause hallucinations, disorganized thinking, paranoia, anxiety, hostility, or incoherent speech, as well as numerous other symptoms or combinations of such symptoms. This issue highlights the need to obtain a thorough medical and psychiatric history. The information will be especially helpful to the nurse in determining whether a change in the client's mental status is related to a deterioration in the person's psychiatric condition or related to a reaction to a change in medication or the onset or exacerbation of a physical illness.

If a client exhibits one or more psychiatric symptoms that had not been previously evaluated, refer the client to his or her primary care provider for evaluation. Some of the symptoms to consider include: hallucinations, slurred or incoherent speech, disorganized thinking, depression, disturbances of sleep, inability to concentrate, acute anxiety, unwarranted hostility, or aggressive acts. This list is not exhaustive and the nurse should report any unusual changes in the client to the primary care provider. This point cannot be stressed enough. Many symptoms, even those that appear relatively benign, can actually be a manifestation of an underlying physical condition. Often such conditions can pose serious health consequences or even be life threatening.

PSYCHIATRIC DIAGNOSES AND SYMPTOMS COMMON TO THE ELDERLY

Whereas it would not be practical to discuss all the various emotional disorders found in the general population, it is important to identify the diagnoses that are prevalent in the elderly population and provide basic information regarding each. By being able to recognize the signs and symptoms associated with these maladies, and how they impact upon the person, the home care nurse is able to understand the needs of the elderly client and what actions to take to best meet those needs.

Although there are exceptions, most elderly people with a mental illness disorder are not aggressive and hostile toward others. They are generally rather passive and fearful. Whereas many will act in a bizarre manner, perhaps talk to themselves, speak incoherently or irrationally, dress oddly, or exhibit unusual behaviors or body movements, these behaviors most often do not result in hostile acts. Most such clients feel awkward around people and have difficulty in social and interpersonal interactions as a result. Many are more fearful around others, than others are around them.

The following information may help to promote a greater comfort level for the nurse so that unnecessary fear will not interfere with the treatment process.

Depressive Disorders

The most prevalent mental illness among the elderly is depression. There are several forms of depression. Depression in elders is associated with withdrawal, listlessness, confusion, loss of appetite, disturbed sleep, irritability, loss of interest or pleasure in the usual activities, feelings of worthlessness, memory loss, confusion, or suicidal attempts or thinking. In some cases, hallucinations may be involved. Clinical depression is not just feeling bad some of the time. It is a bad feeling that just will not go away. It does not improve over a short period of time and generally does not improve merely because a person's circumstances have changed. Depression interferes with the way the person feels, thinks, and behaves. Depressed people cannot concentrate and cannot enjoy normal pleasures. They have a poor self-image, sleep poorly or too much, and feel sad and empty. There is a constant feeling of hopelessness.

Depression is the most common, although most often unrecognized of all mental illnesses. Some forms of depression such as major depression and bipolar disorders (e.g., manic depression) have been known to run in families and therefore are believed to be genetically predetermined. Other theories relate to a biologic etiology caused by hormonal or biochemical disruptions. Still other theories relate to a psychosocial etiology. Although it is unclear why, the prevalence of depression is higher among women than men.

Regardless of the cause, depression can be treated and many of the symptoms alleviated. It has been estimated that approximately 80% of those afflicted with depression can be helped with the proper medications, counseling, and psychotherapy. Unfortunately, many do not receive the help they need and languish in their own chasm of despair. Understandably, it is difficult for those steeped in depression to understand what they are experiencing, and therefore do not realize the need to ask for help. Others have difficulty asking for help because they are too embarrassed. Some feel they are responsible for their own situation, still others do not realize that help is available. Often, depression is unrecognized by the sufferer and by those they come in contact with. Depression is often viewed as a physical problem, such as, tiredness, headaches, and so on. Conversely, serious physical problems are sometimes incorrectly presumed to be depression. The home care nurse should be especially careful to rule out physical maladies, such as stroke, cancer, hormonal imbalances, infections, and so on. Misguided interventions could have serious effects upon the person's health, or even pose life-threatening consequences.

When treating persons with depression, it is important to encourage them to access proper professional interventions such as pharmacotherapy and psychotherapy. Depression must be taken seriously, as the elderly commit suicide at a higher rate than any other age group (approximately 20% of the suicides occur among the elderly population, which makes up 12% of the population). Suicidal clients should be assessed and worked with as various treatment options are available. If a person appears to be in imminent risk of self-harm and refuses to take appropriate steps to obtain help, the nurse should call the person's family if feasible, and emergency medical personnel immediately. Each home health agency has specific protocols identifying appropriate emergency interventions. Never leave the client's home until emergency personnel have arrived.

Dementia

Dementia is an impairment in short- and long-term memory associated with problems in abstract thinking, problems with judgment, other disturbances of brain function, and changes in personality. Dementia is often severe enough to interfere with the person's ability to perform routine activities of daily living and can prevent the person from functioning independently.

Symptoms associated with dementia include memory impairment, anxiety, unwarranted suspiciousness, depression, difficulty with abstract thinking, poor judgment, and brain function disturbances such as the ability to speak effectively, recognize people or objects, perform basic motor tasks, and the inability to engage in the usual social activities. Delusions are common, especially involving a belief of persecution, for example, believing misplaced belongings have been stolen.

All cases of dementia have a physical cause, such as blood vessel disease or small strokes in the brain causing vascular dementia, brain infections, AIDS, metabolic disturbances, neurological diseases, lack of oxygen to the brain, persisting effects of substance use (including toxin exposure), or a buildup of pressure in the brain. Alzheimer's disease (AD), the most common dementia, is believed to be caused by changes in the structure of the brain that may develop as a result of genetics, a chemical imbalance, or viral infection.

Although dementia can begin at any age depending on the etiology, most often the onset is late in life. According to present studies, it is estimated that 5% of the population over the age of 65 have AD, with other dementia types being much less common. The prevalence of dementia increases with age, especially after age 75 and the prevalence rate for AD increases to 50% in people over age 85.

Although there is no cure for vascular dementia or AD, with proper assessment and medical intervention, many of the symptoms can be treated and managed. Medications are available that can reduce anxiety, agitation, depression, impulsive behavior, and sleep disturbances. The degree of success will depend on a confluence of factors, particularly the degree and etiology of underlying pathology, the timeliness of treatment, and the specific treatment provided. The degree of the impairment will depend on the severity of the individual's cognitive deficiencies and the availability of treatment and supports. In advanced stages of dementia the individual may be totally dependent on others and require constant supervision. Such individuals are susceptible to accidents and infectious diseases, either of which could be fatal.

Anxiety Disorders

As with the depressive disorders and dementia, there are several types of anxiety disorders. A brief summary of some of the more prevalent features will be discussed as they relate to the elderly population.

Anxiety disorders may include panic attacks, agoraphobia (anxiety about being in a place from which escape may be difficult or embarrassing), phobias, obsessions or compulsions, and generalized anxiety. At various times (e.g., during a panic attack), anxiety disorders may manifest with a number of somatic symptoms, including palpitations, accelerated heart rate, sweating, trembling, shortness of breath, dizziness or feeling faint, chest pain or discomfort, and so on. The specific causes vary considerably. They may relate to a specific phobia, be posttraumatic, or be due to a general medical condition. Examples of general medical conditions that can cause an anxiety disorder include hyperthyroidism, hyperparathyroidism, pheochromocytoma, vestibular dysfunctions, seizure disorders, and cardiac conditions.

Although it is difficult to establish a direct cause and effect link between an anxiety disorder and general medical condition, laboratory tests can be instrumental in establishing the presence of a medical condition and may help primary care providers formulate the proper treatment plan. Anxiety symptoms may cause significant distress or impairment of social, occupational, or interpersonal functioning. In the event the client reports or otherwise exhibits symptoms that appear to indicate either the onset or exacerbation of an anxiety disorder, it is important that the nurse reports this information to the client's primary care provider and psychiatrist. Many anxiety disorders can be treated effectively with the proper combination of medication and therapy.

In the event the client has an anxiety disorder, it is important to reassure him or her that the nurse is there to help. The client needs to be referred to the primary care provider or psychiatrist for evaluation. Once a treatment regimen has been specified, the client needs to be assisted to follow up with the recommendations. Family members may be helpful in providing additional support and reassurance to the client.

DEFENSE MECHANISMS AND ADAPTIVE BEHAVIORS

Many of the problems and events, such as the death of a spouse, deteriorating health, loss of independence, and so on, that are often associated with advancing age can give rise to the adoption of a number of defense mechanisms that the caregiver should be aware of when providing services. It is important to keep in mind that it is not always easy to identify the relationship between specific behaviors and their emotional basis. The home care nurse may encounter one or more defense mechanisms during the course of providing services. Understanding why these behaviors develop may help alleviate possible frustration that nurses experience as they can at times impede the ability to provide care. Some common defense mechanisms include the following:

Denial. This mechanism is often used to deny the occurrence of a specific event or events, or the possibility of something happening, such as the serious illness of loved ones and the possibility of their dying. Clients might deny their own illness, which could result in their refusing to comply with treatment. They may not allow the nurse into their home and therefore refuse necessary care. In this event, the nurse should notify the nursing supervisor and the client's primary care provider. If the client's refusal to accept treatment poses serious health risks, then a determination must be made regarding the necessary interventions that must be initiated on the person's behalf. If indicated, law enforcement and emergency medical personnel may have to be contacted to render involuntary care.

Regression. Although regression can be subtle and not impede the nurse's ability to provide care, some clients may exhibit pronounced regression and behave in a childlike manner. Sometimes the person appears helpless, easily overwhelmed, and incapable of executing even the simplest of tasks. The person avoids accepting responsibility and routinely looks to others to help them. It is important to assess which tasks the client can realistically be expected to accomplish with regard to his or her own care, that is, attend to personal hygiene needs, comply with medical or psychiatric treatment recommendations, schedule treatment appointments, and so on. The home care nurse should encourage clients to accept tasks that they are capable of, rather than allowing them to become immobilized and completely dependent upon others. A good way to approach this problem is to work with the client on one task at a time, providing guidance, support, and encouragement. This approach will help ease the client back into accepting responsibility for fulfilling some of his or her own needs, without feeling overwhelmed. Each new accomplishment will bring a sense of confidence and pride. Whereas in the beginning, improvement will likely move at a slow pace and be frustrating, ultimately the rewards can be gratifying. It is important that the nurse does not overestimate the client's abilities, as this mistake could lead to unrealistic expectations and further regression.

Selective Memory. The client may have difficulty remembering specific events or information. As discussed earlier, memory loss can be as a result of dementia; however, for some clients, memory can be affected by specific traumatic events or other painful associations. In some cases, remote memories of times when the client was younger, perhaps in better health or more independent and active, are likely to be more pleasurable. As a result, the client may tend to block out recent events or information. Recent information is likely to relate to failing health, loss of loved ones, loss of social supports, and so on. As a result they have a painful association and are therefore forgotten by the client in order to maintain a better sense of self.

The client's tendency to not remember important information related to physical care needs could have serious impact on his or her well being and the nurse's ability to provide care. It is important that the nurse recognize this problem quickly so that it can be promptly addressed. If the client would rather not face aspects of life as a defense mechanism, it may not be advisable nor necessary for the nurse to attempt to prompt a change. What is important is that the client is helped to recognize those aspects of treatment that require attention and action. The nurse may be able to help organize the client so that important items are addressed in a timely manner. Perhaps helping the client to write down a schedule of tasks that must be completed over a specified period of time will help him or her become organized without directly addressing the underlying causes of the selective memory.

Exclusion of Stimuli. This relates to a person blocking out stimuli that are distressing or painful. For example, a person refusing to hear something that would be distressing. Clients may refuse to hear or acknowledge the degree of their illness or the specific treatment recommendations that relate to their illness. As a result, they may refuse treatment because they do not understand why they would need such care, not follow up on medical appointments, or not allow the nurse into their homes for the same reason. The manifestation of this type of problem varies greatly and requires evaluation. The refusal of necessary care has to be addressed according to the severity of the situation. If the client is refusing to allow caregivers into the home, perhaps family members can help explain to the client why care is necessary.

Secondary Gain. This behavior is characterized by the person deriving a benefit that is secondary to the action or inaction being engaged in. For example, it is not uncommon for people to try to prolong medical or psychiatric treatment because it provides the person with an increased level of attention and companionship.

The home care nurse may experience a client who insists on continuing to receive specific home care services, even though there is no clinical basis. Some clients may even manifest an exacerbation of symptoms to demonstrate the need to continue to receive care. This may be a subconscious attempt to continue the secondary gain they are receiving. The symptoms, however, are real and should be taken seriously. One possible way to deal with this dilemma is to try to replace the method by which the client derives the secondary gain with a more acceptable one. For example, if the client is fearful of losing companionship once home care services are reduced or discontinued, perhaps assisting the person to join a local community support organization will help. The organization may be able to provide a volunteer to go to the person's home on a regular basis to provide support and companionship.

Rigid Personality. Generally, people will not develop this trait late in life; however, if a person has been rigid, their rigidity may increase as a defense against a general sense of threat or in response to actual crisis.

The home care nurse may notice a sense of rigidity in one or more of the clients served. This behavior will usually not impede the ability to serve the client, unless the level of rigidity is pronounced and affects the person's ability to comply with treatment recommendations. Often this can be ameliorated by talking to the client in a patient and supportive manner, explaining the benefits of compliance and of taking proactive steps to help themselves.

Regardless of the adaptive behavior or group of adaptive behaviors the client may be engaging in, it is important that the nurse keep in mind that the client's actions or inaction is meant to insulate the client from emotional pain. The client is not reacting to the nurse's personally and not trying to make things difficult. Rather he or she is operating from a desire to maintain a sense of homeostasis and avoidance of that which he or she believes to be painful. Patience and the ability to communicate a sincere desire to help the client will most often determine the degree of success nurses have in providing services.

RECOGNIZING SIGNS OF PSYCHIATRIC DECOMPENSATION

From time to time a home care nurse may notice a negative change in a client's behavior. Such changes may relate to a deterioration of the client's mental status and require careful consideration. It is important to be able to identify signs of psychiatric decompensation, because unless addressed, this can seriously affect the person's ability to function and may lead to hospitalization. Some of the more common changes that should be assessed for include aggressive actions or verbalizations, hallucinations, suicidal or homicidal thoughts or acts, acute paranoia, acute disturbances of sleep, marked and prolonged changes in mood, disturbances of thought, and so on. Although it is important to not overreact, a marked decrease in functioning, or self-injurious or otherwise dangerous actions or threats must be appropriately addressed. If possible the nurse should explore any concerns with the client to try to determine the severity of the problem. Additionally, the information proves helpful when the matter is referred to other caregivers for assessment or treatment.

As part of the assessment of the situation, clients are asked if they have experienced any significant changes that they are concerned about, or if any significant event has happened recently. It is possible that something in particular is precipitating a significant increase in stress and is causing the deterioration. Although the client may not be able to make the connection, the nurse's discussion may provide some insight. If the nurse is able to identify one or more new or increased stressors, he or she may be able to help the client find ways to ameliorate or cope with the problems.

Another possibility is that the client is not taking psychotropic medication(s) properly, or is having a negative reaction to the medication, as previously discussed.

Regardless of the precipitant(s), prompt and appropriate attention to a change in symptoms can often make the difference between the person being able to remain at home or requiring placement in a hospital or other facility.

PRINCIPLES OF HOME CARE PSYCHIATRIC MANAGEMENT

1. Establish a relationship with the client. The ability to "connect" with a client and establish a strong relationship determines the degree of success that the home care nurse has in helping a client. This task is not as simple as it may seem. Many elderly requiring home care, and who have emotional illness, have difficulty with interpersonal relationships. Initially the client may not be receptive to the nurse. However, if the nurse visits on a consistent basis, most clients over time will probably let down their barriers. (In the new managed care environment, numbers of visits may be limited, so the time for relationship development may be shorter than in the past.) For some, a long history of disappointment has left them resistant to establishing trusting relationships. As they see positive results from the nurse's involvement, they will likely seek further help.

2. Foster a sense of self-control and independence. One of the unfortunate results of advancing age is the loss of independence many older adults experience. Increased physical ailments coupled with mental illness can lead to a significant decrease in independent functioning, which can be depressing, and in turn, negatively impacts on the person's ability to function. This can lead to a downward spiral from which it may be difficult to recover. The nurse's ability to capitalize on the person's strengths and encourage an undertaking of even the most basic tasks to promote a feeling of accomplishment, can prove extremely beneficial. As the person completes these tasks he or she will feel more capable, therefore building self-esteem and nurturing independence. This feeling helps improve the person's outlook and reduce feelings of hopelessness and helplessness.

3. Foster a sense of hope and optimism. A hopeful and optimistic outlook is essential for the maintenance of a healthy mind. To the extent that the nurse promotes a positive attitude, he or she contributes to the client's progress. If possible, point out to clients things that they can look forward to. If their health has improved, or they report that they are feeling better, the nurse can take a moment to tell them how pleased he or she is with their progress. If possible, accentuate possible future gains that they should look forward to.

4. Communicate a sense of caring. Many sick people feel that they are a burden on others and feel self-conscious about being dependent on them. This outlook can add to their feelings of worthlessness and despair. Many do not ask for assistance or do not accept offers of help because of this very reason. Communicating a genuine sense of caring and a desire to be of help will serve to ease the client's mind.

5. Respect the client's boundaries. It is important to be sensitive to a client's emotional and physical boundaries. A person who is already feeling vulnerable and not in control of important aspects of his or her own life, for example, health, will likely feel greatly compromised should the nurse venture into areas that the client feels are personal or off limits. Additionally, the client may not feel comfortable telling the nurse how he or she feels, perhaps fearing that the nurse will be angered and discontinue visiting. When asking personal questions, explain the reason for the inquiry, and how the information assists efforts to help the client. Similarly, nurses should keep in mind they are guests in the client's home and they need to ensure that their movement within the client's home is not felt to be intrusive. Also provide assurances to the client that all information will be kept confidential and that family members, neighbors, and others will not be provided with information without the client's consent.

6. Listen, listen, listen. Carefully listening to the client can accomplish more than just the obvious. Of course the nurse hears what the client has to say, however, the nurse often picks up more subtle, yet important information. Frequently, for a variety of reasons, people do not express themselves clearly, leaving a great deal for the nurse to interpret in order to effectively understand their needs. The attentiveness also conveys the nurse's interest in the client and will foster acceptance of the nurse.

7. Involve the client in the solution. The interventions will of course be directly related to the recommendations of the client's primary care provider; however, to the extent the nurse can involve clients in the process of addressing their own needs, the more they are likely to "buy into" the treatment process, and the greater their compliance is likely to be.

8. Effectively communicate the nurse's role in the client's treatment. To avoid confusion, faulty expectations, disappointment, and possibly anger on the part of the client, it is critical that the nurse clearly conveys to clients what services will be provided to them. Clients should know what they can expect from the home health agency and the nurse in particular and how the nurse's role relates to their other care providers.

9. Establish discharge criteria with the client. As early as possible, and preferably during the first home visit, the nurse should establish discharge criteria jointly with the client. This practice provides clear expectations for both the nurse and the client of what must be accomplished prior to discharge. Ongoing discussions should evaluate progress in reaching goals.

10. Be consistent. It is important to be as consistent as possible in all interactions with the client. Inconsistency can contribute to confusion and disorganization, as well as anxiety and apprehension. Often, these are issues that the psychiatric client already needs help with. Adding to the problem by missing appointments, coming late, not following through on commitments, and so on is counter-therapeutic and inconsiderate. It may be helpful to mark down appointments on a calendar for the client. Showing clients how to maintain such a calendar for all of their appointments and important dates to remember may prove to be extremely beneficial.

FAMILY MEMBERS AS ALLIES

Understandably, members of the client's family can be a source of great support for the client. Often family members are in the best position to know the client's special needs and how to address them. Additionally, relatives will generally be readily accepted and trusted by the client. The nurse should let clients decide whether they would like a family member to be present during initial visits.

Family members can also assist the nurse in a number of ways. They can be of help when a client is refusing treatment. The client may not yet accept nursing services or may not fully understand why the services are necessary. A trusted family member may have success in explaining these matters and gain the client's acceptance. In the event the nurse has difficulty understanding the client, a family member, who has obviously known the client a lot longer, may be able to convey the client's communication to the nurse more effectively. Family members can be particularly helpful in providing the nurse with relevant historical information regarding the client's prior illnesses and treatments.

On occasion, the nurse may encounter one or more family members who are not helpful, are negative, and in extreme cases, interfere with the client's treatment. In some cases, family members may consistently sabotage all treatment plans, possibly because they want to maintain the client in the current state. It may be hard to understand the motivation for this kind of behavior; however, the nurse will have to be careful to address the needs of the client while not offending the client's family. Sometimes, family members can be reacting to negative experiences that they, or the client had with previous caregivers. Another possibility is that they do not understand the nature of services provided or the reason for them. Sometimes the person poses opposition for no apparent reason. Regardless, the challenge is to work with the person as well as possible. The nurse's ability to establish a positive relationship with the family will help them to work through their negativism and attend to the client.

As the population ages and a growing number of people need care, the role of families as caregivers and care managers increases. Working closely with family members serves to ensure appropriate, coordinated, and quality care.

SERVICE COORDINATION

Coordinated home care can ensure follow up with medical and psychiatric appointments, optimize the client's ability to function, and prevent recidivism.

1. Home Health Aides: If the client has the need for visits by a home health aide the nurse should speak with the aide to determine whether he or she understand the needs of the client and

whether he or she has encountered any difficulties. The home health aide needs to understand the client's plan of care. When indicated, the nurse participates in training the aide in how to provide specific aspects of care. It is important to consider whether the aide has had training or experience in working with clients who have serious emotional illnesses. If not, the aide may not be adequately prepared to deal with the array of problems and issues that can arise. Depending on the specific nature of the client's psychiatric problems and the level of preparedness of the aide, a problem may or may not develop. In most cases, aides will be effective in appropriately providing services to clients with psychiatric illnesses. If, however, it becomes apparent that the aide is experiencing difficulty, either because the aide shares this with the nurse individually or during a case conference, as a result of something the nurse observes, or the client relates something to the nurse, the nurse should discuss the issue with the aide to see what assistance is needed. If this discussion is either not advisable for some reason, or does not remedy the situation, discussion of the matter with appropriate staff members may initiate placement of a different home health aide.

2. Mental Healthcare Workers and Programs: A client who is experiencing serious mental illness symptoms will usually be receiving services from either a mental healthcare private practitioner or an outpatient mental health program such as a clinic, partial hospital, or day treatment program. Psychiatric home care services may be provided by the home health agency. In this case nurses within the agency need to coordinate care if more than one nurse is visiting the client. Depending on the client's illness, he or she may be receiving a combination of services, likely to include medication therapy, psychotherapy, and possibly socialization and rehabilitation services. If the person is not able to leave home due to a physical disability, he or she will probably be receiving in-home care for the psychiatric illness while homebound. If a home care nurse believes that a client is experiencing new or increased psychiatric symptoms, the mental health professional should be notified immediately of the change. By doing so, the nurse may help avert an exacerbation of the problem and assist in obtaining appropriate and timely care.

3. Community Service Organizations: Many local community service organizations offer a wide range of services to the elderly. Some provide volunteers to go to the homebound and provide

companionship, assistance with shopping, and so on. If a client is not currently receiving such services and the nurse believes the client could benefit from them, the nurse assists in accessing the services. Family members may also be helpful in enrolling the client.

4. Other Medical Care Providers: Depending on the client's physical illness(s), he or she may be receiving in-home care from a number of providers in other fields, such as, physical therapy, podiatry, neurology, and so on. As touched upon previously, a person with a mental illness generally has difficulty dealing with stressors. Although the care delivered by the various providers is important and is appreciated by the client, it is possible that the client may not be able to handle the various aspects of coordination and needs assistance. Although it is not necessarily the nurse's responsibility to coordinate the various aspects of the client's care (unless the nurse is the case manager), cooperation in this process will be important. Once again a calendar may be helpful to the client in keeping track of the many appointments that may be scheduled over the coming weeks or months. The nurse may suggest to the client that the services should be spaced out. For example, only one home visit per day.

5. Family Members: The importance of family members as allies in the overall care of the client has already been explored above. However, the critical role that relatives play in the treatment process and the significance that they often have in the recovery of their loved ones must be underscored. The clinical significance that the love and support family members play cannot be overestimated.

6. Friends and Neighbors: Many clients have the support of neighbors and friends who have known them for a long time and are willing to help them. They can be particularly helpful by visiting the client during meal times to assist, or just to keep the client company. They can also assist by reminding the client to take medication at the required times. Remember to obtain the client's approval prior to talking to friends or neighbors.

SUMMARY

Caring for the elderly psychiatric client can be a wonderfully rewarding experience. The presence of mental illness may add an unfamiliar dimension to the demands of providing treatment. However, the home care nurse's ability to attend to both the physical and emotional needs of clients will be an important factor in their stabilization and recovery.

Establishing a therapeutic relationship is the foundation to the successful home management of elderly psychiatric clients. Understanding psychiatric diagnoses and related symptoms provides the home care nurse with information necessary for beginning caregiving. Nevertheless, many elderly clients have underlying medical problems along with the psychiatric diagnosis and signs and symptoms of these diagnoses may overlap and must be recognized and separated. In addition to established diagnoses, clients may display defense mechanisms and adaptive behaviors that have helped them cope over the years. These must also be recognized and dealt with effectively by home care personnel. At times, stress in a client's life may precipitate a psychiatric decompensation. Recognizing signs of decompensation may be critical to the life of the client and is an important part of the home care nurse's assessment.

Finally, the home care nurse must collaborate with a bevy of other caregivers, family members, and friends. It is important for caregiving to be coordinated and not to become overwhelming to the client. The home care nurse may function in the role of case manager and can help to reduce unnecessary stress by coordinating various visits by professionals and suggest the best ways friends and family members can be of assistance to the client.

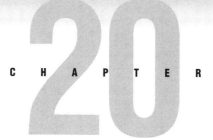

CARING FOR THE ELDERLY CLIENT WITH CANCER

Bettina Bentley Willis

◆ ◆ ◆

This chapter is dedicated to my mother, Mrs. Alice Bentley, who died from lung cancer on August 25, 1997. I hope that our personal experience of living with cancer in the home will benefit other elderly clients.

The diagnosis of cancer is devastating and frightening at any age, but it is even more so for an elderly person. The physical changes that have developed over the years of life often tax both the body and spirit of the aged. The elderly frequently endure decreased mobility, bone and joint pain, lessened muscle tone and flexibility, changes in skin elasticity, loss of memory, and decreased sensations, especially hearing and sight. Some clients may have other chronic illnesses, such as arthritis, diabetes, heart disease, or peripheral vascular disease.

This chapter provides the home care nurse with an update of the latest information about diagnosing cancer, tests ordered, treatment options, and anticipated side effects. This information is essential when working with the elderly cancer client at home. Cancer diagnosing and treatment frequently occurs on an outpatient basis and the home care nurse needs to prepare the client and family for upcoming testing or treatment. The technology of cancer care is always changing and keeping current is key to providing high-quality care.

The healthcare professional who cares in the home for the elderly client with cancer accepts the challenge of combining the skills of both oncology and geriatric nursing in what is often the most comfortable setting for the client and his or her family. This chapter addresses many aspects of that challenge. It can be very rewarding for the nurse prepared to handle the many aspects of the cancer experience.

THE IMPACT OF THE DIAGNOSIS: CANCER

Cancer is not one disease, but consists of several entities. It is unique because whereas cancer may affect different parts of the body (e.g., lung, colon, rectum, brain, blood, and blood-forming organs), it alters the entire existence of the client/family system. Changes in the roles and relationships among family members, disruption of the routine of daily living, additional financial burdens, and the heartache of having a seriously ill family member in the home, comprise extreme stress on the client/family system. Fortunately, the diagnosis of cancer does not carry the stigma of "death sentence" that it did years ago. Many clients not only survive the chronicity of cancer with today's better technology, they possess a full quality life. Yet from diagnosis through treatment and long-term survival to the possibility of recurrence and terminal illness, cancer causes fear and havoc for the whole client/family system.

Family members are considered the primary caregivers in the home setting. For elderly clients, this may be a spouse (who may also be experiencing a chronic medical condition), adult children (who may be elderly and dealing with chronic illnesses of their own), or some other close relative. Family members, primary care providers, nurses, home health aides, and other healthcare workers are part of the multidisciplinary team required to deliver quality care to the client with cancer. Although it is true that the major responsibility in the home lies with the primary caregiver, the home care nurse has the opportunity to offer the guidance and support that is so intensely needed.

ROLE OF THE HOME CARE NURSE

It does not matter at what stage of the continuum of the cancer experience the home healthcare professional enters into the life of the client, it must be remembered that both client and family are suffering throughout the course of this illness. The role of the healthcare professional in the home setting is to assist the client and family in achieving their goal of an optimum quality of life. To accomplish that goal, the strategies and interventions necessary are many. The nurse must use the steps of the nursing process while delivering professional care and provide accurate information to the client and family that dispels fears, myths, and misconceptions. The role includes:

- Assessing any physical changes or side effects, reporting them to the primary care provider, and assisting in their management.
- Monitoring and evaluating interventions, modifying them as needed.
- Providing client/family education throughout the course of the illness.
- Assisting the client and family by making referrals and helping them to access appropriate resources within the community.
- Being an advocate for decision making by the client.

It is important to remember that the elderly client and family system frequently fear loss of control. The nurse, by teaching and encouraging as much self-care as possible, assists in alleviating this fear.

It is absolutely essential that the initial assessment be both comprehensive and thorough when caring for the elderly client with cancer in the home. Many of the effects noted in the elderly may be caused by varying conditions, related or not to the diagnosis of cancer. It is essential to establish initial baseline data to effectively monitor any changes during the course of home care. Several nursing interventions assist in caring for a variety of potential side effects and prevent progression to toxicities or worsening conditions.

THE EXPERIENCE OF CANCER

Diagnosis

The diagnosis of cancer conjures up many different images for both clients and their families. Misconceptions and fears, as well as well-meaning, but misguided and incorrect advice from relatives, friends, and acquaintances suddenly become abundant. Any previous experience with cancer, or even hearsay, looms large in the minds of these clients and their families.

Once the diagnosis has been made, the client may undergo a myriad of tests, hospitalizations, visits to the primary care provider, and trips to the hospital or other institutions for treatments. Biopsies, blood tests, x rays, computerized axial tomography (CAT scans), sonograms, magnetic resonance imaging (MRI), and other procedures become a part of life. They aid in identifying the type and site of cancer, the extent of the disease, and assist in planning the most effective treatment. All too often the client and the family do not understand the necessity of the various examinations and procedures. The home care nurse assists by providing repeated explanations as needed, and assessing the client for possible complications from various procedures.

Blood Work

The home care nurse should be familiar with the normal values of various blood tests in order to identify problems early and interpret the need for the test to the client and family. The bone marrow is the site of hematopoiesis, or blood cell production. The stem cells that are formed in the bone marrow mature into leukocytes (white blood cells), erythrocytes (red blood cells), and thrombocytes (platelets). Leukocytes combat infection by engulfing bacteria (phagocytosis), lysing viruses (cellular lysis), and removing debris. Erythrocytes carry hemoglobin, which transports oxygen and carbon dioxide, and platelets assist in clot formation to prevent bleeding. Normal values to be familiar with are:

Leukocytes 5,000–10,000/mm^3
Erythrocytes 450,000–500,000/mm^3

Thrombocytes (platelets) 150,000–300,000/mm³
Hemoglobin 12–16 gm/dL (female)
                14–18 gm/dL (male)
Hematocrit 38–46 gm/dL (female)
             42–54 gm/dL (male)

Chemotherapy and radiation cause cytotoxic effects on the bone marrow, decreasing its function of cell production (bone marrow depression or myelosuppression). Leukopenia (low white blood cell count), anemia (indicated by low red blood cell count, low hemoglobin, and low hematocrit), and thrombocytopenia (low number of platelets) pose a serious threat to the cancer patient. When all blood cell counts are low simultaneously, the condition is called pancytopenia. Neutrophils comprise 55–60% of white blood cells. Neutropenia, or the decrease in neutrophils, is a dose-limiting factor in cancer treatment. Blood counts are lowest 7–14 days after chemotherapy administration. This period is called the nadir. Most of the antineoplastic drugs are myelosuppressive and subsequently cause neutropenia. Many clients have to be admitted to the hospital during the nadir because of sepsis related to neutropenia.

If the white blood cell (WBC) count falls below 3,000/mm³, cancer treatment may be held or postponed because the client is at high risk of developing an infection. Elderly clients are particularly at risk because of the physiologic changes related to decreased immunity during the aging process. Some elderly clients may normally have a low WBC count or low hemoglobin level. Blood tests are taken at frequent intervals throughout the course of cancer treatment to determine its effects on the bone marrow and avoid the risk of infection for the client. Supportive interventions may include transfusions of blood components, postponement of chemotherapy, or the administration of colony-stimulating factors, which enhance the growth and release of blood cells from the bone marrow.

Other blood tests may also be ordered, and the home care nurse should be familiar with all normal values. Keeping such information available for immediate recall is an impractical expectation for most nurses. It is recommended that the home care nurse keep available a medical dictionary, a nurses' drug book, and a table of laboratory values on all home visits (e.g., keep in the trunk of the car) to refer to as needed. The nurse can be instrumental in identifying problems early, explaining the need for frequent tests to the client or family, and offering them reassurance should supportive measures be required.

Imaging

Diagnostic imaging tests provide important information by visualizing organs and tissues, including both normal and abnormal structures, for the primary care provider to interpret. Many of these procedures are repeated frequently throughout the course of the client's illness. Elderly clients and their families may fear the terms they hear and proposed tests that they do not understand. By explaining the terminology, reasons for these tests, and what to expect, the home care nurse offers the support and reassurance needed.

Ultrasonography

Ultrasound utilizes high frequency sound waves to provide images of internal structures. The test begins by a technician placing a gel on the skin over the area of the client's body to be viewed. A probe is passed over the skin, and the image is viewed on a screen. The procedure is painless and noninvasive.

CAT Scan

CAT scans (also known as CT scans) involve repeated passage of narrow x-ray beams through cross-sections of targeted body tissue and organs. The computer records tissue density and generates a three-dimensional image on a screen. Performance of the scan requires that the client be positioned, motionless, on a radiographic table for approximately 1 h. The procedure is painless and noninvasive; however, older clients with claustrophobia or those who experience pain and discomfort remaining in a fixed position for a lengthy period of time may need sedation for this procedure.

MRI

MRI is another technique frequently used to identify tumor sites or determine the effectiveness of cancer treatment. MRI utilizes electromagnets and radiofrequency signals to provide sharper images of tissues and organs for primary care providers to interpret. The client lies on a moving table that slides into a tubular machine. The MRI machine generates noises that some clients find disturbing and again clients are confined and must remain immobile for a period of time. This procedure is noninvasive and does not involve the emission of x rays.

An oral or intravenous radioactive contrast dye may be administered to clients undergoing some of these procedures to define the vascularity in the area. Care is taken to establish whether clients are hypersensitive to the contrast material prior to the scan. Hypersensitive clients may experience hypotension or hypertension, pruritus, dyspnea, diaphoresis, and possibly anaphylactic shock.

Biopsy

Clients may need to undergo the surgical excision of tissue at some point during their illness to determine or confirm diagnosis or follow the effectiveness of prior treatment. The home care nurse includes the assessment and monitoring of any biopsy sites in the client's care plan and follows up with appropriate documentation and reporting.

COMMON TYPES OF CANCER FOUND IN ELDERLY CLIENTS

The most common types of cancer found in the older population include colorectal, prostate, lung, and breast. Older women are also at risk for gynecological cancers: cervical, vaginal, vulvar, uterine, and ovarian cancers. Skin cancer is the most common form of cancer and is very common among the elderly, but is the most treatable and curable form of cancer. Both clients and healthcare professionals tend to attribute the signs and symptoms of early cancer to normal aging processes. Therefore, often the disease is in an advanced stage by the time it is diagnosed. Metastases to bone, liver, and brain are common by the time the tumor is found in many elderly clients.

Colorectal Cancer

Elderly clients experience a variety of alterations in the functioning and elimination patterns of the intestinal tract due to the aging process. A high fat, low fiber diet has long been associated with the development of cancers in the bowel. Conditions such as polyposis, diverticulosis, and inflammatory bowel diseases are considered to predispose the colon to malignant changes. The decreased activity and subsequent elimination patterns in the elderly are frequently ignored for years. Healthcare professionals are aware of the importance that the elderly often place upon their daily evacuation and the fact that use of laxatives is high among older persons. Symptoms such as changes in the consistency of fecal matter, diarrhea, severe constipation, and fecal incontinence are handled by clients with over-the-counter drugs for years prior to seeking medical assistance. Treatment for colorectal cancer may involve surgery, chemotherapy, radiation, or a combination of treatments.

Prostate Cancer

A similar scenario exists with this male malignancy. Elderly men are frequently diagnosed with a condition known as benign prostatic hypertrophy (BPH), due to changes in the prostate caused by age. Symptoms (post-void dribbling, weak stream, urinary frequency or hesitancy, nocturia) of prostate problems are often not considered serious until the client is truly hindered psychologically or socially by their effects. Some men may avoid seeking medical advice because they realize that the screening method for prostate cancer involves a digital rectal examination. Again, the combination of what may be viewed as normal aging effects and the barriers to seeking medical assistance may cause elderly men to live with an untreated detrimental condition longer than they have to.

Prostate cancer, the most common cancer in American men, can now be diagnosed early through the use of a blood test, the prostate-specific antigen (PSA). PSA becomes elevated in prostate disorders; a level of more than 10 ng/ml may indicate a malignancy. Treatment for prostatic cancer may involve radical prostatectomy, radiotherapy, bilateral orchiectomy, hormonal therapy, or chemotherapy.

The older male client undergoing treatment for prostate cancer needs education, support, and advocacy from the home care nurse. Because of the nature of the surgery or other treatment, sexual functioning may be altered. These changes must be discussed and feelings about them must be allowed to be vented. The home care nurse's client advocacy role is important to access follow-up care. Counseling, psychotherapy, or a penile implant are alternative treatment methods designed to restore the client's ability to have sex or enhance the client's sense of well being.

Lung Cancer

Respiratory changes due to age include decreased muscle tone, loss of elasticity of alveoli, decreased chest cavity volume due to degenerative bone changes (e.g., osteoporosis), and muscle atrophy. The elderly have higher incidences of respiratory disorders such as chronic bronchitis and emphysema. Years of exposure to smoking or second-hand smoke, pollution, and exposure to environmental substances such as asbestos add to the high risk of lung cancer among the elderly. Symptoms such as hoarseness, cough, progressive shortness of breath, chest pain, weight loss, fatigue, and difficulty swallowing are attributed to normal physiological aging changes and are frequently ignored. Thus, unfortunately, lung cancer is often diagnosed in advanced stages in the elderly. If warranted, the client may be a candidate for a lung resection or lobectomy. However, if the disease has metastasized this may not be the best treatment. Other forms of treatment, including chemotherapy and radiation, become the treatment choices.

Breast Cancer

Breast cancer is one of the leading causes of cancer deaths among women today. Women who have not established a pattern of monthly self breast examination (SBE) or following a recommended pattern of mammography after the age of 40 have lost the benefits of these important screening tools. Thus, many elderly clients may be diagnosed with breast cancer late in the progress of the disease and undergo a lumpectomy or mastectomy with less than ideal prognostic expectations. These women require a careful combination of medical, physical, and emotional support.

TREATMENT OPTIONS

Surgery, chemotherapy, radiation therapy, and hormonal therapy represent the main modalities of cancer treatment. Other treatments include biotherapy, bone marrow transplantation, or immunotherapy. The goal of treatment may be cure, control, or palliation of the disease. Modalities may be combined to offer the client the most effective treatment for the disease. To fully assess, monitor, evaluate, and support the elderly client with cancer, the home care nurse needs to possess knowledge about these treatment modalities, their potential side effects, and how to manage them.

Surgery

By the time the home care nurse meets a new client with cancer, that client may have undergone some type of surgery or surgical procedure. Examples include lobectomy for lung tumors, lumpectomy or mastectomy for breast tumors, colostomy or ileostomy for colorectal tumors, cystectomy for bladder tumors, exploratory laparotomy and hysterectomy or pelvic exoneration for female reproductive organ cancers, and tumor debulk-ing prior to chemotherapy or radiation. Other surgical procedures might include thoracentesis to relieve pleural effusion, chest tube drainage, paracentesis to relieve abdominal ascites, placement of an indwelling ve-nous access device for administration of parenteral nutrition or chemo-therapy, or placement of gastric feeding tubes.

The home care nurse needs to manage the wound care and teach the client and family how to manage ostomies or surgical wounds and the various equipment used to treat cancer clients at home. Fluid and elec-trolyte balance must be maintained. Meticulous care in handling the equipment and supplies related to surgical wounds or surgically placed devices is an essential part of cancer care. As always, using universal pre-cautions is paramount in preventing infection and possibly saving lives.

Chemotherapy

Chemotherapeutic agents (also called antineoplastic drugs) are prescribed medications taken by clients with cancer to fight the tumor cells. Where-as these drugs may be administered by various routes (oral, intravenous, intramuscular, subcutaneous, intrathecal, topical), the most common routes for clients at home are intravenously or orally. The client may be receiving chemotherapy at home or may make daily trips to the hospital or clinic for its administration. Careful attention must be given to specific side effects that might be seen frequently or more acutely in the elderly.

Anticancer drugs interfere or damage cell function and cause cell death. Agents that affect cells while they are in the reproductive phase are considered cell cycle specific, while those that act upon cells re-gardless of cycle phase are called cell cycle-nonspecific agents. Cancer cells are characteristically more susceptible to the action imposed by the antineoplastic agents than normal cells. Chemotherapy regimens or pro-tocols may consist of a single agent or a combination of several drugs. Chemotherapy may be administered in special units at a hospital or in a primary care provider's office. It is important for the nurse to learn about each drug the client is receiving. Some of the more common antineo-plastic agents utilized are listed in Box 20-1 and are also discussed in Chapter 8.

Some chemotherapeutic agents cause specific toxicities that may be detrimental to elderly clients, and a few warrant special mention:

Bleomycin. This drug may cause pulmonary fibrosis in cumulative doses, further compromising the respiratory function of the elderly client.

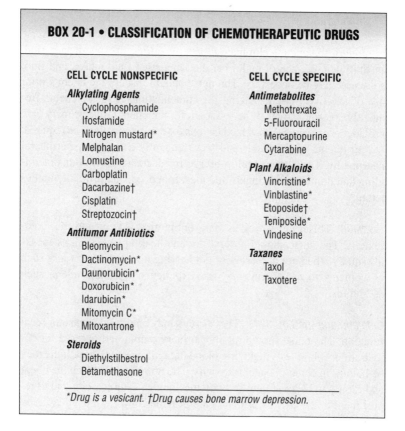

BOX 20-1 • CLASSIFICATION OF CHEMOTHERAPEUTIC DRUGS

CELL CYCLE NONSPECIFIC

Alkylating Agents
 Cyclophosphamide
 Ifosfamide
 Nitrogen mustard*
 Melphalan
 Lomustine
 Carboplatin
 Dacarbazine†
 Cisplatin
 Streptozocin†

Antitumor Antibiotics
 Bleomycin
 Dactinomycin*
 Daunorubicin*
 Doxorubicin*
 Idarubicin*
 Mitomycin C*
 Mitoxantrone

Steroids
 Diethylstilbestrol
 Betamethasone

CELL CYCLE SPECIFIC

Antimetabolites
 Methotrexate
 5-Fluorouracil
 Mercaptopurine
 Cytarabine

Plant Alkaloids
 Vincristine*
 Vinblastine*
 Etoposide†
 Teniposide*
 Vindesine

Taxanes
 Taxol
 Taxotere

Drug is a vesicant. †Drug causes bone marrow depression.

Observe client for respiratory changes such as cough and shortness of breath.

Doxorubicin and daunorubicin. These drugs are anthracyclines and may cause cardiac changes when associated with cumulative doses, resulting in cardiomyopathy or congestive heart failure. The nurse should monitor for irregular pulse and observe the client for signs of congestive heart failure (CHF) such as fatigue, dyspnea on exertion, cough, restlessness, weight gain, anorexia, orthopnea. Clients may experience fluid overload and edema, especially in their lower extremities. Using a tape measure to measure ankles and recording the measurements may be helpful in identifying fluid retention in a timely fashion. The client and family must be taught to report any signs of cardiac changes. Refer to Chapter 16 for information about cardiac changes in the elderly.

Vincristine and vinblastine. These drugs are vinca alkaloids and may cause constipation or peripheral neuropathy. It is important for the nurse to monitor the client's elimination patterns during the treatment period. Instituting a regimen of high fiber diet, increased fluid intake, and stool softeners may be necessary. The nurse should discuss the client's prior use of laxatives before making recommendations. Elderly clients frequently abuse laxatives. If necessary, refer the client to the primary care provider because prescribed medications for constipation may be required.

Erythema of the hands and feet frequently accompany peripheral neuropathy. The nurse should observe for decreased sensations or tingling and numbness in fingers and toes, foot drop, and difficulty ambulating.

Cisplatin. This drug, as well as many antibiotics, is known to cause ototoxicity. The nurse should observe for any hearing loss, such as speaking loudly when not necessary or not hearing higher-pitched tones such as women's voices. Clients may also experience hearing problems such as tinnitus.

Cisplatin and methotrexate. These drugs may cause a decrease in renal function. The nurse should monitor urinary output and observe for dehydration. Blood tests including blood urea nitrogen and creatinine may be helpful in detecting nephrotoxicity. The nurse should teach the client and family to become familiar with the signs of drug toxicity and to report them to the client's primary care provider.

It is not within the scope of this chapter to delineate ALL of the chemotherapeutic agents available today. Information regarding most of these drugs, their indications, dosages, routes of administration, and their specific side effects are readily available from several other sources. This chapter is meant as a general guide for the nursing management of elderly clients experiencing common side effects caused by many of the antineoplastic agents.

Radiation Therapies

Clients with cancer who are entrusted to home care may have completed their radiation therapy treatments. In other cases, the client may still be undergoing treatments. There are various methods of delivering radiation treatments including external radiation, radioactive intracavitary implants, and interstitial radioactive isotope implants.

External Radiation

The very word, radiation, is frightening to elderly clients and families. Understanding how radiation is delivered and what to expect may alleviate their fears. External radiation is given in a hospital or imaging center by linear accelerators or Cobalt machines. The client lies motionless on a radiographic table in a room alone, and the machine rotates around the client. The client is monitored by a technician via a TV monitor screen and intercom. Initial treatment and work up lasts 3–4 h, the follow-up treatments last for approximately 15 min. It may be necessary for treatments to be given at varying angles, and often supportive devices are utilized to assist the client to remain in one position. The treatment is noninvasive but positioning may be uncomfortable for some elderly clients. The course of external radiation treatment is usually daily 5 days per week for up to 6 weeks. Upon the completion of external radiation therapy, the client is expected to return for follow-up visits at varying intervals.

The home care nurse should monitor the client for the side effects of the treatment, some of which may last for weeks posttherapy. One of the most common side effects of radiation is generalized fatigue, which can be particularly disturbing to the elderly client. Inability to continue with the level of activity experienced prior to treatment can lead to anxiety and depression. Encourage the client to balance periods of rest and activity. Reinforce to both the client and family that fatigue after radiation is anticipated, and it will eventually subside. Encourage a high calorie, high protein diet, if not contraindicated. Meals should be of soft consistency or pureed to assist in swallowing if needed. Encourage oral intake of supplements that are commercially available or made at home. The home care nurse can teach the client or family how to season foods that are palatable while avoiding foods that are spicy.

Skin change is another potential side effect of radiation therapy. The older client's skin is already drier, less elastic, and more fragile than that of younger clients. Additionally, circulation in irradiated areas may be compromised and the healing process may be slower. Once radiation therapy is completed, the irradiated areas may demonstrate additional dryness, become darkened, or show signs of breakage. If dry and intact, cornstarch may be applied, or lotions or creams may provide comfort. Leave the area open to air, if possible. If the skin is broken, be sure to keep the area clean. Washing with normal saline before applying any dressing and using nonstick dressings (e.g., Telfa dressings or gel dressings like Vigilon) are usually most comfortable for the client. Several cleansers and gels for irradiated skin are available commercially. Check for any allergy or hypersensitivity before applying a new product to the skin. (Note: do not apply any soaps, creams, or lotions to the skin of clients still undergoing therapy, as this may interfere with the delivery of the radiation treatment.) Clients should be taught to avoid exposure to the sun during and after radiation treatments. Large-brimmed hats, clothes with long sleeves, and sunglasses are recommended. It is important to reiterate to clients and families that once the client who receives external radiation therapy in the hospital returns home, the radioactivity poses no threat to the persons close to the client. Clients may return to their normal activities as tolerated, including playing with the grandchildren.

Because this form of therapy occurs over several weeks, transportation for frequent treatments may be a problem. In general, transportation for elders is an area of concern and when a daily hospital or outpatient visit is required for several weeks, usual sources of transportation, such as family members, friends, or neighbors may become overburdened. The home care nurse can assist in helping the client and family develop a schedule that is agreeable for all involved or initiate services of the community's American Cancer Society or senior services. The home care agency's social worker or hospital's social worker can be of assistance. Sometimes suggestions coming from a neutral outsider to the family are more clearly made and more readily accepted.

Brachytherapy

Implants of radioactive material such as cesium, iodine, or phosphorus are often utilized in clients with breast, prostate, and thyroid cancers. Clients with breast cancer may receive implants during their hospitalization, and once the implants are removed prior to discharge, no radioactivity remains. It is essential, however, to monitor the site for swelling, skin changes, and possible infection, and to report any changes to the primary care provider. Male clients with prostate cancer may have radioactive implants that will remain within the site. The amount of radioactivity is minimal, but special precautions may be indicated. It is imperative for the home care nurse to communicate with the radiation oncologist. Which source has been implanted, what is the half-life of the source, how is the radioactivity metabolized, eliminated, or absorbed, and what precautions are required are crucial questions. Client education must be a large component of the nurse's visit, because there will be some restrictions while the radiation source is in place.

Bone Marrow Transplantation

Bone marrow transplantation (BMT) is actually a supportive measure rather than a modality of treatment itself. Clients who require extremely high doses of chemotherapy or radiation to eradicate their disease may be eligible for BMT. There are two types of BMT: allogeneic and autologous. Allogenic BMT means the bone marrow comes from a donor who is cancer free.

In the autologous BMT the client receives his or her own bone marrow. High doses of chemotherapy are administered that completely destroy the cells in the bone marrow. Unfortunately, both normal and malignant cells are affected. Once the bone marrow is "purged," samples are removed and stored. The client is allowed a rest period, during which tumor cells may reappear. The high dose chemotherapy is repeated, hopefully destroying the malignant cells again, and the purged bone marrow is reimplanted (rescued). The goal of therapy is cure. Clients having undergone a BMT require frequent follow-up visits. Once the BMT client is well enough to remain at home, the side effects to be monitored may be more severe, but are similar to those experienced by clients undergoing conventional chemotherapy regimens or radiation.

Hormonal Therapy

Hormones such as androgens, estrogens, and corticosteroids are frequently used in the treatment of cancer. Drugs such as diethylstilbestrol and flutamide may cause gynecomastia, nausea and vomiting, hot flashes, decreased sexual drive, and impotence in male clients being treated for prostate cancer. Female clients with breast cancer may be treated with Tamoxifen, used primarily in postmenopausal women. Side effects include nausea, hot flashes, fluid retention, and swelling of extremities. Corticosteroids such as dexamethasone are frequently prescribed to reduce the side effects of nausea and vomiting, but cause fluid retention, weight gain, and mood changes. Steroids frequently cause diabetes and some clients have to start on insulin.

The side effects caused by hormonal therapy may be extremely disturbing to the elderly client. It is important to remind the client and family that these side effects will subside once the therapy is completed or the drug is discontinued. Elderly clients who find the side effects distressing may be tempted to discontinue the drugs on their own. They must be encouraged and supported throughout this type of therapy and the

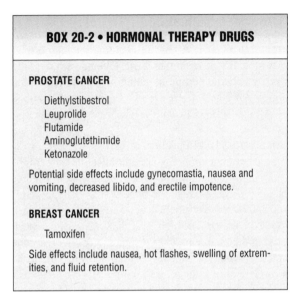

> ## BOX 20-2 • HORMONAL THERAPY DRUGS
>
> **PROSTATE CANCER**
>
> Diethylstibestrol
> Leuprolide
> Flutamide
> Aminoglutethimide
> Ketonazole
>
> Potential side effects include gynecomastia, nausea and vomiting, decreased libido, and erectile impotence.
>
> **BREAST CANCER**
>
> Tamoxifen
>
> Side effects include nausea, hot flashes, swelling of extremities, and fluid retention.

nurse should know which drugs the client is taking and their potential side effects (see Box 20-2).

Biotherapy or Immunotherapy

Biological response modifiers (BRMs) are used to incorporate the assistance of the client's own immune system in battling the disease. Techniques of therapy utilizing substances such as interferon, interleukin, monoclonal antibodies, and cytokines aid in the destruction of malignant cells by the body's own defense mechanisms. Clients receiving this type of therapy may experience flulike side effects, among others. The nurse should maintain close communication with the client's primary care provider to learn which type of BRM the client is receiving and its potential side effects.

In the absence of acute complications, many elderly clients successfully live in remission from their disease. The client and family live with the threat and fear of potential recurrence of disease, and may require psychological support during this period. Support groups, organizations like the American Cancer Society, National Cancer Survivorship, and others provide information, support, and counseling. The home care nurse must be aware of the availability of community resources, and make referrals as needed.

HOME MANAGEMENT OF CANCER THERAPY SIDE EFFECTS

The modalities of cancer treatment, especially chemotherapy and radiation, may induce various side effects. Some of the potential side effects may seem just as injurious as the disease itself to the elderly client experiencing them. Assessment, planning, subsequent interventions, and reevaluation and modification as required, are the earmarks of the home care nurse's role. Clients may experience fatigue, pain, nausea and vomiting (often resulting in decreased food intake), weight loss, anorexia, alterations in taste, cachexia, diarrhea and/or constipation, stomatitis, pruritus, or alopecia. It is easy to appreciate that the entire persona of the individual is affected.

Bone Marrow Depression

Bone marrow depression, also known as myelosuppression, is one of the most common side effects of cancer treatment. It occurs when the antineoplastic agents or radiation therapy cause the marrow stem cells to be destroyed or damaged. As mentioned earlier, bone marrow depression may involve leukopenia, anemia, and thrombocytopenia. Periodic blood tests are required to determine whether treatment may be continued, decreased, or delayed. Thus, it is imperative that clients keep follow-up visits to get blood tests. Blood tests may be also taken by the home care nurse or clinical laboratory technicians in the home. In either case, the nurse should be aware of results in order to provide care. Leukopenia places the client at high risk for infection, erythocytopenia places the client at high risk for anemia, and thrombocytopenia may induce bleeding.

Fevers and Infections

Elderly clients may have a normal temperature slightly higher or lower than 98.6°F. To accurately assess any changes, it is crucial that the nurse's initial assessment include the determination of the client's normal baseline temperature. An elevation of 2° above the client's normal temperature should be considered problematic. During the nadir period, *any* increase in the temperature should be reported to the primary care provider, as this may be a sign of infection.

A variety of factors may cause elevated temperatures in the client with cancer. Fever in the elderly client with cancer may prove more detrimental than in younger persons. Interventions for potential infection should be initiated immediately.

A slight rise in temperature may be a common side effect of certain cancer treatments (chemotherapy or radiation). Tumor growth may cause an increase in temperature in specific neoplasms (malignant growths). Febrile reactions may occur posttransfusion of blood products. Certain medications are affiliated with increased temperatures (e.g., Amphotericin). The nurse should become familiar with all of the potential causes in the individual client, but institute the care plan for infection.

Cancer treatments cause the client's WBC to decrease, impairing the body's ability to fight off bacterial, fungal, and viral infections. The primary care provider may order periodic blood tests including WBC, red blood count (RBC), thrombocyte count (platelets), hemoglobin, and hematocrit. The home care nurse should monitor blood test results for changes, especially the WBC. Whereas an increased WBC may indicate an infection, it is important to remember that clients undergoing chemotherapy or radiation may actually have a decreased WBC (leukopenia). Neutropenia, which is the decrease in a specific type of WBC (neutrophils), is particularly threatening to clients with cancer. The nurse's assessment must encompass a systematic inspection of all potential sites for infection (see Box 20-3). Any increase in temperature or a sore throat are early signs to report to the primary care provider.

The primary care provider should be notified when there is an initial change in temperature, when an elevated temperature persists for more than 24 h, or when an infection is suspected. The home care nurse should instruct the client and family to maintain a daily record of the client's temperature. Rectal thermometers should always be avoided due to risks of infection or bleeding. There is a potential for perforation of the intestinal wall lining, which may cause bleeding in clients with low platelet counts. The digital otoscan thermometers are highly recommended for families to use. The client and family should be taught to observe for the signs and symptoms that might indicate a fever or infection:

Increase in oto/oral/axillary temperature.
Change in skin temperature (e.g., warm or clammy).
Any swelling, pain, or erythema (redness).
Chills.
Increased malaise or fatigue.
Painful, decreased, frequent, or urgent urination.
Complaints of headaches, muscle aches.
Restlessness or confusion.

BOX 20-3 • CLINICAL ASSESSMENT WHEN INFECTION IS SUSPECTED

Monitor blood tests, especially CBC and differential.

SKIN (ALL SKIN-FOLDS)

Breasts	Groin	Pressure points (occipital, shoulders,
Axilla	Perianal	elbows, heels, sacrum)

ORIFICES

Mouth	Nose	Urethra	Rectum
Ears	Throat	Vagina	

Assess for erythema, edema, swelling, rashes, pain, and white patches.

PROCEDURAL SITES

Biopsy	Fingersticks
Bone marrow aspiration	Catheter entrance and exit ports
Venipuncture	

SYSTEMS

Respiratory
  Auscultate lungs for decreased sounds.
  Determine breathing pattern, rate.
  Note cough or change in cough
  Note sputum production, color, and consistency.
Gastrointestinal
  Poor appetite
Genitourinary
  Determine changes such as frequency, hesitancy, painful urination, decreased output.
Neurologic
  Monitor for anxiety, restlessness headache, listlessness, generalized fatigue.

Advise the client's family to notify the home care nurse or primary care provider when the client exhibits any of the above signs or symptoms. It is important that the cause of the rise in temperature be determined. Self-treatment (for example, administering Tylenol, etc.) and home remedies should be discouraged, unless prescribed by the primary care provider. At times this is difficult to accomplish because elders may have a long history of self-medicating, using over-the-counter and folk remedies. Nevertheless, the home care nurse should be aware of the client's self-care practices and intervene when they are in conflict with the current medical regimen. Antibiotic therapy or other medical care may be required, and the nurse should encourage adherence to the medical regimen. However, interventions such as adequate clothing, increased fluids (if not contraindicated), adequate rest, and cold compresses are appropriate. As a final note, it is essential that persons with upper respiratory infections or any other infectious process not come in contact with the client with cancer.

Bleeding

Clients with thrombocytopenia (low platelet count) tend to bleed easily. Elderly clients in poor physical health may not even notice small petechiae or ecchymotic areas on their extremities. Bumping into a chair or table may usually go unnoticed, but may cause bleeding under the skin for the client. Thus, careful assessment of the entire body must be done daily for the elderly client with a low platelet count. Many elderly clients have hemorrhoids and use over-the-counter preparations such as Preparation H. Use of rectal suppositories in clients with thrombocytopenia should be avoided. Sitz baths and commercially available products placed topically should be substituted. Constipation should be avoided. Men should shave with an electric razor only. These clients should also be instructed to avoid medications that include aspirin or ibuprophen (Motrin, Advil). Special attention should be given to mouth care, because this site is prone to bleeding. If bleeding in the mouth does occur, the client should be instructed to:

> Keep mouth and lips moist.
> Rinse mouth every 2 h and after every meal with warm
>   water and baking soda ($1/4$–$1/2$ tsp to 4 oz of water)
> Use soft toothbrush or Toothettes to remove any debris.
> Maintain a diet of high protein, soft foods.
> Drink nutritional supplements, such as Sustacal or Ensure.
> Avoid wearing poorly fitting dentures.
> Avoid hot, spicy, or acidic foods or drinks.
> Use ice chips instead of hard candy.
> Use cold foods (ice cream, frozen yogurt, etc.).

The nurse should teach the client and family to report any signs of bleeding, especially epistaxis, hematemesis, melena, or hematuria.

Stomatitis and Xerostomia

Other distressing side effects of cancer treatments are sore mouth or dry mouth. Elderly clients may wear dentures, and good oral hygiene is essential. Daily assessment of the oral cavity should be a routine part of the client's care. The home care nurse should teach the client or family to report any changes in taste or feeling in the mouth and observe for redness, white patches (which may indicate infection, such as Candida albicans), thick or no saliva, difficulty swallowing, sores or ulcers in the mouth, or difficulty placing dentures. The nurse should perform an oral assessment on the mouth on every visit. In addition to the interventions mentioned above for bleeding in the mouth, clients should be taught to:

Maintain adequate hydration (3,000 cc/day if not contraindicated).
Breathe through the nose and avoid mouth breathing as much as possible.
Moisten lips with Chapstick or water-based gels.
Use artificial saliva for dry mouth.

Fatigue

Fatigue, another common side effect, may result from anemia or from the cancer treatments themselves. Interventions that may assist the client in conserving energy include:

Eating properly.
Alternating rest and activity.
Taking small naps during the day.

Lethargy or any change in level of consciousness must be reported to the primary care provider immediately. The nurse should include an assessment of the client's regular sleeping patterns and note any changes. Anxiety, pain, and other factors often play a role in poor sleeping habits. If sleeping medications are prescribed by the primary care provider, the nurse makes sure that the client uses them appropriately, and monitor their effectiveness.

Pain

Pain is one of the most feared complications of cancer. Most elderly clients have learned to live with a variety of aches and pains. Often the very complaints that would have sent a much younger person to seek healthcare are tolerated by older persons because over the years they have experienced various discomforts, which may have become a "normal" part of their lives. Many elderly clients also have a high level of tolerance for pain. They may not wish to be viewed as "complainers" or "whiners." Their ability to adequately communicate exactly the kind of pain they are experiencing may also be compromised due to conditions such as transient ischemic attacks or difficulty finding the words. These factors frequently make it difficult for the nurse to adequately assess pain in the elderly.

Use of easy-to-understand scales like "Describe your pain on a scale of one (not bad at all) to ten (the worst ever)" can be extremely helpful (see Chapter 22). Analogs with pictures of faces demonstrating smiles or frowns in varying degrees are used with children, but should be considered for the older client also. Finally, careful observation of facial expressions and body language may indicate levels of pain. Active listening and astute watching are skills that must be mastered because elders may express pain, but not in the words expected. Whatever is utilized, a baseline measure of pain is crucial in the initial assessment and valuable in the continuous monitoring of pain. Over-the-counter oral drugs are rarely useful in managing the pain associated with cancer. Narcotic analgesics are the most often prescribed drugs. But in the elderly client, extreme caution must be used when administering these medications. Medicines like codeine and morphine causes changes in mentation, including confusion and lethargy, and these effects may be exaggerated in the elderly client. Dosages should be titrated for every individual. The nurse needs to be knowledgeable about the potential side effects of any pain medication the client is receiving. Thus the nurse can be an advocate for the elderly client, carefully monitoring responses to narcotic analgesics, teaching the family to monitor and report changes, and reporting these changes to the primary care provider so doses may be modified or a different medication may be prescribed.

Administering pain medications via IM or SC injection may not be appropriate because the skin of the elderly client is fragile. Alternative methods of delivering pain medication include liquid morphine PO, transdermal patches, patient-controlled administration (PCA) pumps, and continuous intravenous narcotics. Intravenous use of narcotics is done at home only when hospice is involved or the home health agency is certified to deliver hospice care. The home care nurse must be familiar with both the drug and the mode of administration.

Loss of Appetite and Weight Loss

Elderly clients with cancer suffer from several other side effects that may hinder their eating. Stomatitis, xerostomia, dysphagia, loss of taste, nausea, or vomiting are all possible side effects. The nurse needs to be aware of interventions that will assist the client in attaining adequate calories and protein, vital not only to health but also to the success of the cancer treatments. High calorie, high protein diets are desirable, but often clients are unable to tolerate meats and other high protein foods. Small, frequent meals including favorite foods should be encouraged. Ice cream, puddings, milk shakes, and other high calorie foods are often more tolerable. Foods should not be too hot or too cold. Supplements such as Sustacal, Ensure, or Scandishake may enhance the client's diet. Homemade supplements of orange juice and yogurt can be improvised and client and family creativity should be encouraged. It is important, however, to remind the client and family not to allow meals to become a source of anxiety and distress. Allowing the client to eat what and when he or she chooses is often the most effective way of handling appetite loss.

Clients who are unable to eat may receive total parenteral nutrition (TPN). Nurses who are specially trained may set up the administration of TPN in the home and frequently family members are taught to maintain the system on a daily basis. The home care nurse assists by maintaining the intravenous or central catheter site, monitoring serum glucose, monitoring the client's response to treatment, and reinforcing teaching as needed.

Pruritus

Clients may experience severe itching as a result of the skin changes brought on by their therapy or by the disease itself (common, e.g., in cases involving liver metastases, due to jaundice). Meticulous care of the skin is crucial; however, too frequent bathing can cause skin breakdown. The skin of elderly clients is extremely fragile and constant scratching must be discouraged. Keeping the skin clean and dry and maintaining moisture with creams and lotions will assist in decreasing the itching. The primary care provider may also order an antipruritic agent to be administered.

Alopecia

Caused by chemotherapy or radiation, hair loss is a distressing side effect, and frequently cannot be avoided. Clients may benefit from suggestions to use scarves, wigs, hats, turbans, and other head coverings.

ONCOLOGIC EMERGENCIES

Although these emergencies do not occur with any great frequency, it is imperative to recognize the signs and symptoms so immediate and proper attention may be given.

Superior Vena Cava Syndrome

Elderly clients with a mediastinal lesion are at risk for development of this syndrome, which may result from tumor compression on the superior vena cava. The blood flow through the superior vena cava to the right atrium is hindered. Possible sequelae, if left untreated, could be cerebral edema, respiratory complications, or death.

Most often seen in advanced lung cancer, symptoms that the caregiver of the elderly home care client should be alerted to include dyspnea, coughing, and swelling of the face, neck, upper trunk, and extremities. Signs upon further examination might include neck vein distention, edema of the face or upper extremities, or tachypnea. If this condition is suspected, immediately call the primary care provider and arrange transportation to take the client to the hospital. Medical management may be stent placement to prevent distress, radiation if the client requires immediate attention, chemotherapy, or thrombolysis.

Emergencies increase the fear and anxiety in the client/family system. The home care nurse should provide reassurance and information to the client and family that will help to allay anxiety.

Disseminated Intravascular Coagulation (DIC)

Clotting throughout the system may result in hemorrhage as clotting factors and platelets are consumed. Widespread microvascular clotting occurs. Early symptoms and signs include bleeding from the intravenous site and orifices (gingival bleeding, nose bleeds, hematuria, hematemesis, melena), petechiae, headache, anxiety, restlessness, and tachycardia. Later symptoms include altered level of consciousness, joint pain, and frank bleeding from orifices. Diagnostic blood tests include prolonged prothrombin time, activated partial thromboplastin time, and thrombin time. DIC is very difficult to manage medically and much support is needed.

Syndrome of Inappropriate Antidiuretic Hormone (SIADH)

SIADH results from antidiuretic hormone being released in an excessive amount. The syndrome may be induced by the disease process, some antineoplastic drugs, or other conditions. Early signs may include: thirst, headache, muscle cramps, and lethargy. Late signs include: nausea and vomiting, weight gain, and confusion. The nurse must assess and determine if these signs are new for the client, and report them to the primary care provider immediately. Large amounts of fluid intake cause increased urination and sodium levels may become elevated (above 165 mEq/L or higher), which places the client at risk for seizures. Also, altered mental status is common in SIADH. The client is put on extreme fluid restrictions to help the sodium return to a normal level.

PAYING ATTENTION TO DETAILS

From the client's perspective, quality of life may be measured by the capability to function minimally: eating, sleeping, ability to perform activities of daily living, and pain control. It is important to remember that the client with cancer may also suffer from a variety of other medical conditions and symptoms that impact upon his or her ability to perform or function. Not all of these symptoms will be due to the cancer, yet they must also be addressed.

It may be helpful to advise the client and family to maintain a daily journal or record of various daily events and activities in the home. Anyone providing care to the client should be encouraged to record in the journal. Details may be forgotten when one is involved in the daily care of the client. This helpful tool provides a chronicle for reference and aids in the continuity of care. An intact notebook may provide permanence, but a sheet of loose leaf paper placed on a wall or refrigerator provides visibility for all caregivers. Loose papers may then be placed in a folder. Items to be recorded include:

Temperature, pulse, and blood pressure.
Intake of foods and fluids (include foods particularly enjoyed for future reference).
Elimination patterns.
Additional instructions.
Complaints and any changes.

Client's emotional state (e.g., periods of depression, times or events of being especially happy, etc.).

Any other relevant information (e.g., dates of client's visits to hospital or primary care provider's office for treatment, visits by physical therapist or social worker, etc.).

Documentation of this type in the home may serve to alert the primary caregiver of events to report to the home care nurse. A daily record documenting name, dosage, and time of medications administered by all caregivers in the home should also be maintained.

Pressure Ulcers

Many elderly clients have fragile skin and decreased fat stores to absorb pressure, and their healing capacity may already be compromised. An elderly client experiencing decreased mobility runs the risk of developing pressure ulcers. This risk is particularly relevant for those clients who become bedridden. Pressure ulcers may lead to infections and sepsis, which may become life threatening to clients with cancer. It is important to practice preventive strategies: decrease pressure, avoid skin moisture (from incontinence of urine or feces, wound drainage, perspiration, emesis, or food spills), and prevent friction (pulling patient against bedding). See Chapter 12 for prevention and care of pressure ulcers.

Body Image

Alterations in body image may range from hair loss to surgically removed body parts. It may become necessary for the nurse to intervene to assist the client in adjustment. The home care nurse must acknowledge the feelings of the client and encourage the verbalization of feelings. Verbalization of feelings assists in coping.

Deep Vein Thrombosis (DVT)

DVT is another potential effect of decreased immobility. Discuss prevention and/or treatment with the client's primary care provider and teach the client and family about the efficacy and appropriateness of the use of specialized elastic stockings or ace bandages. Appropriate use of an anticoagulant (e.g., SQ injections of heparin or coumarin [warfarin]) as ordered by the primary care provider may be administered by the home care nurse or taught to the client's primary caregiver.

Mobility and Falls

Elderly clients with cancer are susceptible to pathological fractures due to the brittleness that both old age and cancer may cause in bone tissue. Careful assessment of the home environment is essential (see Chapter 5). All areas where the client might ambulate should be clear of small furniture, wires, scatter rugs, toys, and anything that might hinder mobility. The client should wear nonskid shoes at all times while ambulating. If a walker, cane, or other assistive device is utilized, it must be measured and adjusted appropriately for the individual client.

Sexuality

Elderly clients have needs for closeness and intimacy much as younger persons do. Physical intimacy may not be as available for the elderly client who has cancer. Family and friends may withdraw from the client to protect themselves from the pain of seeing a loved one suffer or undergo bodily change. The client may withdraw from others, lacking strength or fearing rejection. The home care nurse should be prepared to assess needs and make recommendations. Behaviors such as hugging, sharing, being close, kissing, etc. should be encouraged. Counseling and making referrals may be beneficial. See Chapter 7 for important information on encouraging expressions of sexuality among elders.

The Spirit and Spirituality

Those clients possessing a strong spiritual faith fair better psychologically during the course of their illness and disease process. The home care nurse can do much to enhance the client's spiritual connectedness. At times the family or caregivers are at a loss as what to do when they are alone with the client. Often just being there, reading to the client or praying with the client is important.

The home care nurse should encourage the client and family to continue as many of their regular activities as possible. Diversional therapy techniques that the client enjoys such as reading, relaxing music, watching favorite TV programs, taking a ride in the country, etc. should be encouraged.

Elderly clients who enjoy going to senior citizen centers, movies, visits to neighbors, and so on, and are well enough to do so, should continue. If the client is not well enough to go out, visits from the clergy, neighbors, and friends may assist in lifting the client's spirits and contribute to a feeling of connectedness with the greater environment. Often, family and friends visiting and sharing stories about activities and happenings among people they know makes the client feel less isolated.

COMMUNITY RESOURCES

Clients and families are often unaware of resources in their own communities. The client and family may not be aware of the extent of agencies and supports available for the elderly client with cancer. The home care nurse in an advocacy role can provide community resource information as well as encouragement and support. Referrals to social workers can help clients meet a variety of needs related to their health status and financial situation.

Organizations such as the American Cancer Society are available locally and can help the client with direct services. They can obtain help with the cost of medications, transportation, and dressing supplies.

Local public libraries and hospital medical libraries are good sources of information about cancer, from basic to very technical. Depending on the client and family either or both types of libraries may be good resources.

The hospital oncology department and outpatient department are also good resources of information and should have pamphlets available for clients and families. At a more general level, The National Cancer Institute provides answers to questions when healthcare professionals are not available (call 1-800-4-CANCER).

PALLIATIVE CARE AND HOSPICE PROGRAMS

Hospice care is palliative management of the terminally ill client, and the objective is death with dignity for the client. Pain should always be avoided, but at the end stage of life, it becomes the most important factor. The nurse may be helpful in such discussions by explaining the goal of hospice care and facilitating the transition through referrals when hospice care becomes necessary.

Criteria for acceptance into hospice include a prognosis of 6 months. Acceptance into a hospice program requires a primary care provider referral and can be continued if the client lives longer than 6 months. Some client/family systems may benefit by hospice care in the home and many home health agencies are certified to provide hospice care.

A team of healthcare professionals (primary care provider, nurses, social workers, clergy, and trained volunteers) will assist the family during this difficult time. Counseling and bereavement services are made available. When the client or family decide that care in the home is no longer possible or manageable due to the client's condition, hospice care in a hospital may be initiated. The nurse may be supportive by making appropriate referrals. Whatever decision is made by the family, the nurse may play an important role by helping to expedite the plans and make the transition as smooth as possible.

The skill of listening to clients and their families when caring for the elderly client with cancer in the home is paramount to all other tasks and talents the home care nurse must have. It is easy to get caught up in performing the technical duties and functions required. Remember, the family and the client are the best sources of information regarding how the client is doing. The family, as primary caregivers, are with the client more than anyone else involved in the care, and as such, are frequently the first to notice minor changes that may precede more serious conditions. Often, the elderly client may experience difficulty in expressing what he or she really wants to communicate. Both healthcare professionals and family members may be tempted to ignore the client, and do what they feel is best. Yet, it is the client who knows exactly how he or she is feeling. It is important to hear what the client has to say. It may be the only indicator of whether a plan of care is actually working for the individual. The home care nurse should practice and develop the habit and skill of listening. The few extra minutes it takes will prove invaluable in administering quality care to the client. It may be possible to incorporate interventions that the client and family recommends, if it is not medically contraindicated.

The nurse needs to be familiar with the stages of grieving and the tasks that may need to be completed by the client. Tasks may include writing a will, giving precious mementos to special people, expressing love to all the family, in addition to being able to talk about the dying experience. Frequently, family members are unable to listen effectively and negate these feelings. The nurse can be present with the client at these times and encourage ventilation of feelings.

SUMMARY

Caring for the elderly client in the home is a rewarding experience. Elderly clients have the advantage of having lived a long life, achieving an age of wisdom deserving of the best that life has to offer, no matter where they are on the continuum of the experience of cancer.

Providing holistic care to the client experiencing the diagnostic procedures for cancer and then dealing with the diagnosis of cancer is one of the greatest challenges for home health nurses. The nurse must face his or her own feelings about the diagnosis and possible ramifications of a cancer diagnosis.

To be most helpful to the client with this diagnosis, much information is needed, information about diagnostic procedures, treatment modalities, side effects clients encounter, and dealing with the psychosocial aspects of the disease with the client and family members. Teaching the client and caregivers how to manage the day-to-day care and what signs and symptoms to be aware of is an important part of the home care nurse's role.

Finally, if aggressive treatment is ineffective, palliative caregiving opportunities must be focused on and some of the home care nurse's most rewarding moments are experienced when working with clients during such an emotionally intense period in life. The home care nurse who enters the life of the elderly client with cancer encounters a golden opportunity to deliver quality care to one of life's phenomenal gifts—the older adult.

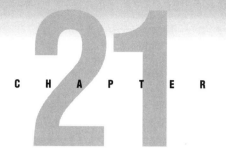

CARING FOR THE ELDERLY CLIENT WITH ALZHEIMER'S DISEASE AND RELATED DEMENTIAS

Anne Walsh

◆　◆　◆

Delirium
Depression
Primary Degenerative Dementia
Stages of Dementia
Developing a Nursing Care Plan
Caregiver Needs
Summary

Although the community health nurse will frequently encounter elderly clients with varying degrees of cognitive impairments, including confusion, disorientation, and short-term memory loss, these disabilities must never be considered a normal part of aging, but rather symptoms of an underlying disease. The etiology of the disease needs to be determined before appropriate treatment can be initiated.

Benign forgetfulness is a condition that everyone experiences from time to time. Misplacing keys or forgetting someone's name are examples. With age, forgetfulness may increase, but it is not considered problematic unless it interferes with the ability to conduct normal activities of daily living. When this occurs, a true cognitive impairment exists.

Most often, the cause of cognitive impairment will fall under one of the following disorders: delirium (attention disorder), depression (mood disorder), or primary degenerative dementia (memory disorder).

DELIRIUM

Delirium is an acute confusional state that is often mistaken for dementia. Delirium constitutes a medical emergency requiring prompt diagnosis and treatment to ensure a complete recovery. The onset of delirium is rapid and the client quickly becomes confused and disoriented. The client is not alert, but rather, alternates between stuporousness or lethargy and periods of extreme agitation, which often becomes worse at night. The client may experience hallucinations and is unable to focus attention on any task.

There are many causes of delirium. Frequently, it is the result of an acute illness, such as infection. The elderly often present with nonspecific signs and symptoms, such as confusion, weakness, and loss of appetite. Pneumonia and urinary tract infections are common infections that often precipitate delirium.

Delirium is a common symptom of an adverse drug reaction in the elderly. Even when prescribed at "therapeutic levels," drug intoxication may occur, resulting in delirium. High levels of digoxin, dilantin, or prednisone are common causes, but delirium may be caused by many other medications, as well.

Drug–drug interactions may also cause delirium, and for many elderly clients, polypharmacy is a major problem. It is not unusual for elderly clients to have several chronic diseases for which many medications are prescribed. If a client is being treated by more than one primary care provider, or utilizes different pharmacies, there is a greater risk for potential drug interactions to be overlooked.

The home care nurse will be able to reduce this risk substantially by careful review of all medications the client is taking, including over-the-counter medications. It is necessary to conduct a medication review at every visit to the client and check that medications are being taken as prescribed. The primary care provider must be informed of all medications that are prescribed by specialty primary care providers and clients and their caregivers should be advised to bring all their medications with them whenever they visit a primary care provider. See Chapter 8 for more information on medications common among elders and specific concerns.

Other conditions that may cause a confusional state are brain tumors, pernicious anemia, endocrine disorders, electrolyte imbalance, and head injuries. Subdural hematomas can present in just a few days or 2–3 weeks after a head trauma. The elderly are also known to develop spontaneous subdural hematomas. Normal pressure hydrocephalus, which is caused by an accumulation of fluid in the ventricles of the brain, is another cause of delirium of somewhat rapid onset. Often, gait disturbance and urinary incontinence will precede the onset of mental status changes.

The home care nurse needs to conduct a careful assessment of the elderly client's mental status and be sensitive to both sudden and subtle changes. A thorough physical assessment helps identify early symptoms of urinary or respiratory infections, drug toxicity, changes in diabetic status, and other conditions that when treated promptly can halt the progression of, or even reverse, the cognitive impairments.

DEPRESSION

Many elderly clients have *depression* and exhibit cognitive impairments that may produce dementia. The dementia of depression used to be referred to as "pseudo" or false dementia. Depressed clients perform poorly on cognitive function tests because they are poorly motivated. Depression-induced cognitive impairment fully resolves with successful treatment of the depression. However, there is some evidence that a first episode of major depression late in life may "signal" an incipient dementia.

Depression commonly coexists with the following neurological conditions: Alzheimer's disease, cerebral vascular accident (CVA, particularly of the left front brain), Parkinson's disease, multiple sclerosis, and Huntington's disease. Depression may be brought on by critical life events, such as the death of a spouse or other close family member, loss of friends, and loss of independence due to physical impairments and illness. Bipolar affective disorders or manic depression may also affect the elderly client. Symptoms of depression in the elderly include change in appetite, loss of self-esteem, somatic complaints, social isolation, loss of motivation, and self-report of cognitive decline (see Chapter 19).

When assessing an elderly client who exhibits mental status changes, the home care nurse should also consider the possibility of alcohol abuse, which is a problem that is increasingly affecting those over age 65. While taking a client's history, the nurse needs to ask about the use of alcohol, which in combination with certain medications can precipitate delirium. Chronic alcoholism may also lead to depression and dementia.

PRIMARY DEGENERATIVE DEMENTIA

Primary degenerative dementia is a progressive disease, insidious in onset, characterized by decreased decision-making capacity, poor judgment and insight, and short-term memory deficits. It is a chronic, irreversible deterioration of mental function. Alzheimer's disease is the leading cause of primary dementia. It is responsible for 70% of all dementias and the incidence increases exponentially with age. It affects about 4% of the population between the ages of 65 and 74 years, 19% between the ages of 75 and 84 years, and nearly 50% of the population over the age of 85. Since the over-85 age group is the fastest growing population in this country, Alzheimer's disease poses a significant health problem.

Vascular dementias occurs as the result of small vessel ischemic disease (for example, secondary to hypertension) resulting in multiple cerebral infarcts. Multi-infarct dementia (MID), more generally referred to as ischemic vascular dementia (IVD), accounts for about 10–15% of all dementia. Medical intervention to control blood pressure and other risk factors for atherosclerosis is important to the prevention and progression of vascular dementia. A combination of Alzheimer's disease and vascular dementia is not unusual. Other causes of primary dementia are Parkinson's disease, alcoholism, AIDS and more rarely, Creutszfeld–Jacob disease (CJD).

Alzheimer's disease is a progressive, degenerative neurological disease that causes memory, thinking, and behavioral deficits. Gradual nerve cell death occurs in the brain. The disease can take anywhere from 4 to 15 years to run its course. There is no cure and the cause is yet unknown, however, researchers have made many advances in recent years.

Only a few risk factors for developing Alzheimer's disease have been identified. Age is the most significant risk factor. The older one gets, the greater the risk. Recent research has identified genetic markers on chromosomes 12 and 19–21. A family history of Alzheimer's disease may also increase risk, especially for early onset dementia, sometimes referred to as *presenile dementia*. This type of Alzheimer's disease occurs before the age of 65 years and researchers have identified a genetic link to chromosomes 1 and 14. A history of head trauma has also been identified as a possible risk factor.

Assessment

At present, the only way to make a definitive diagnosis of Alzheimer's disease is by autopsy, when neuritic plaques and neurofibrillary tangles are seen in a particular distribution in the brain. These are the hallmarks of the disease. A differential diagnosis can be made by ruling out all other possible causes of dementia.

Early diagnosis of a dementing illness is essential to be sure the client receives the appropriate treatment and to help clients and families plan for the future. The home care nurse should be alert to symptoms that may signal the onset of dementia and the need for a complete assessment by the primary care provider.

All further discussion refers to primary degenerative dementia, of which Alzheimer's disease is the leading cause. The progression of the disease process may vary from client to client and depends on the type of dementia.

At the onset, the client may have difficulty in one or more of the following areas, identified by the Agency for Healthcare Policy and Research (Costa, 1996), as triggers that should prompt an assessment for dementia:

1. Learning new tasks and retaining new information. The client may begin to forget appointments, frequently misplace things, and shy away from unfamiliar environments and people.
2. Handling complex tasks such as carpentry or advanced sewing projects. If the client is still employed, he or she may have difficulty performing at work. The client may no longer be able to manage finances.
3. Reasoning ability. The client may experience difficulty problem solving and making simple decisions. The client may begin to show signs of impaired judgment.
4. Spatial ability and orientation. The client may get lost, even when taking familiar routes.
5. Language. The client may be unable to follow the flow of conversation, especially when several people are talking at the same time. The client may have trouble finding the right words to express him or herself or may easily lose a train of thought.
6. Behavior. Personality changes may appear, such as increased irritability, decreased energy levels, apathy, or suspiciousness.

Once the home care nurse or family member has identified one or more of these triggers, a full assessment by the primary care provider should be performed. This assessment includes a history and physical examination as well as assessment of functional and mental status, and may include laboratory tests and imaging studies. Use of a collateral informant is essential as the client often has diminished memory or insight as to changes.

The focused history includes information regarding onset, progression, and duration of symptoms. A medical history is needed to possibly identify underlying systemic disease, psychiatric illness, or neurological disorder. Any history of head trauma or substance abuse should be noted.

A family history will alert the clinician to any genetic conditions that may predispose the client to dementia, such as early onset dementia or Huntington's disease. A social and cultural history is needed because these factors affect performance on mental status examinations. Reviewing the clients medications will help to identify toxicity or polypharmacy as possible causes of cognitive changes.

After performing a physical examination, the primary care provider may order laboratory testing if a specific medical condition is suspected. A brain imaging study, such as magnetic resonance imaging (MRI) or a computed tomography (CT) scan, is needed if a brain tumor or ischemic vascular disease is suspected.

Tools

The **Functional Activities Questionnaire (FAQ)** is a standardized test that is particularly useful in identifying early dementia; however, it must be based on information provided by a reliable source, such as a close family member or friend (see Box 21-1).

The **Folstein Mini-Mental State Examination** is the most widely used mental status test. By itself, it is not a diagnostic tool, but used in conjunction with all the other components of a dementia workup, will help to complete the clinical picture. It also is used to establish a baseline to measure changes in cognitive function over time. Sometimes the primary care provider will recommend that the client consult with a neurologist or neuropsychologist for further neuropsychological testing (see Box 21-2).

STAGES OF DEMENTIA

As many as seven stages of Alzheimer's disease have been identified; however, for most practical purposes, the disease progresses from early, to middle, and late stages. Progression of the disease may vary from client to client, and sometimes the stages overlap. A precipitating factor, such as a cerebral ischemic attack, may hasten the otherwise slow progression of the disease.

BOX 21-1 • FUNCTIONAL ACTIVITIES QUESTIONNAIRE (FAQ)

ADMINISTRATION AND SCORING

The FAQ is an informant-based measure of functional abilities. Informants provide performance ratings of the target person on 10 complex, higher-order activities.

INDIVIDUAL ITEMS OF THE FAQ

1. Writing checks, paying bills, balancing a checkbook.
2. Assembling tax records, business affairs, or papers.
3. Shopping alone for clothes, household necessities, or groceries.
4. Playing a game of skill, working on a hobby.
5. Heating water, making a cup of coffee, turning off the stove.
6. Preparing a balanced meal.
7. Keeping track of current events.
8. Paying attention to, understanding, discussing a TV show, book, or magazine.
9. Remembering appointments, family occasions, holidays, medications.
10. Traveling out of the neighborhood, driving, arranging to take buses.

The levels of performance that are assigned range from dependence to independence, and are rated as follows:

- Dependent = 3
- Requires assistance = 2
- Has difficulty but does by self = 1
- Normal = 0

Two other response options can also be scored:

- Never did (the activity), but could do now = 0
- Never did and would have difficulty now = 1

A total score for the FAQ is computed by simply summing the scores across the 10 items. Scores range from 0 to 30; the higher the score the poorer the function, i.e., the greater the impairment. A cutpoint of "9" (dependent in three or more activities) is recommended.

Pfeiffer, R. I., Kurosaki, T. T., Harrah, C. H., et al. (1982). Measurement of functional activities of older adults in the community. Journal of Geronotology, 32, 323–329. Reprinted with permission.

In the early stages of dementia, the client is physically able to perform essential activities of daily living but requires supervision with instrumental activities of daily living, such as cooking or balancing a checkbook. The client is slower to respond and may be unable to

BOX 21-2 • FOLSTEIN MINI-MENTAL STATE EXAMINATION

Maximum Score	Score	
		Orientation
5	( )	What is the (year) (season) (day) (month)?
5	( )	Where are we: (state) (county) (town) (hospital) (floor)
		Registration
3	( )	Name 3 unrelated objects, allow 1 second to say each. Then ask the patient to repeat all 3 after you have said them. Give 1 point for each correct answer. Repeat them until he learns all 3. Count trials and record.
		Trials: _____
		Attention and calculation
5	( )	Ask patient to count backwards from 100 by sevens. 1 point for each correct answer. Stop after 5 answers.
		Alternatively, spell "world" backwards.
		Recall
3	( )	Ask patient to recall the 3 objects previously stated. Give 1 point for each correct.
		Language
9	( )	Show patient a wrist watch; ask patient what it is. Repeat for a pencil. (2 points).
		Ask patient to repeat the following: "No ifs, ands or buts" (1 point).
		Follow a 3-stage command: "Take a paper in your right hand, fold it in half, and put it on the floor" (3 points).
		Ask patient to read and obey the following sentence, which you have written on a piece of paper: "Close your eyes" (1 point).
		Ask patient to write a sentence (1 point).
		Ask patient to copy a design (1 point).

_____ Total Score

Assess level of consciousness along a continuum: _____
                                                  Alert   Drowsy   Stupor   Coma

Folstein, M. F., Folstein, S. E., & McHugh, P. R. (1975). Mini-mental state: A practical method for grading the cognitive state of patients for the clinician. Journal of Psychiatric Research, 12, 189–198. Reprinted with permission.

initiate an activity but will perform with verbal cueing. Periods of confusion, disorientation, and memory loss may alternate with periods of mental clarity and lucidity. The client may withdraw from social situations and become self-absorbed. Personality changes and difficulty with language are other early signs.

Physical functioning begins to decline in the middle stages. The caregiver may now need to assist with activities of daily living, such as bathing, dressing, and feeding. Short-term memory loss is more pronounced, although long-term memory may still be intact. The client may have difficulty recognizing people and confuses one family member for another. It is during the middle stages that clients often exhibit behavioral problems with which caregivers have great difficulty managing and coping. Some of the behaviors common to dementia clients are: wandering, pacing, sleep disturbances, paranoia, hallucinations and delusions, anxiety, agitation, and repetitive speech and behavior patterns.

In the late and final stages of the disease, the client no longer recognizes the primary caregiver and continues to decline physically. Weight loss is evident, bladder and bowel incontinence occurs, and the client eventually loses the ability to speak and to ambulate. If the client lingers, the ability to sit, swallow, and communicate will be lost.

DEVELOPING A NURSING CARE PLAN

Care plans must be developed by the home care nurse in conjunction with family caregivers, taking into consideration their needs and concerns as well as the client's current level of physical and cognitive functioning. The care plan needs to be reevaluated frequently to accommodate for disease progression and the individual client's level of physical and cognitive decline.

Safety

Whenever caring for a client in the community, an assessment of the home environment is necessary to identify potential safety hazards. For the client with dementia, safety considerations are based on more than obvious concerns, such as frayed wiring or scatter rugs. The environment must be evaluated in terms of the client's physical and mental status, taking into account the current stage of the disease. A social history also helps to identify issues specific to the individual client.

In early dementia, when the client is still fully ambulatory and may be left alone for periods of time, he or she should be encouraged to wear a Medic Alert bracelet. These clients may get lost even in the familiarity of their own neighborhood. If possible, close neighbors should be made aware of the situation, so they can be of assistance should they see the client wandering around the neighborhood.

In the home, observe the client going up and down stairs. Dementia clients have difficulty negotiating stairs because of visual–spatial disturbances and may not see the edge of the steps. Using fluorescent tape at the edge of each step can help in this situation. If not, the family may consider using a gate at the top of the stairway, especially if the client wanders during the night.

Is the client able to use kitchen appliances safely? If the client is left alone at times, the knobs on gas stoves may need to be removed and appliances unplugged. Cleaning products should be stored out of reach, because of the danger of the client ingesting them. Sharp knives should also be put away. All medications should be kept securely out of reach and supervised by a caregiver. Clients may forget that they already took their medication and take it again. Male clients who are still able to shave themselves, should use electric shavers and not razors with blades.

In the bathroom, again spatial disturbances will affect the client's ability to get in and out of the tub safely. A tub rail and grab bars should be installed. Use nonskid mats in and out of the tub. If door sills are high, they may need to be removed. Dementia clients have difficulty adjusting to changes in the environment, so that moving furniture may result in disorientation and pose a threat to safety. If there is any possibility that the client may attempt to drive, car keys must be hidden or the car disabled (see Chapter 4).

Behavioral Management

Difficult behaviors, such as wandering, pacing, restlessness, agitation, and paranoia, may be the cause of greatest distress for family caregivers. These behaviors usually peak during the middle stages of the disease. Letting the caregivers know that these behaviors are common in dementia clients is often reassuring. Family members may feel that the client's behavior is deliberate. They need to understand that it is part of the disease process and that the client has no control over it. Referral to a support group is essential at this stage.

Dealing with behavior problems is extremely difficult but with some common sense and creativity, they can often be minimized. Using medications to control behavior should only be considered as a last resort. Physical restraints, which not only rob a client of dignity, but also increase agitation in an already agitated client, should never be used. Physical restraints can be dangerous, as well, causing injury to wrists or entangling the client.

Some behaviors may be a direct result of the client's impaired ability to communicate. The client may have physical or emotional needs that he or she is not able to express, causing anxiety and frustration. Trying to determine what the client needs should be the first step in planning an intervention. To make this determination, certain strategies for improving communication should be used.

First, consider any sensory deficits the client may have. If a client has eyeglasses, make sure that they are kept clean and worn. If the client wears a hearing aid, check the batteries and see that it is properly positioned.

When trying to determine a need, the family or caregiver should be taught to ask the client a question that can be responded to with a "yes" or "no" answer, such as, "Do you need to use the bathroom?" If necessary, repeat the question, but use the same words. If the question is rephrased, the client will have to start processing the information all over again. Always allow the client sufficient time to respond. Although the client may not always understand the spoken word, he or she will respond to the emotional tone. The client can detect when a caregiver is angry or irritable.

Some clients exhibit "catastrophic reactions," which are exaggerated responses to what would normally be considered minor stressors. They may scream, cry, or even become physically aggressive. Causes of catastrophic reactions may be physical discomfort, frustration with the inability to perform a task or communicate effectively, or may be triggered by an environmental situation that frightens or confuses the client. A client in the midst of a catastrophic reaction should be quietly reassured, and if possible, distracted and gently removed from the stressful situation.

Living with a *wanderer* can be stressful. These clients require constant supervision. As mentioned before, they should wear an identification bracelet in the event that they leave the home alone. For the client who wanders at night, extra precautions need to be taken. Locks on the door should be placed very high or very low. Sometimes disguising the doorknob, or covering it with a towel, is sufficient to thwart the client. The caregiver may rest easier by using a room monitor at night. For the really persistent wanderer, bed alarms, door alarms, and light sensors may need to be used.

Wandering may increase at certain times of the day, usually in the evening. This phenomenon is known as "Sundowner's Syndrome." Instituting a regular exercise program during the day may decrease the wandering and help the client sleep better at night.

Sudden wandering or pacing may indicate the client is trying to locate the bathroom or is hungry or thirsty. The client may also be suffering from boredom and lack of sensory stimulation. Engaging the client in some activity may stop the behavior for a time. Clients who continue to wander regardless of any intervention should not be prevented from doing so, because this will only increase agitation. Supervise the client and provide enough space to allow wandering safely. Caregivers should keep things that they do not want the client to disturb in a room that is not accessible to him or her.

Agitation, restlessness, and pacing are problems for many clients with dementia. These behaviors may be initiated because of physical discomfort or pain. The client may be irritable because of sleep loss and fatigue. The client may be hungry or thirsty or may have pain due to arthritis, a headache, or toothache. The client may be suffering from constipation. Most elderly clients who are cognitively intact routinely take analgesics for chronic conditions, particularly arthritis. Clients with dementia have these same types of conditions but are unable to express their discomfort or to manage them. A client who suddenly becomes agitated may be acutely ill with an infection. Trying to determine the cause of behavior will help to identify the appropriate intervention.

Sensory overload is sometimes the cause of agitation. A very noisy environment or one in which there is a lot of activity can be disturbing to a client with dementia. Sensory deprivation can have the same effect. A lack of stimulation promotes boredom and will increase restlessness.

Some clients exhibit *paranoid behavior*. They may accuse the caregiver of stealing. They may believe that a spouse is having an affair. Families become very upset when the client with dementia suddenly starts using profanities or engages in inappropriate sexual behavior. Visual and auditory hallucinations accompanied by delusions may also occur. These hallucinations may be intensified if the client has poor vision or hearing loss. Hallucinations can be very frightening to the caregiver but can often be stopped if the client is engaged and redirected. If they become excessive, antipsychotic medication is helpful. Medication may also be needed if the client becomes physically aggressive or combative.

Whatever the behavior, caregivers should not attempt to physically prevent or stop it, but rather try to distract the client, lower expectations, and always offer comfort and reassurance.

When behavioral problems become truly unmanageable, certain medications may be prescribed. Antipsychotic medications such as Haldol, Mellaril, Clozaril, or Risperidol are helpful in controlling hallucinations and delusions. Antidepressants such as Prozac, Zoloft, or Paxil sometimes decrease agitation associated with depression. Antiseizure medication such as Tegretol and Depakote have been shown to decrease agitation in some clients. A sedating agent such as Trazodone may help with sleep.

Many of these medications have undesirable side effects. The home care nurse must be alert to signs of gait disturbances, Parkinsonian symptoms, tardive dyskinesia, depression, tremor, dry mouth, and hypotension. Clients should be started on low doses and gradually increased. It may take several weeks for the medication to reach therapeutic levels. Instruct the family to be patient and not to increase doses because they do not see an immediate improvement in behavior.

Nutrition

The home care nurse must teach and provide anticipatory guidance to family members and caregivers to prevent nutritional problems as the client progresses through the dementia stages. Maintaining proper hydration and nutrition can be a real challenge in each stage of dementia. In the beginning, clients may have forgotten that they already ate, and will eat again. If they are still preparing their own meals, they may only be able to prepare very simple meals that may not be nutritionally well balanced. For example, they may rely on eating cold cereal for dinner or eating bread or crackers, frozen dinners, or take out food. For these clients, enrolling them in a local meals delivery program may be a way of ensuring that they eat at least one nutritious hot meal a day.

Caregivers should make sure that healthy foods are available and within easy reach for the client. They will need to shop for the client and inspect their cupboards and refrigerator. The client may not recognize when a food item has spoiled and needs to be discarded.

In the middle stage, particularly in the presence of behavioral problems, getting the client to eat a complete meal can be difficult. The client may be unable to sit long enough to eat, and will wander away from the table. The client may be frustrated by the difficulty getting food from the plate onto a fork and into his or her mouth successfully. The client may spill things or mix food items inappropriately, like putting orange juice in the oatmeal instead of milk. Meal time should be made as pleasant as possible. The environment must be calm and quiet with little distraction. The client should not feel rushed. Offer the client one food item at a time so he or she does not have to think about what to eat first. Give the client the right utensil for the item being offered and prepare it to the extent required, for example, cutting the meat before it is brought to the table. If the client has difficulty managing utensils, try to serve as many finger foods as possible. It may be better to offer several small meals throughout the day rather than three larger meals. A colorful place mat under the plate may help the client to locate the dish and also distinguish the edge of the table, which will help to prevent spills. A cup that has a cover on it is easier for the client to manage.

Keep healthy snacks like fresh fruit available. At this stage, dementia clients often prefer sweets, but it is important that they get all the nutrients they need and not just empty calories. If weight loss is evident, nutritional supplements such as Ensure, Sustacal, or Carnation Instant Breakfast should be given. Some supplements come in liquid or pudding form.

Clients with dementia do not like to try anything new or unfamiliar. Offering the client favorite foods will be more successful. Fluids should be offered at regular intervals to ensure adequate hydration, especially in hot weather. Make sure enough fiber is included in the diet to prevent constipation.

Substantial weight loss is inevitable in the late stages. Many of these clients, often bedbound, now have difficulty swallowing and are at risk for aspiration. Some may require gastrostomy tubes for feeding. If they are still able to take food by mouth, the family needs to observe for signs of dysphagia and to be aware of the dangers of aspiration pneumonia. Instruct the family to puree foods in the blender and make sure the client is in semi-Fowler's position for feeding. They should avoid foods like grapes, nuts, and candies that could cause choking. (See Chapter 6 for further information on nutrition.)

Personal Care and Activity

Appropriate activity is essential in maintaining and stimulating remaining physical and cognitive functioning. The goal of intervention is to help the client remain as independent as possible for as long as possible.

Although it is often easier and faster for the caregiver to do things for the client, it will increase the client's dependency and lower self-esteem. There are ways the home care nurse can encourage independence with activities of daily living that will benefit both client and caregiver.

The client with dementia will have more success at dressing if the procedure is made less confusing. Clothes that go together can be put on the same hanger, so that selecting what to wear will not be a difficult decision. Clothes that are easy to put on will lessen the client's frustration and anxiety. Choose pants with elastic waists and avoid clothes with a lot of buttons. Women may find it difficult to put on bras and pantyhose. Undershirts and socks may be a better choice, if the client is comfortable in these.

The caregiver can lay out the clothes in the order in which they should be put on. Giving verbal cues is helpful as well as demonstrating what to do next. Put the right shoe next to the client's right foot. Sneakers with Velcro closures are not only easy to put on, but they also offer good support and safety in walking.

Bathing is frightening to many dementia clients. Tub rails, tub chairs, and the use of a hand-held shower will make the client feel more secure. If the client becomes severely agitated in the bathtub, sponge baths may need to be substituted. Allow the client to wash independently, giving verbal instruction or demonstration as needed.

Grooming is important to both the client and the caregiver. Women should be taken to the beauty parlor regularly if this is what they are used to, or have a beautician come to the house. If she routinely used make-up or nail polish, the caregiver can continue to assist her with these activities. The client must be reminded to brush his or her teeth or the caregiver may have to perform this task. More frequent visits to the dentist for cleaning may be useful in maintaining dental hygiene. Foot care is an important part of the daily routine, especially in the presence of diabetes or vascular disease.

Incontinence of both bladder and bowel inevitably occurs in the late stages of dementia, but if the client begins to have accidents earlier, look for a cause. Urinary incontinence may develop as a result of a urinary tract infection or be due to urgency brought on by diuretics. Or incontinence may occur simply because clients miss body cues or cannot find their way to the bathroom.

Incontinence can be minimized by establishing a regular toileting schedule. (See Chapter 11.) Specific techniques can be taught to the family members or caregiver. Taking the client to the bathroom every morning after breakfast, for example, may help to establish regular bowel habits. The client should be taken to the bathroom every 2–3 h during the day to urinate. In the evening, limit fluids after dinner and toilet the client right before bedtime. Limit the client's intake of caffeine. If the client requires toileting at night, consider using a bedside commode and leave a night light on for safety. Caregivers will feel more secure if they use an incontinence pad for the client when going outside the home.

In the early stages, visual cues may remind the client to go to the bathroom independently. Leaving the bathroom door open may make it easier for the client to locate the bathroom, or a picture or sign could be put on the door.

The client's ability to continue to perform some household tasks is not be discounted and he or she should be encouraged to continue them as long as possible. Caregivers can take advantage of the client's past talents or interests, such as gardening. Folding laundry, setting the table for dinner, drying dishes, or dusting helps the client to feel like a useful and productive member of the family.

Stimulating remaining cognitive abilities is important to preserving the client's self-esteem and may slow the progression of the disease. Lack of stimulation and subsequent boredom may also contribute to behavioral problems, like wandering.

There are two drugs currently available that have been shown to slow the progression of memory impairment and deterioration of daily functioning in some clients with mild to moderately severe Alzheimer's disease. They are tacrine (Cognex) and donepezil (Aricept). These drugs slow down the degradation of acetylcholine in the brain. Acetylcholine is a neurotransmitter essential to memory. Tacrine can have adverse effects on liver functioning and clients on this drug need to be monitored carefully, having blood tests performed regularly. Donepezil is easier to administer and has few side effects. There is some evidence that donepezil may be useful in the management of difficult behaviors like agitation.

Planning meaningful recreational activity for the client with dementia must be based on the client's interests and present abilities. Activities should be blocked into short periods of time because of the client's limited attention span. Establishing a daily routine provides structure and familiarity that is comforting to the client.

Physical exercise is just as important to the total care of the dementia client as it is to any other client and should be incorporated into the daily routine. Exercise increases oxygen perfusion to the brain, which may improve cognition. It produces a feeling of well-being and is an acceptable substitute for inappropriate behaviors that some clients with dementia may exhibit. In some cases, exercise may inhibit wandering and promote better sleep patterns.

Walking is an exercise that most clients can perform safely with supervision. Properly fitting shoes are all that is required. Movement to music is another enjoyable form of exercise for most clients. Whatever form of exercise is chosen, it should be done on a regular basis and preferably at the same time so that the client adjusts to the routine.

Listening to music may benefit the client in many different ways. Some studies have shown that music can decrease agitation, lessen feelings of depression, and stimulate memory. Selecting music that is meaningful to the client has the most beneficial effect. When listening to music, there should be little outside distraction. The room should be quiet and the music played at a comfortable level. When provided regularly, music adds structure to the daily routine. Music can also be used, when needed, as an intervention for undesirable behaviors.

Music is a universal language with the ability to evoke emotional responses even in those who are cognitively impaired and with deficits in the ability to communicate verbally. Musical selections should be based on the client's ethnic and cultural backgrounds and preferences regarding style of music.

Lively tunes will sometimes prompt physical responses like dancing, singing, humming, or foot tapping. These physical responses increase alertness in a client who may otherwise be withdrawn or apathetic. Soothing music may have a calming effect. Music that is nostalgic may relieve depression by reminding the client of happier times, by helping to recapture lost identity and reengage with others. Music that has meaning for the client can stimulate memory and provide a vehicle for reminiscence.

Opportunities for reminiscence can be provided by initiating other activities, as well. Looking at old family photos and organizing them into albums is a good activity for clients and caregivers to share. Watching old, favorite movies is another pastime that may be enjoyable. Family should be aware that certain movies and television programs may not be appropriate for clients with dementia because they may have difficulty distinguishing what they see from reality. Violent programs can be frightening to some clients.

Art is a form of nonverbal communication that many cognitively impaired clients can appreciate. Providing paper, pencils, crayons, and coloring books can offer the client a much needed form of self-expression.

All family members should be encouraged to provide recreational activities for the client. Young children can offer to play simple card games, or play catch with a sponge ball. The client has a short attention span and no one activity will interest him or her for too long. The client needs to be included in family gatherings, as well; however, he or she may become agitated or frightened in the presence of too many people or too much noise.

CAREGIVER NEEDS

Approximately 70% of the care that is required for clients with dementia over the course of the disease is provided by family caregivers. When evaluating the needs of the client, the home care nurse must also evaluate the needs of the caregiver. Family caregivers often experience grief, depression, social isolation, financial hardships, and physical exhaustion.

Grieving occurs as the caregiver witnesses the slow death of the loved one's personality. With increasing loss of memory, clients with dementia become shells of their former selves. The grieving process occurs slowly over time, and then when the client dies, the process begins again.

Caregivers sometimes become so involved in client care, that they neglect their own physical and emotional needs. They isolate themselves from friends and often give up their former social and recreational activities. Many of these caregivers, especially the spouses, are elderly, and are at great risk for developing serious health problems of their own.

The home care nurse can be instrumental in providing these family caregivers with the emotional support and guidance they so desperately need. The role of the home care nurse includes helping caregivers develop effective coping skills by educating them about the disease, formulating a care plan, and helping them to access community resources.

Providing families with information about the disease process is crucial to the development of coping skills. They need to know what to expect as the disease progresses so that they can establish short-term goals and initiate long-term planning.

At the onset of dementia, the family should be advised to consult an elder care attorney who can assist with important legal issues. While the client is still competent, he or she can appoint a healthcare proxy and write a living will. Establishing a power of attorney can make it easier for family members to handle the client's financial affairs when the client is no longer able. The attorney can also advise them concerning transfer of assets and current Medicaid eligibility requirements. Caregivers should be encouraged to make alternate arrangements for the client's care in the event that they become ill and are hospitalized or otherwise not able to care for the client.

Home care nurses should provide information, a bit at a time, so caregivers do not become overwhelmed. Give written information whenever possible so that the caregiver can refer to it at his or her leisure. Education should include simple explanations of what the disease is, how it progresses, and some of the behavioral problems that may occur and how to manage them.

The home care nurse may find that the caregiver is having difficulty managing the care of the client alone and still is reluctant to ask for help. The nurse must help the caregiver realize that he or she does not have to do it all and that it is essential to ask for help to protect his or her own health and well being.

If there are other family members, the primary caregiver should ask for help in specific ways. Family members are often willing to help but do not know what to do. The caregiver can say, for example, "I would like you to stay with Dad on Saturday mornings for a few hours while I run some errands." or, "Why don't you take Mom on Sunday afternoons so I can rest?"

Another option for the caregiver is to hire a home health aide or companion for at least a few hours a week. The nurse can determine if a home health aide from the home health agency can be of assistance and if the services are covered by Medicare or Medicaid or if the services of a home health aide or companion can be provided at an hourly rate for as much time as the family needs or can afford.

When hiring a companion, the family should make sure that the companion is given a clear assignment to ensure continuity of care, and that the client's daily routine is not upset. The client may be resistant to care by a stranger, at first, and will need time to adjust to this new person. A home health aide or companion is not only able to provide physical care, but also to provide recreational and social activities, as well. The companion should not be considered a baby sitter, but a member of the healthcare team and must be directed to consider all aspects of client care.

Adult day care programs for dementia clients can be of invaluable assistance to the primary caregiver and provide the client with professional care. While the client is at the day care center, the caregiver is free to take care of his or her own needs. The client also benefits by being given the opportunity for socialization with peers, and to participate in specialized programs for clients with dementia.

Caregivers can also take advantage of respite care. Respite allows the client to stay in an assisted living or skilled nursing facility for a short time, usually for a few days, weeks, or up to a month. The caregiver can utilize this service if he or she wants to go away on vacation, needs to be hospitalized for a short time, or just feels overwhelmed.

For those clients with limited family support, a care manager may be employed in the early stages to arrange for the client's daily care needs and to provide intermittent supervision. Sometimes, a referral to a social worker may be indicated to help access community resources and services.

The home care nurse should also refer the caregiver to a local support group. Caregivers need to share their experiences with others who understand their situation. It is helpful for them to learn that their loved one is not the only one who behaves in a certain way, for example, and often they learn effective caregiving skills from others who have had to deal with the same problem. In a supportive group environment they can freely express emotions like anger, guilt, or frustration, which they would otherwise not verbalize. *The 36 Hour Day* by Nancy L. Mace and Peter V. Rabins, MD (1991), is an invaluable resource book for family caregivers.

There may come a time when the caregiver is no longer able to care for the client at home, and may be considering placement in an Alzheimer's disease center especially designed to meet the needs of the person with dementia. Some clients with skilled nursing needs benefit by a nursing home placement. This decision is very difficult for many primary caregivers. They may experience feelings of guilt, or failure, or have difficulty letting go of their caregiving role. The home care nurse needs to support caregivers at this time and assure them that they did the best they could, for as long as they could.

Often, a nursing home placement is the best choice when the client needs skilled nursing care. The nurse should encourage caregivers to visit several nursing homes and to choose one that they feel comfortable with, and that is close by, so that it will be convenient for them to visit on a regular basis. Assure caregivers that they are not abandoning the client, but rather, are making sure the client is receiving the best care possible. The caregiver can still be involved in the client's care by visiting often and participating in the nursing home care plan, family conferences, and recreational activities.

The healthcare professional and the client, family, and caregivers need to be aware of community resources. National organizations are available for disease and referral information. Many regional and local agencies are available where direct services are provided such as diagnosis, treatment, counseling, and support. The more informed the home care nurse is about Alzheimer's disease and the needs of all involved, the better the client and the caregivers can be helped (see Table 21-1).

SUMMARY

Home care clients may undergo a variety of behavioral and cognitive changes. Some are caused by medications, infections, or life events and are reversible. Others are caused by physical, age-related changes beyond

TABLE 21-1 • RESOURCES FOR HEALTH PROFESSIONALS, CLIENTS, AND FAMILIES

Name of Organization	Explanation
Administration on Aging 330 Independence Avenue, SW Washington, DC 20201 (202) 619-1006 Fax: (202) 619-7586 Internet: http://www.aoa.dhhs.gov	The Administration on Aging (AoA) coordinates delivery of services specified by the Older Americans Act. Services are coordinated and provided through 57 State agencies and 657 areas. The range of services provided by these Area Agencies on Aging (AAA) varies, but all include nutrition, access, in-home, and community services. Addresses and phone numbers of State and local AAAs are available from the national office. The Elder Care Locator (800-667-1116) provides a toll-free access number to locate State agency networks.
Alzheimer's Association 919 North Michigan Avenue Suite 100 Chicago, IL 60611-1676 (312) 335-8700 800-272-3900 for information and local chapter referrals nationwide (24-hour telephone line) Internet: http://www.alz.org	The Alzheimer's Association is a national voluntary organization with 220 local chapters and more than 2,000 support groups. The Alzheimer's Association funds research, promotes public awareness, advocates legislation for patients and families, and provides support services, including support groups, adult day care programs, respite care programs, and telephone helplines through its national, chapter and volunteer network.
Alzheimer's Disease Centers (Access through ADEAR; see next entry)	The National Institute on Aging, part of the National Institutes of Health, supports 28 Alzheimer's Disease Centers across the county. This program provides clinical services, conducts basic and clinical research, disseminates professional and public information, and sponsors educational activities. A growing number of satellite clinics associated with this program are helping to expand diagnostic and treatment services in rural and minority communities and collect research data from a more diverse population.
Alzheimer's Disease Education and Referral Center P.O. Box 8250 Silver Spring, MD 20907-8250 800-438-4380 Fax: (301) 495-3334 Internet: adear@alzheimers.org	The Alzheimer's Disease Education and Referral (ADEAR) Center, a service of the National Institute on Aging, provides information and publications on Alzheimer's disease for health professionals, people with Alzheimer's disease and their families, and the public. The ADEAR Center serves as a national resource for information on diagnosis, treatment issues, patient care, caregiver needs, long-term care, education, research, and ongoing programs. In addition, the Center provides referrals to national and state resources.

(continued)

TABLE 21-1 • Continued

Name of Organization	Explanation
The Corporation for National Service Office of Public Liaison 1201 New York Avenue, NW Washington, DC 20525 (202) 606-5000 Fax: (202) 565-2794	The Corporation for National and Community Service is a public corporation that administers Federal service programs, including AmeriCorps, the Foster Grandparent Program, and the Senior Companion Program (SCP), which provides supportive services to adults with physical, emotional, and health limitations. A major SCP emphasis is preventing or delaying institutionalization. Foster Grandparent volunteers work with children, including those with disabilities. AmeriCorps members address a range of local health issues.

OTHER RESOURCES

American Association of Retired Persons
 (AARP)
Washington, DC
(202) 434-2277
800-424-3410

AARP Pharmacy Price Quote Center
800-456-2226
(open 24 hours a day)

American Bar Association Commission on
 Legal Problems of the Elderly
Washington, DC
(202) 662-8690

Children of Aging Parents
Levittown, PA
(215) 945-6900

Consortium to Establish a Registry for
 Alzheimer's Disease (CERAD)
Durham, NC
(919) 286-6406 or 6405

Insurance Consumer Helpline
Washington, DC
800-942-4242

Medicare Beneficiaries Defense Fund
New York, NY
(212) 869-3850
800-333-4114

Medicare Hotline
Baltimore, MD
800-638-6833

the client's control. Each must be identified and treated or managed accordingly. Often the home care nurse is the first healthcare professional to recognize these changes in the client. Sometimes behavioral changes are from nonreversible disease entities.

Although researchers have made many advances in their search for a cause and toward identifying interventions to possibly delay the onset or progression of the disease, at this time, the goals of the home care nurse should be focused on improving the quality of life for clients with dementia and their caregivers. The nurse must help family members to develop effective coping skills, stimulate remaining physical and cognitive abilities of the client, and help the client and caregiver enjoy their time together, to whatever extent that is achievable.

REFERENCES

Costa, P. T., Jr., Williams, T. F., Somerfield, M., et al. (1996). Early identification of Alzheimer's disease and related dementias. *Clinical Practice Guideline, Quick Reference Guide for Clinicians, 19 (AHCPR Pub. No. 97-0703)*. Rockville, MD: U.S. Department of Health and Human Services, Public Health Service, Agency for Health Care Policy and Research.

Mace, N. L. & Rabins, P. V. (1991). *The 36-Hour Day*. Baltimore: Johns Hopkins University Press.

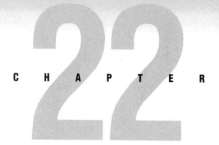

PROVIDING PALLIATIVE CARE FOR THE DYING ELDERLY CLIENT

Vivian Schulkin

◆ ◆ ◆

Palliative Care Versus Cure
Stages of Death and Dying
Planning the Care
Implementing the Care
Comfort Measures and Pain Control
Tools for Successful Pain Management
Religious and Cultural Beliefs
Client and Caregiver Teaching
Community Resources and Hospice Programs
Summary

Healing a person does not always mean curing a disease.
Dame Cicely Saunders, Hospice Founder

For many elderly clients there is no possibility to cure their diseases or illnesses. The body is unable heal itself from trauma or to fight the invasion of infectious organisms. A lifetime of reserves has been depleted. The course of treatment must be altered from curing to caring. How is a plan introduced to alter the course of treatment for the older, terminally ill client in home care? When an illness cannot be treated successfully (to achieve a "cure"), altering the treatment plan becomes necessary. In this situation, focusing on "care" may be more appropriate than continuing the search for a "cure." The successful outcome for the client may be death with dignity, while remaining in his or her own home. How does a home care nurse help the client and family achieve this goal? The nurse advocates for the client and becomes a source of strength, offering caregiving and information, and is a purveyor of resources. Each role is discussed in this chapter as the home care nurse as provider of palliative care is explored.

PALLIATIVE CARE VERSUS CURE

When the home care nurse introduces "palliative care" to the family and primary care provider of an elderly client, the nurse is moving the focus away from the medical concept of "cure" toward the nursing concept of "care." Often the primary obstacle is that all those involved are attempting to avoid any discussion of death. Family members and medical providers might express concern about the client's inability to handle "the news." It generally is not "news" to the client. Ill people will often say that they knew they were terminally ill before they saw the doctor, or before they were given the results of any tests. People who are dying, often times, wish to discuss their dying, but may choose not to. Clients explain that they do not open this discussion because it makes others cry and become upset.

When talking about death, the specifics of what is said, and how it is said, must be understood as this can impact the openness of communication. Hope can be enhanced or destroyed and hope is often what keeps people alive. Hope may also be responsible for making any life, no matter how short or long, meaningful.

Elizabeth Kubler-Ross, an expert on death and dying, was asked in an interview (1990) how to tell someone who is dying, about the fact that they are dying. She replied that "you have to be honest, but you don't have to be totally honest. You have to answer their questions, but don't volunteer information for which they have not asked, because that means they're not ready for it yet." Continuing on, she said that you can help a person without offering a cure. "You never, ever, ever take hope away from a dying client. Without hope nobody can live . . . . Because we do not know what the future holds, we cannot predict what is in store for anyone . . . ." None of us can judge how meaningful the time left to the dying client may be. So, Kubler-Ross warns, ". . . you don't just go and drown them in 'truth.'" She tells about a teacher who once said that of his clients, 50% live 1 year, another 35% live 2 years, and another so-and-so many percent live 2^1/2 years, and so on. When all the percentages were added up, there was always 1% left. The class would note this and say to the teacher, "Hey, you forgot, what about that last one percent?" He always said, "The last percent is for hope."

Palliative care is advocated for older clients who are in the final stages of life. In the process of their dying they need respectful and dignified care in which pain is minimized and comfort maximized. Because home care nurses work in a person's home, the plan should always encompass the needs of the "family system." Introducing the idea of palliative care is begun with the client. The client needs to be assured that a nurse will still visit, and that medical treatment will still be available, as needed. Clients will always have choices about what they wish to have done, and what they do not want. Talking about these options may present new hope for the client.

Sometimes the client clearly expresses the wish to die at home, but the family is terrified at the thought. The nurse needs to open this discussion so that the wishes of all parties can be expressed. If there is time to come to a decision with everyone's input understood, then the outcome will be more comfortable for all. People must be informed, additionally, that all choices made are always open for revision, or retraction.

At times the primary care provider needs education about palliative care as well. The home care nurse discusses this on the phone, and perhaps follows up by mailing literature on hospice caregiving offered by the home care agency or general pain management techniques used with terminally ill clients. This discussion gives the primary care provider information that allows him or her to become actively involved with the client's decision making. The primary care provider can also continue to develop medical interventions that are congruent with this concept.

STAGES OF DEATH AND DYING

As in all theories that are depicted as stages through which people move, the stages of death and dying presented by Kubler-Ross are not "pure" nor is movement through them unidirectional. People are multidimensional, and do not progress in a linear fashion. All people individually take longer or shorter time periods to accomplish various tasks, and some may not accomplish all tasks. Thus, to expect that any client who is coping with end-of-life issues will go from denial (at time of diagnosis) to acceptance (before they do die) would be erroneous and naive. People use learned coping techniques that have served well in the past, and this is certainly the case when they learn of their own terminal prognosis. They will probably go through these stages, in somewhat the order presented by Kubler-Ross, but there is no "right" way to die and each individual works through the dying process differently.

Denial and Isolation. When people are confronted with a situation that they cannot process, they use the defense mechanism known as denial. In this way, they do not take on the knowledge with which they are unable to cope. They will sometimes say outright, "This is not true . . . . They must be wrong . . . ." The diagnosis of a terminal/fatal illness is questioned, often leading the person to seek third, fourth, and fifth opinions of primary care providers. In obtaining these many medical diagnostic tests and opinions, the person may get the confirmation required to assure the truth of the initial diagnosis. He or she will also gain the time needed to process, and to come to terms with such a prognosis. Many people will also isolate themselves, also allowing time to process the information. Having "time out" is used by many people when they are unable to tolerate the stimulation they are receiving. Usually the person will at least acknowledge, if even momentarily, that his or her state of mortality is real. Most people will retain some degree of denial throughout their last days or months, allowing space for hope and pursuit of life.

The home care nurse needs awareness of how denial can interfere with, or destroy, the treatment plan. People who believe they have not been given the correct diagnosis will also believe they require no treatment. They will see no need for medication, follow-up testing, or special diets.

Anger. When the reality that the person actually is at the end of life makes itself clear, anger, rage, envy, and resentment replaces the denial. The anger is often displaced and projected. The client resents others for being well, is angry at healthcare professionals for causing pain, and blames the government for decreased services that he or she "deserves . . . worked a lifetime for . . . ." It is at this stage that the home care nurse is required to have unending patience. The family and the nurse may not only be the target of the displaced anger, but they may also experience rejection from the person they wish to help. At this point the nurse may be called upon to appease the client and comfort the family. All of the "family system" will be experiencing emotional pain and suffering. An objective professional mediating may be of utmost importance for the success of the whole home care plan.

Bargaining. In terminal illness the stage of bargaining is usually short lived. People will often ask caregivers to just help them be well enough to see a child married, or see a grandchild graduate from school. These "deals" that are struck are often doomed to failure. If they see their oldest child married, why not the youngest?

Home care, with all its intimacy, makes for a strong desire on the part of many nurses to try to help make these wishes, and "repayment" tags, realities. It is very important to understand what the home care nurse's part of the deal is meant to be. The nurses may feel powerless and conflicted. They understand the need of clients to complete certain "passages," but also know of the futility in these "deals." They do not wish to destroy hope, but they understand that fulfilling these bargains and promises are not within their control.

Depression. When the client's physical status deteriorates to the point that he or she can no longer deny that the illness is terminal, and he or she is too tired to fight, the client will become depressed. The costs (physical, emotional, and financial) have taken their toll, and have the appearance of being all consuming. This reality can cause depression. The ill person can no longer believe he or she will become well. The client may be helped, at this point, to receive encouragement that some of his or her favorite activities are still available. Providing financial assistance, through entitlement programs and community resources, may alleviate some serious worries.

When clients start to mourn their losses, it is the door to acceptance and accompanying peace that is starting to open. The nurse will need to be aware that this depression, the anticipatory mourning of the client, is not an emotional stage to hasten or reshape. The nurse needs to be present, although it is often very uncomfortable, and allow the process to move forward. The end product will be a client, and following not too far behind, a family, who will accept the anticipated death with less anxiety and fear.

Acceptance. The client who has had the opportunity of moving through the other stages, will now frequently be "ready for the final journey." This client is not resigned, nor just "too tired to fight any more," but is prepared and waiting for the end to come. The wait is not in pain, nor desperate to escape the discomfort of illness. There is often a peace that allows the person to "leave" quietly. During this period, the client will show a process of withdrawing from this world and its people and objects. Verbalizations are minimized, the TV and radio are turned off, and visitors are enjoyed for short periods of time only. The client will sleep frequently, and for long periods of time. It is not the same as the avoidance associated with depression, nor the sleep used to escape from pain.

At this point the home care nurse can best guide the family through coping with their losses, and helping them understand what the client needs. What is helpful for the client is having a person present, merely there to hold a hand and assure the client that he or she will not be alone at the final moment.

PLANNING THE CARE

Assessment of the needs of the client and family system will provide the home care nurse with the appropriate nursing diagnoses for each client. The nurse then should prioritize these needs. When the prioritized needs are established, specific goals and methods to achieve these goals are developed. Knowledge of what problems can be anticipated should generate plans to meet these problems, within boundaries of available resources and the specific payers and community resources available to the client.

Looking into what resources will be needed, what services different organizations may offer, and their costs, will help develop how care will be implemented. When the nurse is planning care, the client and family will need to be given specifics of what will be involved, so that they may make an informed decision. Specifics of who will be responsible for the different facets of the client's care should be outlined, in advance. For example, using a patient-controlled analgesia (PCA) pump involves costs of the pump and the medication. There is the added responsibility of frequently changing the apparatus (cassette, tubing, and needle). All of these details must be explained to the client and caregivers. The training of the caregivers also requires that the home care nurse assess their ability to learn and perform the highly technical skills needed to use such a pump. Good planning will avoid some very unpleasant surprises, when the plan is actually implemented.

Planning care for any client requires that the nurse maintain open, ongoing communication with the primary care provider. Effectively using resources from all disciplines requires that each professional be kept apprised of changes in the client's status, and what is being done to address these changes. Home care nurses need to show responsibility in oversight and case management skills when there are other professionals involved in caring for a person who remains at home.

IMPLEMENTING THE CARE

Assuming the planning was done well, the home care nurse can begin to delegate to appropriate family members and ancillary personnel. The nurse delegates care based on individual level of ability, as well as the client and family needs. Monitoring routinely for any changes in the status of the client, and the family, will allow the interventions to be well timed. Assessment and planning will have anticipated what may need to be done at any given point. Formulating and developing teaching goals and methodology that are consistent with the needs of the client and the caregivers is done as the plan is being put into place. This is the time when the home care nurse can obtain the services of interagency professionals from the appropriate disciplines. The nurse should be documenting all changes in the client's status, all teaching done and outcomes, and the communications among the multidisciplinary team members.

COMFORT MEASURES AND PAIN CONTROL

When palliative care is indicated, comfort measures and pain control are primary interventions. Removing sources of suffering, and easing pain and distress requires a complete nursing assessment. The actual and potential roots of these problems must be uncovered before beginning to remove or lessen the discomfort.

Suffering may be emotional, spiritual, psychological, or physical. It may come from any of the first three, but manifests as physical symptoms. All of these possible roots of suffering can be addressed by the home care nurse. However, many times an older person will have a lifetime of problems to work through, and age and illness confounds these issues. For these reasons the nurse may consider several options as deemed appropriate. The assessment can be completed on two or more visits, with mental health specialists or the clergy consulted. These professionals can address the psychosocial and spiritual needs of the dying client. The family, too, may benefit by having their suffering eased, using the modalities of these professionals.

Nursing interventions may be most appropriate for discomfort related to sleep disturbances and insomnia, fear and anxiety, and physical pain. For muscle pain and tension, using cutaneous stimulation (e.g., superficial application of heat or cold, massage, pressure, or vibration) may be helpful. Techniques such as progressive muscle relaxation, visualization, and guided imagery, and distraction are excellent means to ease discomfort. Having soft, gentle background music, and taking "time out" (time in a quiet space away from the "sick room") can also aid in relaxation. Stress reduction may involve use of water (shower or bath), reading books or watching TV, or "romance" (with or without a partner). A romantic mood may be engendered by enjoying a delicious meal, using a fancy table cloth, place mats, candles, and flowers. Laughter increases endorphins (natural narcotics), which cause muscle relaxation. Laughter can change one's mood, as well as reflecting the mood one is in.

Older people who are dying often fear death will come at night, so they avoid sleeping (especially at night). Leaving a light on, or a radio playing softly, works well to allow relaxation, and even sleep. Another person sleeping in the room can also relax the client, allowing sleep to come. People also fear certain types of dreams. Dreaming of a dead relative can lead to severe anxiety, and even panic. Techniques may be taught that help control dreams. It may be helpful to have someone in the room, or immediately nearby, if the client has a frightening dream.

A snack available at the bedside is a comfort measure for many older people. Fears of being unable to get something to eat or drink, of being hungry, and of being alone, are addressed with this gesture. Comfort often takes the form of food.

Terminal illness and physical pain are often inextricably tied together in the mind. A diagnosis of cancer to most people means dying in unending, uncontrolled, and severe pain. This image may engender the ultimate primal fear. To be dying, to be alone in the process of dying, and to die in pain, constitute a most dreaded triad. Refer to Chapter 20 for more information on cancer management at home.

TOOLS FOR SUCCESSFUL PAIN MANAGEMENT

The home care nurse can be assured that there are tools available that may ease the impact of the events leading to death. Death cannot be prevented. It is a natural part of any life. But the client does not have to be alone.

INITIAL PAIN ASSESSMENT TOOL

Date: _____

Patient's name: _____   Age: _____

Address: _____   Physician: _____

Diagnosis: _____   Primary nurse: _____

  I. Location:
      Patient or nurse
      marks drawing

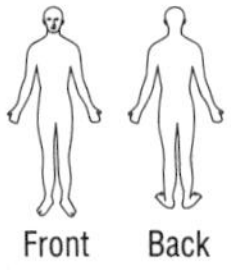

        Front   Back

 II. Intensity: Patient rates the pain. Scale used: _____

     Present: _____

     Worst pain gets: _____

     Best pain gets: _____

     Acceptable level of pain: _____

III. Quality: (Use patient's own words, e.g., prick, ache, burn, throb,
     pull, sharp) _____

IV. Onset, duration, variations, rhythms: _____

 V. Manner of expressing pain: _____

VI. What relieves the pain? _____

VII. What causes or increases the pain? _____

VIII. Effects of pain: (Note decreased function, decreased quality of life.)

     Accompanying symptoms (e.g., nausea) _____

     Sleep _____

     Appetite _____

     Physical activity _____

     Relationship with others (e.g., irritability) _____

     Emotions (e.g., anger, suicidal, crying) _____

     Concentration _____

     Other _____

IX. Other comments: _____

 X. Plan: _____

     _____

FIGURE 22-1 • Initial Pain Assessment Tool

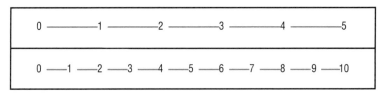

FIGURE 22-2 • Pain Rating Scales

The family and hospice home healthcare team members are there for the client throughout this time. The hospice team is also there for the family after the client's death, making their grief a shared process. The pain caused by the illness can also be palliated. The role of the home care nurse is particularly vital in this area. It is essentially the skills and expert knowledge of the professional nurse that can assure pain control for the client.

The nursing process phase of assessment, followed by the implementation phase, is used to understand and help to alleviate the pain experience. Assessment involves determining the location, onset and duration, intensity, and factors that alleviate and aggravate the pain. Figure 22-1, The Initial Pain Assessment Tool, provides a guide for assessing pain and associated factors that will be used to develop an appropriate plan of care.

Pain intensity should be quantified in some way, thereby allowing comparison and evaluation of the effectiveness of the interventions that are being used. Commonly used scales are numeric (often written on a graphlike visual), whereby it is determined that a "0" means the client is experiencing no pain, and "10" is symbolic of the greatest pain possible. A "0" to "10" scale is most effective for persons who need more exact means to describe their pain. However, a scale based on "0" to "5" is easier to conceptualize, and thus may be more meaningful to see what methods are effective in palliation (Figure 22-2).

The Pain Management Log (Figure 22-3) is used to quantify pain just prior to the pain control intervention and then 1 h after the intervention. This allows optimal evaluation of effectiveness of the pain control interventions being implemented. The log shows the caregivers and the client what is occurring, and this feedback itself may be a means of decreasing pain and fear. Further, the evaluation process is often perceived, correctly, as the nurse taking seriously the significance of the pain the client experiences in the process of dying.

A flow sheet that includes the physiologic responses that occur with the use of opiates is of value to the home care nurse and the prescribing primary care provider when the medication is being titrated. The flow

PAIN MANAGEMENT LOG

Pain management log for: _____

Please use this pain assessment scale to fill out your pain control log.

```
L___|___|___|___|___|___|___|___|___|___|
0   1   2   3   4   5   6   7   8   9   10
No                                      Worst
pain                                     pain
```

Date	Time	How severe is the pain?	Medicine or nondrug pain control method	How severe is the pain after 1 hour?	Activity at the time of pain

Note: May be duplicated for use in clinical practice.

Pain rating: A number of different scales may be used. Indicate which scale is used and use the same scale each time.

Possibilities for other columns: bowel function, activities, nausea and vomiting, and other pain relief measures. Identify the side effects of greatest concern to patient, family, physician and nurse.

Source: McCaffery & Beeb. (1989). *Pain: Clinical Manual for Nursing Practice.* St. Louis: Mosby.

FIGURE 22-3 • Pain Management Log

sheet for pain management documentation allows for documentation of vital signs, level of arousal, the pain level experienced, and a place for the plan and any modifications that are needed.

Pain and suffering have a strong association with aging and dying. Suffering implies an extended sense of threat to self-image and life, a perceived lack of options for coping, a sense of personal loss, and no existing basis for hope. Suffering can be defined generically, as the state of severe distress associated with events that threaten the "intactness" of the person. Often, the suffering of clients in pain can be relieved by demonstrating that their pain can truly be controlled.

Pain can exacerbate individual suffering by worsening helplessness, anxiety, and depression. Nurses can enhance the individual's personal control through allowing the exercise of choice; enhancing access to and use of relevant information; and assisting with access and use of social support. Pain often reduces clients' options to exercise control, diminishing psychological well being and making them feel helpless and vulnerable. Therefore, clinicians should support active client involvement in effective and practical methods to manage pain.

The obligation to alleviate suffering is an essential component of the clinician's broader ethical duties to benefit and not harm; it dictates that health professionals maintain clinical expertise and knowledge in the management of pain. Physical pain is further impacted by factors other than pathophysiology. These factors may include past experience with pain (both directly or indirectly), the image/meaning of pain, beliefs about pain control, perceived secondary gains associated with the presence of pain, social and cultural influences on pain and pain control, personal goals for controlling pain, and the expectation that pain will occur as part of the diagnosis.

When the plan is being developed to control pain, all these factors must be assessed. The plan of care will depend on attending to the physical *and* psychosocial needs of the client. Adequate pain control cannot be achieved without addressing both. Ongoing exploration of the impact of these influences on pain perception is essential for ultimately controlling the pain of the terminally ill client. Discussion of the psychosocial factors requires the input of the family system and the client. It may be that external stimuli in the environment need to be removed or modified to achieve comfort for the client. This often requires that activities of family members be modified. Planning interventions will be utilized more effectively if they are made with the client and the family. Goals that are realistic and achievable should also be developed with all those involved with client care.

Pain control, itself, is best if medical, surgical, and pharmacological interventions are used along with noninvasive, nondrug pain relief techniques. Surgical interventions may include interfering with nerve pathways, as in a nerve block, sensory rhizotomy, or cordotomy procedures. Surgical debulking of tumors, or use of chemotherapy and radiation to decrease tumor size, can reduce pain. This is useful when the pain results from pressure of the tumor on other organs, or the obstruction of a hollow viscus (e.g., the bowel or bladder).

There are multiple analgesic and narcotic medications available for use. Of course there are also side effects and toxic effects associated with their use. As in the management of any client's care who is taking medications, compliance and satisfaction result from limiting these "negative" effects.

Pain management is often needlessly suboptimal. Healthcare professionals may not be comfortable with their pain management skills, may not realize the importance of pain management, or may not recognize that a client is in pain, and may fear prescribing opiate medications. Like some clinicians, clients and families may shun the use of opiates. Because of their fears of addiction and worries about tolerance, they may not complain about pain or about poor pain relief. These fears and concerns must be addressed, thereby allowing the client to receive adequate doses of medications and thus successful control of pain.

Depression and grieving are other possible sources of distress in the geriatric population. For persons with a terminal illness, the chances are even greater for these stressors having a negative impact. Depression is accompanied by psychological and physical symptoms. Changes in sleep and appetite, fatigue, poor concentration, and social withdrawal are symptoms of depression that can significantly further impair the functional ability of these clients. Illness that saps strength and causes loss of function, and the treatments for the illness, may be a cause of depression. Multiple losses experienced by many older clients, with the addition of anticipatory grieving of their own death, make geriatric clients who are dying at very high risk for depression. The home care nurse needs to assess clients for depression, and then make referrals to mental health professionals, support groups, or the clergy so the problem can be addressed appropriately. (See Chapter 19 for further discussion.)

RELIGIOUS AND CULTURAL BELIEFS

Death and religion are inherently tied together through the concept of spirituality. Culture provides a guide as to how one implements spirituality and also guides how the elders of the group are treated. How individuals are treated when they become older is also guided by cultural mores and family dynamics. In groups where more traditional values prevail, the extended family takes responsibility for the care of the elders.

These families may express strongly their desire to keep a dying member at home. They may arrange their entire work and social time schedules so the ill person will always be cared for by the family. People with these common beliefs may also ask for involvement from members of a religious group, who become available to spend time with the dying person, allowing family members some respite.

Religious and cultural beliefs will provide the rites of this passage from life to death. These rites may include types of food and fluid the dying person should have. What may be spoken of in the presence of the dying person may be prescribed by culture, as may appropriate dress, and even specific kinds of light and music. Many of these beliefs are determined by how cultures and religions view death. When death is thought to bring the "spirit" to a better place, or a higher level, death may not be feared. It may be seen as a reward for a life on earth that was filled with toil. If there is a belief in "afterlife," there may be "reunions" with those who went before to look forward to. It may be that "death" is a new beginning, a place to learn and improve, for the next incarnation. When the body is considered a vessel to carry the soul, spirit, or mind, death of the body is not critical. This soul/spirit/mind will live on, again on a higher plane.

On the other hand, death may be seen as a time when one is judged by "The Creator." The concept of judgment is often frightening. Human behaviors are often seen as errors, or "sins." One who sins is believed to be doomed to "everlasting Hell." A belief in these concepts may cause a person to fear "crossing over" to death. As one's life is viewed by the older dying person, the scale used to weigh the sins against the good will be skewed by anxiety and remorse. Death in this type of belief system carries a heavy penalty. Dying then is no longer a "passage" but a one-way downward "fall."

Whatever beliefs the client and family follow, the home care nurse must show sensitivity and respect. Each person has an individual set of beliefs and customs, but the American Nurses' Association's Code of Ethics mandates that nurses provide for the spiritual needs of clients. When involved with terminal care of any client, nurses are there to make the client's transition to death as comfortable as possible. Any related rituals that brings comfort to an older person should be encouraged. The elderly have usually held beliefs about death for a lifetime and they developed meaning beyond the religious interpretation from which they originated. Many older clients have been preparing for their death, consciously or unconsciously, for many years. Their years of living have added layers to the original tenets, as did their experiences with others who have "gone before."

The home care nurse's sensitivity to the client's belief system will be a source of comfort to the client and family. The client's specific customs surrounding dying may be foreign to the home care nurse; however, through observation of what is being done and validation of the meaning of these behaviors helps the nurse plan interventions in light of that knowledge. A family who wants to have an older member die at home should be given the appropriate information and tools available, so that this may be accomplished. It may mean calling the family's clergy, and advocating for members of the congregation to assist with the client's care. Perhaps the family should be encouraged to contact the leaders of the client's congregation to inform them that this person is dying and requires clerical assistance to follow the religious mandates, for this "passage."

CLIENT AND CAREGIVER TEACHING

Family caregivers need sleep and respite from the burdens of caregiving and may have socioeconomic needs and fears related to the costs of providing care. Sophisticated pain management strategies may require clients and families to manage complex medication regimens, involving parenteral or epidural infusions in the home. Some family caregivers may hesitate to give adequate doses of pain medications out of fear that the client will become addicted, tolerant, or develop respiratory depression. Teaching caregivers and clients about the need for continuous administration of pain medications, what can be done to relieve side effects, and how and when to use nonmedical techniques is a vital component in assuring client comfort.

Teaching the client and caregivers should also be focused on comfort measures, which may include methods for increased physical comfort, limiting emotional pain, and explaining anticipated events. For instance, it may be suggested that a client have radiation as a method to reduce pain. The client may fear this treatment, anticipating the discomfort experienced with chemotherapy. The home care nurse can explain the procedure and benefits of it so the client makes an informed decision and will not fear the treatment itself. Increasing knowledge decreases fear of the unknown.

Frequently, family members can handle the terminally ill client at home but the actual act of dying and knowing when this is or what the family should do causes stress and concern for families. Educating caregivers about changes they may observe in the client will relieve some anxiety. Reassuring them that they can call the home care nurse or agency and the nurse will visit them or arrange for a home health aide to be available more frequently near the end provides additional comfort. Many home care nurses have incorporated into the plan of care that the client's family is to call them if death is imminent or has just occurred so they can be there with the family.

Some physical changes that occur in a dying person include the following:

- Consciousness: The client may be unconscious for days, or may remain alert and with a clear mind until the last moments. Clients can hear and feel, even with the loss of awareness. There may be increasing confusion over the last days or moments. The client may experience decreased pain.
- Temperature: Due to decreasing circulation, extremities become cool, and the color becomes pale or dark. Although the skin is cool, the person does not experience being cold.
- Breathing: The respiratory pattern may change. There may be gurgling, or a "rattle" sound, but the person is usually not uncomfortable.
- Reflex-related movements of the body: There may be some reflexive movements, usually of the extremities. When the heart stops, and the person stops breathing, the pupils become fixed and dilated.

Letting the family know what they can anticipate after the client dies will also help them know what to do and that grief is normal. This includes the community practices regarding pronouncing the client's death, transportation of the body, and contacting the final arrangement service of choice. When describing the stages of grief and the process of bereavement, the home care nurse should include the following information:

- Shock: The family members may feel numb as a protection against becoming overwhelmed by the loss and this reaction is normal.
- Pining: Experiencing feelings of guilt and anger. Concerns for "What if . . .?" or "Why didn't I . . .?" They may also express anger at the person for dying, or at God for the

death. This is a time when everything seems to call up the memory of the dead person.

- Depression: Realization of the loss of the person. This step has several stages and is needed for full return to recovery. The immediate depression may last days or weeks and becomes less intense, completing by the end of 1 year. Most people need to experience the anniversary of the loved one's death and go through a year of customary celebrations, in the loved one's absence, to help develop new patterns, before experiencing full recovery.
- Recovery: The mourner experiences the return of energy, interest in daily life events, and has established new patterns of living without the presence of the deceased family member. The memory of the deceased person is not lost, but is experienced with decreased pain.

Families should be reminded of techniques that foster healing. Memorial services, spiritual rituals (e.g., candle lighting), sharing memories, and use of formal or informal support groups are examples of aids that can be used during the bereavement period. Every cultural and religious group has their own practices, which should be encouraged.

COMMUNITY RESOURCES AND HOSPICE PROGRAMS

Informational resources are abundant. Some are more appropriate for the professional and others for the client and family members. Many home health agencies are certified as hospices and provide hospice care through professional and paraprofessional staff especially trained in hospice caregiving philosophy and techniques.

For issues related to pain control the American Academy of Pain Management and the International Association for the Study of Pain (IASP) are professional resources. The American Academy of Pain Management is focused on clinical and pure research on medical and nonmedical interventions for pain control. IASP is an international, multidisciplinary, nonprofit professional association dedicated to furthering research on pain and improving the care of clients with pain. IASP is a Nongovernmental Organization (NGO) affiliate of the World Health Organization (WHO).

The National Hospice Organization (NHO) is an excellent resource for professionals and others who have interest in the care of people who wish hospice care. More than 4,400 hospice professionals and volunteers have joined NHO as members of the National Council of Hospice Professionals (NCHP). Membership includes subscriptions to *HOSPICE Magazine*, the *Hospice Journal*, and *The Hospice Professional*. Members also receive significant discounts on NHO educational programs and NHO store purchases. They may also obtain technical assistance from staff and colleagues and free access to the NHO Job Bank Hotline. The NCHP provides individuals an opportunity to participate in the NHO and the hospice community, through the development of programs, publications, and activities that focus on the individual hospice professional within the hospice disciplinary team.

Telephone numbers and addresses of hospices near the client can be obtained by contacting the NHO Helpline at 1-800-658-8898. Similar information may be obtained by contacting the Hospice Foundation of America at the following addresses:

777 17 St. #401
Miami Beach, FL 33139
TEL: 1-800-854-3402
FAX: (305) 538-0092;

or

2001 S St. NW #300
Washington, DC 20009
TEL:(202) 638-5419
FAX:(202) 638-5312

Support groups are helpful to clients and their families by having peers or professionals who can provide ongoing information and emotional support through the whole dying process. The groups will most often offer bereavement counseling to the family after the client has died. Groups are offered by The American Cancer Society and many hospitals that treat the terminally ill. The hospital social worker can be contacted for specifics of these meetings.

Hospice care neither speeds up nor slows down the dying process. It does not prolong life and it does not hasten death. It merely provides its presence and specialized knowledge of medical care, psychological, emotional, and spiritual support during the dying process in an environment that includes the home, the family, and friends. Hospice programs are intended to get the people involved through the dying process. Often called "palliative" (comfort- oriented) care, hospice care does not employ artificial life support systems or medical/surgical heroics when there is no reasonable hope of remission of the disease. Hospice clients typically are in their last 6 months of life. Hospice is the "something more" that can be done for the client and family when the illness or disease itself cannot be cured.

If the home health agency does not provide hospice care, the client or family needs to have information that can direct them to receiving this care if so desired. Most communities have access to hospice services and in some communities there are inpatient hospice programs to help clients who are experiencing temporary problems that are managed more effectively as an inpatient, such as wound treatment, electrolyte imbalance, pain control, or as respite care for overburdened family members. In addition, some clients (and family members) fear dying at home or dying at home is culturally inappropriate. In these instances, the inpatient hospice setting is very comforting. Some features of hospice care include:

- The unit of care is the client and the client's family. Family is defined as *anyone* the client views as part of the family network.
- The client and family are encouraged to participate in caregiving and decision making.
- Care is offered in the client's home more often than in an institution. The primary caregiver is frequently a family member of the client.
- A multidisciplinary team, which most often includes a primary care provider, registered nurse, social worker, homemaker, clergy, and volunteer, supports both the client and family.
- Although hospice does not provide 24-hours-a-day care in the home, staff is on call 24 h a day, 7 days a week.
- The client should be as pain free as possible. At the same time, clients should remain as alert as possible or desired.
- Death with all the implications is openly discussed with hospice team members, should the client and family desire.
- Hospice team members are specially trained to deal with the loneliness and fears of abandonment experienced by both the client and loved ones. Hospice programs typically offer bereavement counseling to loved ones for a year after the client's death.

- Trained volunteers are an important part of the hospice service.
- Most hospices are Medicare and Medicaid certified. That means they meet specific standards of care and provide a specified range of services that are financially reimbursed by Medicare or Medicaid.

SUMMARY

Caring for the terminally ill at home can be a rewarding experience for the home care nurse. Home is where most clients want to be for all caregiving if the needed support and services are available. Providing palliative care creates new challenges for nurses whose caregiving practices usually focus on curing clients. Caregiving embodies the traditional role of nursing in which the nurse provided comfort measures due to the limited curative practices available. In the hospice philosophy, this caregiving role of the nurse is focused on and allows the nurse the privilege to be a part of a very personal and intense experience in the client and family's life.

For the home care nurse to participate effectively in providing quality palliative care, the nurse must be familiar with the stages of death and dying, end-of-life comfort measures, and aggressive and creative pain management techniques. Caregiving at the end of life considers the holistic needs of the client and family and includes incorporating cultural and religious beliefs. Teaching and anticipatory guidance become important roles for the home care nurse and these roles are enhanced by being knowledgeable about local, state, and national resources of information and services useful to the dying client and his or her family.

REFERENCE

Kubler-Ross, E. (1990). Interview with Dr. Daniel Redwood. Available at: http://www.wholeliving.com/redwood.

I N D E X

Page numbers followed by *f* refer to figures; those followed by *t* indicate tables.